Enhanced Palliative Care

A Handbook for Paramedics, Nurses and Doctors

Disclaimer

Class Professional Publishing have made every effort to ensure that the information, tables, drawings and diagrams contained in this book are accurate at the time of publication. The book cannot always contain all the information necessary for determining appropriate care and cannot address all individual situations; therefore, individuals using the book must ensure they have the appropriate knowledge and skills to enable suitable interpretation. Class Professional Publishing does not guarantee, and accepts no legal liability of whatever nature arising from or connected to, the accuracy, reliability, currency or completeness of the content of *Enhanced Palliative Care*. Users must always be aware that such innovations or alterations after the date of publication may not be incorporated in the content. Please note, however, that Class Professional Publishing assumes no responsibility whatsoever for the content of external resources in the text or accompanying online materials.

The information presented in this book is accurate and current to the best of the authors' knowledge. The authors and publisher, however, make no guarantee as to, and assume no responsibility for, the correctness, sufficiency or completeness of such information or recommendation.

Printing history

First edition published 2021.

The authors and publisher welcome feedback from the users of this book. Please contact the publisher:

Class Professional Publishing,
The Exchange, Express Park, Bristol Road, Bridgwater TA6 4RR
Telephone: 01278 427 826
Email: post@class.co.uk
www.classprofessional.co.uk

Class Professional Publishing is an imprint of Class Publishing Ltd

A CIP catalogue record for this book is available from the British Library

Paperback ISBN: 9781859598757
eBook ISBN: 9781859598764
Cover design by Hybert Design Limited, UK
Designed and typeset by PHi Business Solutions Limited
Printed in the UK by Short Run Press

This book is printed on paper from responsible sources. Please refer to local recycling guidance on disposal of this book.

Contents

2: Ethical and Legal Considerations   21

Jenny Doig, Sandra McConnell and Jill McKane with Lorna Frame,
Stuart P Milligan and Katie Pears

Contents

David Carroll with Alistair Duncan, Gordon Linklater,
Frances MacIvor, Claire McGee, Tim Morgan and Kirsty Thorpe

*Alexandra Little with Shalini Bhola, Andrew Collier, Claire A Douglas,
Alice Radley, Michael K Sullivan, Fiona Finlay, Gillian Foster, Karen J Hogg,
Alistair McKeown, Yvonne Millerick and Ian Morrison*

Contents

Disclaimer

Please note that any prescribing information in this program will be compliant with the Scottish Palliative Care Guidelines. These are regularly reviewed and the online guidelines updated when required. The details and dosages in this book are presented for information purposes only and any guidance, although accurate at the time of publication, may be subject to change. For the purpose of the case studies in the manual, or where symptom control is specifically related to, please check the current advice at: https://www.palliativecareguidelines.scot.nhs.uk/.

Practitioners should always work to local protocols, and within their own level of governance and experience.

Acknowledgement

The idea for an *Enhanced Palliative Care* educational programme grew from many years learning and teaching on several different courses based on the well-established model of a pragmatic and evidenced manual, underpinning a short interactive course. This was catalysed following feedback on the Scottish Palliative Care Guidelines highlighting that many colleagues would appreciate broader and more detailed teaching. A proposal was taken to Macmillan Cancer Support to fund the development of a practical course for paramedics, nurses and doctors to enhance their knowledge and skills in palliative care. They generously agreed to this. I would like to thank all the Macmillan team, and specifically Jean Sargeant who has been a stalwart from the start.

The programme adheres to the principals of the NHS Education for Scotland (NES) framework for Palliative and End of Life Care, and follows the general structure and the drug regimens of the Healthcare Improvement Scotland (HIS) Scottish Palliative Care Guidelines. I am grateful for the support given by HIS, NES, the Scottish Partnership for Palliative Care and the College of Paramedics.

Almost 100 colleagues, from across the professions, gave freely of their time in writing the manual and preparing the course. This was made more demanding due to the pressures on time and resources caused by the COVID-19 pandemic. I owe an enormous debt of gratitude to everyone who is named in the list of contributors. I would like to especially thank the lead chapter authors, and the members of the steering group.

The team at Class Professional Publishing have been excellent with their guidance and drive to keep the project moving forward in difficult times. A mention in particular of Lianne and Katherine for their patience, dedication and hard work.

Finally, I want to thank my wife, Louise. A general practitioner working in a small ex-mining town, she keeps me grounded in the practicalities, demands and pleasures of daily medicine and care at the coal face.

About the Authors

Editor

Neil Pryde graduated from Edinburgh University Medical School in 1982. He trained as a General Practitioner (GP) registrar in South Yorkshire, returning to Scotland in 1987 where he was a GP Principal in Fife for 26 years. During this time he developed an interest in palliative medicine and since 2009 he has worked for the Fife Specialist Palliative Care Service. In 2013 he was appointed to the post of Macmillan Lead Cancer GP for NHS Fife. He chaired the revision of the Scottish Palliative Care Guidelines that were released in 2019. Neil's other area of interest in medicine is motorsport and trauma. He was Chief Medical Officer at Knockhill Racing Circuit for 25 years and has taught on trauma courses in the UK and Europe. This led to the idea of developing a similar style of course for palliative medicine. He retired from clinical medicine in 2019.

Lead Chapter Authors

Paul Baughan – General Practitioner and Clinical Lead with Primary Care Faculty

George Beuken – Head of Pastoral Care and Education

Kirsty J Boyd – Macmillan Reader in Palliative Care

Paul Brown – Consultant Liaison Psychiatrist

Deans Buchanan – Consultant in Palliative Medicine

Sandra Campbell – Macmillan Nurse Consultant for Cancer and Palliative Care

David Carroll – Associate Specialist in Palliative Care

Jenny Doig – Macmillan Cancer and Palliative Care Educator

Mark R Evans – Head of Spiritual Care and Bereavement Lead

Marie Fallon – St Columba's Hospice Chair of Palliative Medicine

Charlie C Hall – Higher Specialist Trainee in Palliative Medicine

Trisha Hatt – Strategic Partnership Manager

Alexandra Little – Strategic Planning and Commissioning Manager

Sandra McConnell – Consultant in Palliative Medicine

Jill McKane – Specialty Doctor in Palliative Medicine

James Neil – Palliative Care Social Worker

Maire O'Riordan – Consultant in Palliative Medicine

Teri Perry – Volunteer Service Manager, Palliative Care

Kim Steel – Consultant in Palliative Medicine

Fiona Walker – Retired Associate Specialist in Palliative Medicine

Paul Wilson – Senior Pharmacist, Palliative Care

Chapter Contributors

Alison Allan – Centre Head at Maggie's Fife

Gail Allan – Macmillan Lead Nurse, Cancer and Palliative Care

Mairi Armstrong – Macmillan Nurse Facilitator, Primary Care

Shalini Bhola – Medical Registrar in Endocrinology and Diabetes

Jane Boyden – Specialty Doctor in Palliative Medicine

Kirsty Brightwell – General Practitioner and Medical Director

Alana Brown-Kerr – Specialty Registrar in Palliative Medicine

Claire Clark – Specialty Doctor in Palliative Medicine

David Clark – Professor Emeritus

Andrew Collier – Consultant Endocrinologist

Fiona Crowther – Complementary Therapist

Sharon Dick – Palliative Care and Bereavement Counsellor

Claire A Douglas – Consultant in Palliative Medicine

Alistair Duncan – Specialist Palliative Care Pharmacist

Emma Dymond – Consultant in Palliative Medicine

Fiona Finlay – Consultant in Palliative Medicine

Roger Flint – General Practice Specialty Trainee and Founder of SPOT

Gillian Foster – Consultant in Palliative Medicine

Lorna Frame – Specialty Doctor in Palliative Medicine

Joanna Franz – Consultant in Old Age Psychiatry

Liz Henderson – Minister: Richmond Craigmillar Church of Scotland

Karen J Hogg – Cardiology Consultant and Honorary Clinical Associate Professor

Scott Jamieson – General Practitioner

Margaret Rose Key – Lymphoedema Clinical Nurse Specialist

Nicola Lewthwaite – General Practice Partner

Gordon Linklater – Consultant in Palliative Medicine

Frances MacIvor – Consultant in Palliative Medicine

Catriona Macpherson – Children and Families Practitioner, Specialist Palliative Care

Fiona McFatter – Consultant in Palliative Medicine

Claire McGee – Specialist Dietitian in Palliative Care and Oncology

Holly McGuigan – Specialty Doctor in Palliative Medicine

Alistair McKeown – Consultant in Palliative Medicine

Lesley Middleton – Marie Curie Clinical Nurse Manager

Denise Millar – Lead Complementary Therapist

Yvonne Millerick – Nurse Consultant and Senior Lecturer

Stuart P Milligan – Lecturer in Palliative Care

Sarah E E Mills – Academic Clinical Fellow in General Practice

Tim Morgan – Medical Director and Consultant in Palliative Medicine and Visiting Professor

Ian Morrison – Consultant Neurologist and Honorary Reader

Allison O'Donnell – Practice Development Nurse Specialist, Learning Disability Services

Katie Pears – Palliative Medicine Specialist Trainee

Leza Z Quate – Specialty Doctor in Palliative Medicine

Alice Radley – Specialty Trainee in Renal and General Medicine

Joy Rafferty – Specialty Doctor in Palliative Care

Fiona Reid – Macmillan Specialist Physiotherapist, Team Leader

Margaret Rice – Lymphoedema Clinical Nurse Specialist

Michelle Salmon – Lymphoedema Clinical Nurse Specialist

Liz Smith – Practice Educator

Elaine Stevens – Lecturer in Cancer and Palliative Care

Michael K Sullivan – Clinical Research Fellow

Kirsty Thorpe – Consultant in Palliative Medicine

Marie Todd – Clinical Nurse Specialist Lymphoedema

Paul Watson – Project Lead, End of Life Care

Nicola Watt – Higher Trainee in Psychiatry

Ruth Yates – Palliative Medicine Registrar

Steering Group

Paul Baughan – General Practitioner and Clinical Lead with Primary Care Faculty

George Beuken – Head of Pastoral Care and Education

Kirsty J Boyd – Macmillan Reader in Palliative Care

Deans Buchanan – Consultant in Palliative Medicine

Karen Campbell – Macmillan

Sandra Campbell – Macmillan Nurse Consultant for Cancer and Palliative Care

David Carroll – Associate Specialist in Palliative Care

Gerry Egan – Executive Director College of Paramedics

Marie Fallon – St Columba's Hospice Chair of Palliative Medicine

Mark Hazelwood – Chief Executive Scottish Partnership for Palliative Care

Claire O'Neill – Macmillan Lead Nurse Palliative Care

Iona Philp – Macmillan TayPEOLC MCN Manager

Lorna Porteous – Macmillan National Lead

Neil Pryde – Lead Cancer and Palliative Care GP NHS Fife

Jean Sargeant – Macmillan Quality Lead

Lianne Sherlock – Senior Editor, Class Professional Publishing

Foreword

It is well known that the field of modern palliative care developed from modest beginnings, was led by a small band of enthusiasts, and often operated outside or on the margins of the mainstream health and social care system. But as hospice founder Cicely Saunders famously said, 'we moved outside the NHS in order to let new ideas and practices come back in.'

This training manual is an eloquent testimony to the success of that ideal.

In the last half century, huge strides have been made to bring about the recognition of palliative care as a specialist activity. We have seen the growth of clinical centres of excellence, accredited training programmes, academic research groups and professional societies that support the local, national and international development of palliative care.

There is much to celebrate.

Yet at the same time, evidence of the growing need for palliative care continues to mount. It is estimated that the current number of 56 million deaths worldwide each year will rise to 92 million by 2050 (Clark et al., 2017). One recent calculation from a Lancet Commission suggests that every year 50 million people could benefit from palliative care (Knaul et al., 2018). At the same time, we know from global mapping studies that just 30 countries, accounting for only 15% of the global population, have access to the highest levels of palliative care provision (Clark et al., 2019). Even within those jurisdictions, we recognise there remains a significant problem of access to the care which is required.

A major and badly needed shift in orientation is therefore under way.

Specialist palliative care, research, education and clinical services will continue to have an important role. But increasingly we must look to raise overall standards of palliative care competence and confidence across the entire care system. This means palliative care enhancement in the practice of people working in many areas and specialisms, new collaborations with other fields, and the strengthening of palliative care in community and primary care settings.

Here in Scotland, we are fortunate to have a group of people who are massively committed to these ideals of 'generalist' palliative care. This manual is packed full of evidence-based wisdom and insight that will prove invaluable to so many people wishing to improve their palliative care practice. The optional accompanying one day course adds further depth and detail. Put together by contributors with high hopes and feet firmly on the ground, the *Enhanced Palliative Care* programme will be an invaluable resource to many and a direct benefit to many, many more who will receive care that has been influenced and improved by it.

David Clark Professor Emeritus

References

Clark D et al. (2017) Interventions at the end of life – a taxonomy for 'overlapping consensus'. *Wellcome Open Research,* 2:7.

Knaul FM et al. (2018) The *Lancet* Commission on Palliative Care and Pain Relief – findings, recommendations, and future directions. *The Lancet Global Health*, 6(Special Issue): S5–S6.

Clark D et al. (2019) Mapping levels of palliative care development in 198 countries: the situation in 2017. *Journal of Pain and Symptom Management*, 59(4): 794–807.

Chapter 1

Principles of Palliative and End-of-Life Care

Paul Baughan, Sandra Campbell and Neil Pryde

Learning Objectives

At the completion of this chapter, you will:

- Be able to describe the philosophy that underpins the principles of palliative and end-of-life care
- Be able to define what is meant by 'palliative care' and 'end-of-life care'
- Be able to describe why early identification of those who may benefit from a palliative approach to care is important, and the tools that can support this
- Understand the importance of anticipatory care planning and the various tools which support this.

The Origins of Palliative Care

The transformation of end-of-life care in the modern era began in 1967, thanks to Dame Cicely Saunders, founder of St Christopher's Hospice in London. Since then, the hospice movement has grown, and the field of generalist and specialist palliative care has evolved. Today there are still variations in how those who require palliative and end-of-life care receive it, with inequity of service provision evident across settings. One of the key aims of this book and the associated course is to reduce these inequalities.

Dame Cicely Saunders trained as a nurse in the 1940s. During her time as a registered nurse at St Luke's Hospital in London she learned a great deal about pain control via the administration of morphine on a four-hourly basis (Doyle, 2002). This would eventually become the foundation model for the treatment of chronic and terminal pain. She then studied to become a doctor, qualifying in 1957, and later became the first modern physician dedicated to palliative and end-of-life care (Stevens et al., 2009).

At her memorial service in 2006, Robert Twycross quoted her philosophy as:
(St Christopher's Hospice, 2021)

> *'You matter because you are you, and you matter to the end of your life. We will do all we can not only to help you die peacefully, but also to live until you die.'*

Definitions of Palliative Care

The term 'palliative care' can mean different things to different people. It is important for health and care professionals to have a firm understanding of what palliative care is and what it is not.

The World Health Organization (WHO) definition of palliative care

The World Health Organization (WHO) defines palliative care as:

'An approach that improves the quality of life of patients and their families facing the problems associated with life-threatening illness, through the prevention and relief of suffering by means of early identification and impeccable assessment and treatment of pain and other problems, physical, psychosocial and spiritual. Palliative care:

- *Provides relief from pain and other distressing symptoms;*
- *Affirms life and regards dying as a normal process;*
- *Intends neither to hasten or postpone death;*
- *Integrates the psychological and spiritual aspects of patient care;*
- *Offers a support system to help patients live as actively as possible until death;*
- *Offers a support system to help the family cope during the patient's illness and in their own bereavement;*
- *Uses a team approach to address the needs of patients and their families, including bereavement counselling, if indicated;*
- *Will enhance quality of life, and may also positively influence the course of illness;*
- *Is applicable early in the course of illness, in conjunction with other therapies that are intended to prolong life, such as chemotherapy or radiation therapy, and includes those investigations needed to better understand and manage distressing clinical complications.'*

(NICE, 2021)

The Scottish Government definitions of palliative care

Palliative care is an approach that improves the quality of life of patients (adults and children) and their families who are facing problems associated with life-threatening illness. It prevents and relieves suffering through the early identification, correct assessment and treatment of pain and other problems, whether physical, psychosocial or spiritual.

Non-specialist palliative care and support is provided by professionals across health and social care in a variety of different settings. This care may be delivered alongside active treatment, where this is appropriate. Such care can be delivered with varying degrees of specialist palliative support throughout the health and social care system.

Specialist palliative care can help people with more complex palliative care needs. It is provided by specially trained multi-professional palliative care teams, who are generally based in a hospice, an NHS specialist palliative care unit or an acute hospital. Specialist palliative care has a particular role in providing support, advice and education to the rest of the health and care system.

End-of-life care is care of the person living through the dying phase of life. This phase could vary between weeks, days or hours, the exact timing often being unpredictable. Changes and deterioration may occur suddenly and unexpectedly. It is helpful to explore and address individuals' needs concerning end-of-life care, and not assume it is covered within the remit of palliative care. End-of-life care should be seen as everyone's responsibility.

Bereavement is understood as 'the experience of losing someone important to us. It is characterised by grief, which is the process and the range of emotions we go through as we gradually adjust to the loss' (Mind, 2019). Bereavement care may be defined as any care provided formally or informally, through statutory or voluntary services or by members of the community to those affected. The need for support will apply to those affected by both expected and unexpected loss and death.

(Scottish Government, 2018)

The Four Dimensions of Palliative Care

In assessing needs, and planning how the full breadth of those needs will best be met sustainably, the following four dimensions of palliative care should always be considered (Figure 1.1). Attending to spiritual, social and psychological and emotional, in addition to physical ones, is not an optional extra, and doing so may impact positively on the physical supports a person needs. Palliative care involves all of these dimensions.

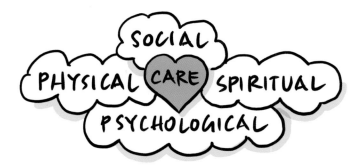

Figure 1.1   The four dimensions of palliative care.
Source: Image by Hazel White, Open Change.

Realistic medicine

From these definitions it is clear that effective palliative care should be available to anyone with an incurable, life-threatening disease. Their need should be identified at the appropriate time, with care and support provided to the patient and their 'family'. This practical and holistic approach sits well with the concept of 'Realistic Medicine', as outlined by Dr Catherine Calderwood in her 2017 report, 'Realising Realistic Medicine'. In the report, Calderwood surmises that:

> 'Realistic Medicine puts the person receiving care at the centre of decision making and creates a supported, personalised approach. It aims to reduce harm, waste and unwarranted variation, whilst acknowledging and managing the inherent risks associated with all healthcare, and championing innovation and improvement. These concepts are essential to a well-functioning and sustainable NHS for the future.
>
> Realistic Medicine is about supporting people using healthcare services, and their families, to feel empowered to discuss their treatment. It is not about failing to offer treatments that are likely to have benefit. That's why changing our style to sharing decisions with our patients is one of our priorities. A move away from the 'Doctor knows best' approach to shared decision making between the professional and patient will require more meaningful discussions about the treatment options available as well as their risks and benefits.'

The Importance of Dignity

It is helpful to approach palliative care issues in a way that has a dignity conserving approach. The following ABCD approach is a useful tool to adopt.

Attitudes
Behaviours
Compassionate **D**ialogue

In situations of distress, or in shared decision making, it is important to ensure **Attitudes** held and expressed are empathetic, demonstrate a sense of calm, and communicate the aim to work together positively to improve the situation. The **Behaviours** exhibited by the health professional, in word and deed, should evidence this attitude and intent. This foundation should set the right tone to enter into purposeful **Compassionate Dialogue**, and will underpin the gaining of therapeutic benefit from interventions. Dialogue allows for symptom experience to be described, heard, understood, acknowledged and managed.

Dr Harvey Max Chochinov, Director of the Manitoba Palliative Care Research Unit, CancerCare Manitoba in Winnipeg, and his team developed a dignity-conserving model of care as a succinct way of thinking about, and addressing, the issue of dignity. As part of this they use the following question to help them provide care: 'What do I need to know about you as a person to give you the best care possible?' (Chochinov et al., 2005).

The Palliative Care Generalist and Specialist

It is important that there is clarity of role, with a clear understanding of who is doing what, with and for the patient and their family. The terms 'generalist' and 'specialist' are often used but can be confusing for people and therefore unhelpful (Phillips et al., 2020). However, studies have shown the positive impact of a specialist nurse on patient outcomes (Leary et al., 2018). In palliative and end-of-life care, access to specialist advice and support should be available if and when required. From the patient and family perspective it is important to understand who does what, how and when rather than if they are a 'generalist' or a 'specialist'. A simple checklist of 'who to contact if ...' is a helpful tool for patients and carers. To take a very pragmatic approach, caring for dying people is everyone's responsibility, and teams must understand their contribution and responsibility to deliver safe and effective care at the end of life. A mutual understanding, and respect, for each other's roles is also integral to seamless care provision.

From a nursing perspective, there has been an evolving model of advanced practice, with a growing number of advanced nurse practitioners (ANPs) within healthcare who are now supporting the provision of palliative and end-of-life care. This model, shown in Figure 1.2, is also applicable to doctors, paramedics and other allied health professionals.

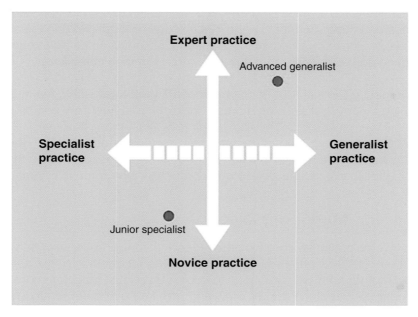

Figure 1.2   Relationship between specialist and advanced practice.

Source: NHS Education for Scotland, 2018a. Reproduced with permission.

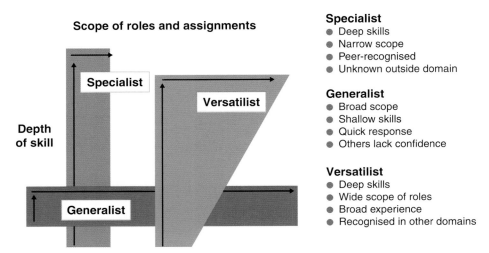

Figure 1.3 Specialist, generalist and versatilist.
Source: Gartner, 2005.

The Merriam-Webster (2019) dictionary's definition of a generalist is *'a person who knows something about a lot of subjects'*. A specialist is defined as *'a person who has special knowledge and skill relating to a particular job, area of study'*. The distinction between them is highlighted by the specialist having *'deep skills and a narrow scope'* compared with the generalist having a *'broad scope with shallow skills.'* In 2005, Gartner introduced the concept of the *versatilist* (Figure 1.3) arguing the benefits of the ability of certain individuals to develop their competence and apply depth of skill to a rich scope of situations and experiences. This could be how we describe what we expect of 'generalist' teams: to be able to embrace the detail of managing palliative and end-of-life care as part of their core skills.

However, this model by Gartner (2005) can be applied to all roles within the multidisciplinary team in describing the level of skills on a broad spectrum and how care can be provided.

Lawler et al. (2019) argue that a lot of the work and support undertaken by generalists, for people living with cancer in the community, goes unrecognised. Whether working as a generalist or specialist, ensuring a skilled and competent workforce is essential.

Cancer and Non-Malignant Disease

Historically, specialist palliative care was developed to support people with a cancer diagnosis, but in recent years there has been increasing recognition of the need for people living with other medical conditions to access specialist palliative care and advice. Increasing numbers of people in the UK are living with frailty and dementia, and many will benefit from a palliative approach to their care (Boland and Johnson, 2013; Zheng et al., 2013). Palliative care is now available to all, regardless of diagnosis, and there has been a very significant shift towards embracing the needs of those with non-malignant disease. Teams should have a knowledge of the requirements that are pertinent to specific medical conditions, but there are many similarities when it comes to providing good palliative and end-of-life care, regardless of diagnosis.

Identifying Those Who May Benefit from a Palliative Approach

> ### Key points
> - It is important to understand who might benefit from a palliative approach to their care.
> - There are a variety of 'tools' which can aid earlier identification.

In order to provide effective, holistic, person-centred palliative care it is important to know and understand the population group who might benefit. This involves an understanding of the definition of palliative care outlined above, with a recognition that it is not just for those approaching the very end of life or with a specific diagnosis.

Earlier identification of those who could be helped by a palliative approach to their care can allow people to make informed choices about what medical treatments they would like to receive, and to prioritise things that are important to them when their remaining length of life may be short.

Studies estimate that 82% of all people in developed countries will die from a progressive medical condition which would have been amenable to a palliative approach to care (Murtagh et al., 2014). It is difficult to know what proportion of people will actually receive a palliative approach to their care, but it is possible to estimate this from general practitioner (GP) practices' palliative care registers. Most GP practices in the UK hold a register or list of people within their practice who are at a palliative phase of their illness. Details of the palliative care register can be found in Appendix 1.1.

In a study examining 684 patients from nine general practices who were on the palliative care register, around 75% of patients with cancer were formally identified for palliative care; but for those with non-malignant disease, only 20% were formally identified (Zheng et al., 2013). In both cases identification was often in the last weeks of life, particularly so for the non-cancer group.

Identification tools

There are a number of different tools which have been developed to facilitate the earlier identification of people who might benefit from a palliative approach to their care. Many of these have been summarised and published by Healthcare Improvement Scotland in their 'Palliative Care Identification Tools Comparator' resource (2019). These tools are all designed for slightly different population groups. Some of these identification tools (for example, electronic Frailty Index) are electronic and designed for use at population level. Other tools can be used with a specific individual to identify particular factors in their medical condition or functional status which might indicate that the person is approaching the palliative stage of their illness (for example, SPICT™). More information on SPICT™ and the electronic Frailty Index is included in Appendix 1.2.

Identification tools must be used in conjunction with clinical or professional judgement and assessment (Figure 1.4). They can help professionals identify who may benefit from a palliative approach to their care and who might benefit from being added to the palliative care register. This in turn must lead to timely, focused conversations and assessments to discuss and plan care.

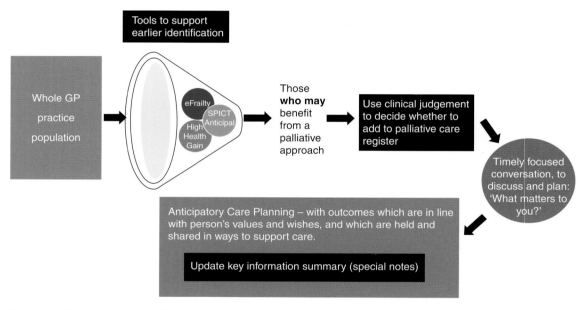

Figure 1.4 Using identification tools in practice.

Source: Scottish Government, 2019.

Anticipatory Care Planning

Key points

- Anticipatory care planning is an approach which focuses on 'What matters to you'.
- These care planning conversations should evolve over time, rather than being a one-off event.
- Good communication skills are essential to support this process.
- There are a variety of 'tools' which can help care planning.
- Sharing information within care plans is essential.

Anticipatory care planning (ACP) is a person-centred, proactive, 'thinking ahead' approach to care. It involves health and care professionals engaging with individuals, their families and carers to have the right conversations about what matters to them. It promotes a shared decision-making approach to care and helps individuals, their families and carers, to set personal goals so that the right thing is done at the right time, by the right person with the best outcome. Anticipatory care planning is also sometimes referred to as advance care planning.

What is anticipatory care planning?

Anticipatory care planning is not a one-off event. It is a process that starts with a conversation and which can develop and evolve over time. It is particularly helpful for people who are living with long-term progressive and incurable medical conditions where there is the potential for a change or a deterioration. Care planning allows people to consider and make choices about how they would like to be treated, and who they would like to be involved in helping them to make decisions about their care, should a change in health occur (Figure 1.5). Whenever possible and appropriate it is helpful to include family members, carers and any legal guardian or person holding a power of attorney in these discussions.

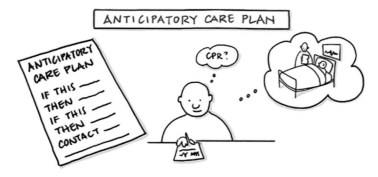

Figure 1.5   The anticipatory care plan.

Source: Image by Hazel White, Open Change.

A summary of these conversations can be captured in an anticipatory care plan. People should have the opportunity to add information to their care plan, and to change their mind or amend details as appropriate.

This plan is a dynamic record of the preferred actions, interventions and responses that care providers should make following a clinical deterioration or a crisis in a person's care or support. It can be reviewed and updated as the patient's condition or personal circumstances change, and different things take priority.

There is consistent evidence from several systematic reviews for the benefits of anticipatory care planning in terms of improving patient and family knowledge, shared decision making, documentation of care preferences, and patient and family satisfaction with end-of-life care provided (Brinkman-Stoppelenburg et al., 2014; Martin et al., 2016). There is also limited evidence of benefit in terms of improving patient outcomes including quality of life or reducing health service utilisation.

Tools to support anticipatory care planning

A variety of tools have been produced to support shared decision making and anticipatory care planning. Systematic reviews provide evidence that such tools can improve patient and family knowledge related to end-of-life decision making (Austin et al., 2015; Cardona-Morrell et al., 2017; Oczkowski et al., 2016).

Some of the different resources and tools to support shared decision making and anticipatory care planning are listed below.

ACP Toolkit, Healthcare Improvement Scotland

A 4-step approach to support anticipatory care planning has been produced by Healthcare Improvement Scotland. During the coronavirus pandemic of 2020, this was supported by a more concise 'Essential ACP' (Healthcare Improvement Scotland, 2020a; Healthcare Improvement Scotland, 2021).

Recommended Summary Plan for Emergency Care and Treatment (ReSPECT)

ReSPECT is a process that supports the creation of personalised recommendations for a person's clinical care in a future emergency in which they are unable to make or express choices. The ReSPECT form is designed to summarise the wishes of individuals and the resulting recommendations about their care. An electronic version of the ReSPECT form is being developed (Fritz et al., 2017).

Anticipatory care planning in three questions

This questionnaire developed by NHS Lothian is given to relatives of new care home residents who lack the capacity to make decisions about their welfare. It asks how they think a resident would like to be treated in the event of the following (Royal College of General Practitioners, 2020):

- A sudden collapse
- An infection not responding to antibiotics
- An inability to eat and drink due to illness.

Talking about care planning: RED-MAP

RED-MAP is a useful six step approach to support anticipatory care planning conversations. This tool helps guide discussions about ACP. It provides prompts under the following headings: Ready, Expect, Diagnosis, Matters, Actions, Plan. For further information on RED-MAP see Chapter Three – Communication.

NHS Education for Scotland (NES) shared decision making training

NES has developed an e-learning module, 'Realistic conversations – shared decision making in practice', which is suitable for all health and care professionals. It provides a

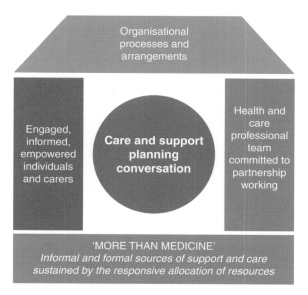

Figure 1.6 Components of Scottish House of Care.

Source: House of Care framework (The ALLIANCE, 2016) adapted from Year of Care Partnerships (2016), used with permission.

foundation in the skills, terminology and evidence base for shared decision making, as well as practical hints and tips that professionals can use in practice (NHS Education for Scotland, 2021).

Scottish Social Services Council open badges

Scottish Social Services Council (SSSC) offers training through their 'Open badges' scheme in a number of topic areas, including communication and relationships in care settings and palliative and end-of-life care awareness (Scottish Social Services Council, 2020).

The House of Care

The House of Care is a model of care provision that is built around a care and support planning conversation (Figure 1.6). It aims to ensure that health and care systems are responsive to the needs of people with long-term conditions (The ALLIANCE, 2016).

Sharing of anticipatory care plans

Anticipatory care plans are of limited use if the professionals delivering care are unaware of them. For this reason, it is important that any decisions around future care choices are shared with those that might be involved at the time. To facilitate this sharing of preferences for care, Electronic Palliative Care Coordination Systems (EPaCCS) have been developed (Petrova et al., 2018). Across the UK, regional systems include Coordinate My Care (London); the South-West EPaCCS; and the Leeds EPaCCS. In Scotland, the Key Information Summary was introduced in 2013 as an electronic care coordination system for anyone who might have urgent care needs, not just those identified for palliative care.

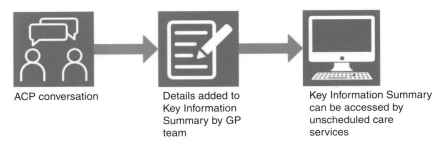

ACP conversation

Details added to Key Information Summary by GP team

Key Information Summary can be accessed by unscheduled care services

Figure 1.7   Sharing of ACPs in Scotland.

Source: Healthcare Improvement Scotland, 2020b. Reused with permission.

The Key Information Summary (KIS) is an electronic clinical tool, which can be used to share components of an anticipatory care plan. The KIS is linked to the electronic clinical systems used within general practice in Scotland, and so is created and updated by professionals working within general practice, and then can be viewed by providers of unscheduled care (including NHS24, GP out-of-hours services, Scottish Ambulance Service and emergency departments throughout Scotland) (Figure 1.7). People who have a KIS in place at the time of death are 3.7 times more likely to die in the community rather than hospital (Finucane et al., 2019). However, the KIS has limitations, as it can only be updated through primary care electronic systems, and some professional groups, including social care, are unable to access it. In Scotland a national digital platform is being developed to replace KIS and address these issues.

Multidisciplinary Teamworking

After the development and sharing of care plans, it is important that teams work closely together to coordinate and provide the care required.

The six step approach as defined by NHS England is a useful framework to support service development (Figure 1.8).

Good teamwork and collaborative working are critical factors on the provision of safe and effective care that ensure optimum outcomes for patients and carers. Being able to

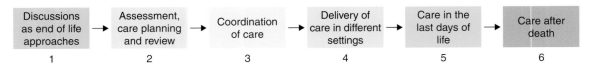

Discussions as end of life approaches	Assessment, care planning and review	Coordination of care	Delivery of care in different settings	Care in the last days of life	Care after death
1	2	3	4	5	6

Figure 1.8   Six step approach.

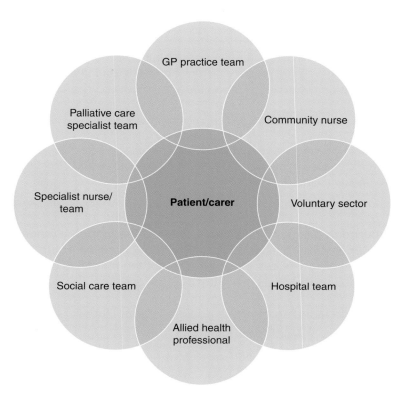

Figure 1.9   Danger of patients feeling overwhelmed by different teams involved in their care.

articulate the outcome of assessment and care planning between teams is a core element of seamless care. This is where it is essential for all the professionals involved, whether generalist or specialist, to work together to provide holistic care.

However, the patient can have so many teams involved that it may feel suffocating and, indeed, intrusive. A balance is therefore needed to ensure that the right team is there at the right time (Figure 1.9).

Good coordination regarding care provision is necessary. Sometimes, as the person nears the end of life, families refuse additional support due to a lack of understanding of how needs can increase significantly in the last days of life. Sensitive communication is required to prepare families for what to expect. The benefit of support with personal care at this time can often prevent an unnecessary admission to hospital.

Care must continue after death, with support for the next of kin, family and carers. The grieving process affects people in many different ways.

Living and Dying Well

The overall goal in providing good palliative care should be to support the person to live as well as possible for as long as possible. There has been an increasing emphasis on rehabilitation with Hospice UK defining rehabilitative palliative care as:

> *'a paradigm which integrates rehabilitation, enablement, self-management and self-care into the holistic model of palliative care. It is an interdisciplinary approach in which all members of the team, including nurses, doctors, psychosocial practitioners and allied health professionals, work collaboratively with the patient, their relatives and carers to support them to achieve their personal goals and priorities.'*

(Tiberini and Richardson, 2015)

Atul Gawande in his book *Being Mortal* (2014) describes the natural changes and adaptions to life that can be made within families to accommodate changing needs as individuals progress through the ageing process. He suggests that the following questions are incorporated in the assessment and care planning process:

1. What is your understanding of where you are in your illness?
2. What are your fears or worries for the future?
3. What are your goals and priorities?
4. What outcomes are acceptable to you – what are you willing to sacrifice or not?
5. What would a good day look like?

This approach is person-centred and in accordance with the 'What matters to you' agenda across the UK. The latter question is very useful for goal setting near the end of life, to help facilitate achievement of what is important to the person (for example, bringing the dog into the hospital ward or sitting in their garden).

Education and Training

All providers of palliative and end-of-life care should undertake regular education and training to maintain their competence and enhance their skills. The educational framework 'Palliative and end of life care: enriching and improving experience' developed by NHS Education for Scotland in partnership with Scottish Social Services Council (NHS Education for Scotland, 2018b) provides guidance as to the skill/ knowledge level expected for our health and social services workforce. It outlines five domains of care:

- Domain 1: Fundamentals of palliative care
  - Reviews the philosophy of palliative care
- Domain 2: Communication and conversation
  - Emphasises the importance and significance of effective communication

- Domain 3: Loss, grief and bereavement
  - Includes the potential impact on those caring for people with palliative and end-of-life care needs
- Domain 4: Care planning and delivery
  - Embraces shared decision making in the care planning process
- Domain 5: Care in the last days of life
  - Includes the need for good symptom control and comfort care.

There are four distinct levels of practice within each domain. These are:

1. Informed
   - For all staff
2. Skilled
   - For those who regularly care for people with palliative and end-of-life care needs
3. Enhanced
   - For those who regularly provide, coordinate and manage palliative and end-of-life care
4. Expert
   - For those who provide specialist care.

The Enhanced Palliative Care (EPC) manual and course will cover each of the five domains of care and is aimed at the enhanced level of practice.

Summary

Palliative care is an approach which aims to improve the quality of life for people and their families when faced with progressive, incurable, life-limiting illness. As well as controlling physical symptoms, the holistic needs of an individual are assessed, taking into account social, psychological and spiritual aspects of care. Every health and care professional has a role to play within palliative care, with expert support from specialist palliative care services.

It is important to be able to identify those people who would benefit from a palliative approach to their care. There are many different tools that have been developed to aid this process. Once someone has been identified, careful care planning can take place with good communication between all those involved. A proactive 'thinking ahead' or 'anticipatory care planning' approach is helpful, and there are many resources available to enable this.

Care plans should be coordinated and delivered through multidisciplinary team working. The patient and their family must be aware how and when to access support. This support should be available in a responsive manner throughout the period of deterioration, and after death for the bereaved.

Throughout the period of care, a person-centred and dignity preserving approach should be adopted. Regular education and training is required for all professionals involved in supporting people who are approaching the end of their life. The Enhanced Palliative Care (EPC) manual and course will help those practising at an enhanced level, as defined within the educational framework produced by NHS Education for Scotland and Scottish Social Services Council.

Further Reading

Fallon M and Foley P (2012) Rising to the challenge of palliative care for non-malignant disease. *Palliative Medicine*, 26(2): 99–100.

Johnston B et al. (2015) The person behind the patient: a feasibility study using the Patient Dignity Question for patients with palliative care needs. *International Journal of Palliative Nursing*, 21(2): 71–77.

Kingston AEH, Kirkland J and Hadjimchalis A (2019) Palliative care in non-malignant disease. *Medicine* 48(1): 37–42.

Maas EAT et al. (2013) What tools are available to identify patients with palliative care needs in primary care: a systematic literature review and survey of European practice. *BMJ Supportive and Palliative Care*, 3(4): 444–451.

Mannix K (2018) *With the End in Mind: How to Live and Die Well*. London: William Collins.

Mohammed S et al. (2020) 'I'm going to push this door open. You can close it.' A qualitative study of the brokering work of oncology clinic nurses in introducing early palliative care. *Palliative Medicine,* 34(2): 209–218.

Scottish Government (2014) Caring for people in the last days and hours of life – guidance. Available at: https://www.gov.scot/publications/caring-people-last-days-hours-life-guidance/

Scottish Government (2015) Palliative and end of life care: strategic framework for action. Available at: https://www.gov.scot/publications/strategic-framework-action-palliative-end-life-care/

Scottish Government (2017) National dementia strategy: 2017–2020. Available at: https://www.gov.scot/publications/scotlands-national-dementia-strategy-2017-2020/

Sims S, Hewitt G and Harris R (2015) Evidence of a shared purpose, critical reflection, innovation and leadership in interprofessional healthcare teams: a realist synthesis. *Journal of Interprofessional Care*, 29(3): 209–215.

Stern N (2015) *Hope in Small Doses*. USA: Ruthenia Press.

Weathers E et al. (2016) Advance care planning: a systematic review of randomised controlled trials conducted with older adults. *Maturita*, 91: 101–109.

White N et al. (2017) How accurate is the 'surprise question' in identifying patients at the end of life. A systematic review and meta-analysis. *BMC Medicine*, 15, 139.

References

ALLIANCE (2016) The House of Care Model. Available at: https://www.alliance-scotland.org.uk/health-and-social-care-integration/house-of-care/house-of-care-model/

Austin CA et al. (2015) Tools to promote shared decision making in serious illness: a systematic review. *JAMA Internal Medicine*, 175(7): 1213–1221.

Boland J and Johnson MJ (2013) End of life care for non-cancer patients. *BMJ Supportive and Palliative Care*, 3(1): 2–3.

Brinkman-Stoppelenburg A, Rietjens JAC and van der Heide A (2014) The effects of advance care planning on end-of-life care: a systematic review. *Palliative Medicine*, 28(8): 1000–1025.

Calderwood et al. (2017) Realising realistic medicine. *Scottish Government*. Available at: https://www.gov. scot/binaries/content/documents/govscot/publications/progress-report/2017/02/chief-medical-officer-scotland-annual-report-2015-16-realising-realistic-9781786526731/documents/00514513-pdf/00514513-pdf/govscot%3Adocument/00514513.pdf

Cardona-Morrell M et al. (2017) A systematic review of effectiveness of decision aids to assist older patients at the end of life. *Patient Education and Counseling*, 100(3): 425–435.

Chochinov H et al. (2005) Dignity therapy: a novel psychotherapeutic intervention for patients near the end of Life. *Journal of Clinical Oncology*, 23(24): 5520–5525.

Church Times (2006) Recollection: 'You matter because you are you'. *Church Times*. Available at: https://www. churchtimes.co.uk/articles/2006/17-march/gazette/recollection-you-matter-because-you-are-you

Doyle D (2002) *Volunteers in Hospice and Palliative Care: A Handbook for Volunteer Service Managers.* Oxford: Oxford University Press.

Finucane A et al. (2019) Electronic care co- ordination systems for people with advanced progressive illness: a mixed-methods evaluation. *British Journal of General Practice*, 70(690): e20–e28.

Fritz Z et al. (2017) ReSPECT is a personal emergency care plan summary. *BMJ*, 357: j2213.

Gartner (2005) The IT professional outlook: where will we go from here? Available at: https://www.ee.iitb. ac.in/~hpc/.old_studs/hrishi_page/outlook/report.pdf

Gawande A (2014) *Being Mortal: Medicine and What Matters in the End*. New York: Macmillan.

Healthcare Improvement Scotland (2019) Palliative care identification tools comparator. Available at: https://ihub.scot/media/6484/palliative-care-identification-tools-comparator.pdf

Healthcare Improvement Scotland (2020a) Anticipatory care planning toolkit. Available at: https:// ihub.scot/project-toolkits/anticipatory-care-planning-toolkit/anticipatory-care-planning-toolkit/ tools-and-resources/documentation-and-sharing/my-acp/

Healthcare Improvement Scotland (2020b) Anticipatory care planning in Scotland: supporting people to plan ahead and discuss their wishes for future care. Available at: https://ihub.scot/ media/7073/20200214-acp-v031.pdf

Healthcare Improvement Scotland (2021) Anticipatory Care Planning in the context of COVID-19. Available at: https://ihub.scot/project-toolkits/anticipatory-care-planning-toolkit/ anticipatory-care-planning-toolkit/anticipatory-care-planning-in-the-context-of-covid-19/

Lawler J et al. (2019) Uncovering the hidden workforce in cancer care in the community. *Primary Health Care*, 30(2): e1610.

Leary A and Dix A (2018) Using data to show the impact of nursing work on patient outcomes. *Nursing Times,* 114(10): 23–25.

Martin RS et al. (2016) The effects of advance care planning interventions on nursing home residents: a systematic review. *Journal of the American Medical Directors Association*, 17(4): 284.

Merriam-Webster (2019) Definition of a generalist. Available at: https://www.merriam-webster.com/ dictionary/generalist

Mind (2019) Bereavement. Available at: https://www.mind.org.uk/information-support/ guides-to-support-and-services/bereavement/about-bereavement/

Murtagh FE et al. (2014) How many people need palliative care? A study developing and comparing methods for population-based estimates. *Palliative Medicine*, 28(1): 49–58.

NHS Education for Scotland (2018a) Specialist and advanced practice. Available at: https://www. advancedpractice.scot.nhs.uk/uk-progress/specialist-and-advanced-practice.aspx

NHS Education for Scotland (2018b) Palliative and end of life care: enriching and improving experience. Available at: https://learn.nes.nhs.scot/2452/palliative-and-end-of-life-care-enriching-and-improving-experience/palliative-and-end-of-life-care-enriching-and-improving-experience

NHS Education for Scotland (2021) Realistic conversations: shared decision making in practice. Available at: https://www.nes.scot.nhs.uk/nes-current/realistic-conversations-shared-decision-making-in-practice/

NHS England (2021) Electronic Frailty Index. Available at: https://www.england.nhs.uk/ourwork/clinical-policy/older-people/frailty/efi/#the-contract-requires-general-practice-to-use-an-appropriate-tool-for-example-the-electronic-frailty-index-efi-what-is-the-efi

NICE (2021) What is palliative care? Available at: https://cks.nice.org.uk/topics/palliative-care-general-issues/background-information/definition/#:~:text='Palliative%20care%3A,to%20hasten%20nor%20postpone%20death.

Oczkowski SJ et al. (2016) Communication tools for end-of-life decision-making in ambulatory care settings: a systematic review and meta-analysis. *PloS One*, 11(4): e0150671.

Petrova M et al. (2018) Crash course in EPaCCS (Electronic Palliative Care Coordination Systems): 8 years of successes and failures in patient data sharing to learn from. *BMJ Supportive and Palliative Care*, 8(4): 447–455.

Phillips J, Johnston B and McIlfatrick S (2020) Valuing palliative care nursing and extending the reach *Palliative Medicine*, 34(2): 157–159.

Royal College of General Practitioners (2020) Anticipatory planning in three questions. Available at: https://www.rcgp.org.uk/clinical-and-research/resources/bright-ideas/anticipatory-care-planning-in-three-questions.aspx

Scottish Government (2018) Palliative and End-of-Life Care by Integration Authorities: advice note. Available at: https://www.gov.scot/publications/strategic-commissioning-palliative-end-life-care-integration-authorities/pages/4/

Scottish Government (2019) The primary medical services directed enhanced services (Scotland) 2019 palliative care scheme. Available at: https://www.sehd.scot.nhs.uk/pca/PCA2019(M)06.pdf

Scottish Social Services Council (2020) SSC Open Badges. Available at: https://www.badges.sssc.uk.com/

St Christopher's Hospice (2021) Tributes to Dame Cicely Saunders. Available at: https://www.stchristophers.org.uk/about/damecicelysaunders/tributes

Stevens E, Jackson S and Milligan S (2009) *Palliative Nursing across the Spectrum of Care*. Oxford: Blackwell Publishing Ltd.

Tiberini R and Richardson H (2015) *Rehabilitative Palliative Care: Enabling People to Live Fully until They Die: A Challenge for the 21st Century*. London: Hospice UK.

University of Edinburgh (2021) Using SPICT™ and RED-MAP. Available at: https://www.spict.org.uk/using-spict/

Year of Care Partnerships (2016) The house. Available at: https://www.yearofcare.co.uk/house

Zheng L et al. (2013) How good is UK primary care at identifying patients for generalist and specialist palliative care: a mixed methods study. *European Journal of Palliative Care*, 20(5): 216–222.

Appendix 1.1   The General Practice Palliative Care Register

What is a palliative care register (PCR)?

The palliative care register is a list of people who may benefit from a palliative approach to their care. It is usually an electronic list held by the GP practice on the GP clinical system (EMIS or VISION in Scotland).

How are people added to the PCR?

People are added to the PCR by the addition of a specific Read code into their primary care electronic medical record. This Read code can be added by community-based staff by:

1. typing the specific alphanumeric code into the medical record of the patient, or
2. through a template on the GP clinical system (for example, a palliative care template), or
3. clicking the appropriate box within the Key Information Summary.

What are the codes that need to be used to add a person to the PCR?

Any of the following Read codes will add a person onto the PCR:

ZV57C	Palliative care
8H7g	Referral to palliative care service
8BAP	Specialist palliative care
8BAT	Specialist palliative care treatment – outpatient 8H6A. Refer to terminal care consultant
8CM1	On gold standards palliative care framework
8HH7	Referred to community specialist palliative care team 8BJ1. Palliative treatment
8BA2	Terminal care
8H7L	Refer for terminal care
8BAS	Specialist palliative care treatment – daycare
9EB5	DS1500 Disability living allowance completed
1Z01	Terminal illness – late stage.

How can the PCR be used?

Many GP practices use the PCR to highlight people to discuss at their multidisciplinary team meetings. These are sometimes called Gold Standards Framework meetings after the initiative by the same name. At these meetings the GP practice multidisciplinary team will meet to discuss the needs of people on their PCR. This will involve considering what proactive and anticipatory care may be required to make it easier to manage future decline in health or function.

Appendix 1.2   Tools to Support Earlier Identification

Electronic Frailty Index (eFI)

The eFI uses existing electronic health record data to detect and assess the severity of frailty. It uses a cumulative deficit model of frailty, in which frailty is defined through the accumulation of deficits, which can be clinical signs, symptoms, diseases and disability.

The eFI comprises 36 deficits, which have been developed using GP Read codes. A person's frailty score is calculated by dividing the total number of deficits that they have by the total number of possible deficits. The score is a reliable predictor of those who are at risk of adverse outcomes, such as care home admission, hospitalisation and death.

The eFI enables services and treatments to be targeted on the basis of people's frailty status, rather than their chronological age, and has the potential to transform care for older people living in the community (NHS England, 2021).

The Supportive and Palliative Care Indicators Tool (SPICT™)

The Supportive and Palliative Care Indicators Tool (SPICT™) can support the identification of people with advanced health conditions who are at risk of deteriorating and dying. It lists general indicators of deteriorating health to look for, and advises looking for clinical indicators of one or more advanced conditions:

- Cancer
- Dementia/frailty
- Neurological disease
- Heart/vascular disease
- Respiratory disease
- Kidney disease
- Liver disease.

It also makes recommendations to review current care and care planning.

SPICT™ can help to identify people at risk of deterioration or dying at an earlier stage so that they can benefit from well-coordinated, supportive and palliative care, combined with appropriate treatment of their illnesses (The University of Edinburgh, 2021).

Chapter 2

Ethical and Legal Considerations

Jenny Doig, Sandra McConnell and
Jill McKane with Lorna Frame,
Stuart P Milligan and Katie Pears

Learning Objectives

This chapter will help you to:

- Demonstrate the importance of person-centred care and an understanding of personal and family values in palliative care
- Deliberate on the legal, ethical and communication issues surrounding ceilings of treatment and 'Do not attempt cardiopulmonary resuscitation' (DNACPR) discussions
- Discuss the assessment of capacity and how to care for people who are unable to make decisions for themselves in the four countries of the United Kingdom
- Understand how the use of advance directives, advance decisions and powers of attorney vary between the three UK legal systems
- Appreciate the complexity and skills involved in managing depression and anxiety in a person with a life-limiting illness
- Understand the governance and legal issues in relation to the use of unlicensed medications and the challenges of travelling abroad with a life-limiting illness and controlled drugs
- Establish an understanding of the issues surrounding a request for physician-assisted dying.

Scenario

Background

Fiona, aged 60, has motor neurone disease and has recently had several severe recurrent depressive episodes. She lives with her husband Gino who is her main carer. They don't have children or other family nearby and rely on social care support four times daily. Fiona's priority is maintaining her independence. Gino is becoming exhausted with caring for his wife as her motor neurone disease progresses and her ability to function deteriorates.

Key points

- Fiona's capacity to make decisions fluctuates such as during episodes of acute illness.
- Discussions with Fiona and Gino about the role of an advance decision and power of attorney are especially relevant as Fiona's capacity fluctuates.
- As Fiona's disease progresses, questions arise for the multidisciplinary team, such as 'What matters most to Fiona now?', 'How can we best meet her needs?', and 'How can the team work with her fluctuating capacity to enable and respect her wishes?'
- Cardiopulmonary resuscitation (CPR) may be considered in the context of anticipatory care planning discussions with Fiona and Gino.
- Fiona has a controlled drug prescription. It is important to have an understanding of safe clinical governance structures regarding prescribing requirements relevant to your scope of practice.

Timeline

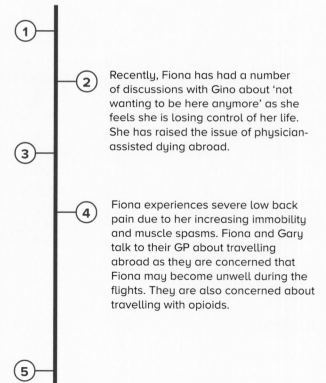

1 Fiona is having frequent chest infections which are treated with antibiotics and her mental capacity tends to fluctuate during these episodes. She has expressed clear views to Gino and her GP about her disease and what treatments she would find acceptable as her condition progresses.

2 Recently, Fiona has had a number of discussions with Gino about 'not wanting to be here anymore' as she feels she is losing control of her life. She has raised the issue of physician-assisted dying abroad.

3 Fiona's GP uses a person-centred approach to enable Fiona and her husband to discuss Fiona's priorities, hopes and fears and plans for her future care. Fiona wants to have a last holiday abroad with Gino and doesn't want future chest infections treated with antibiotics. Fiona decides to write an advance decision refusing life-sustaining treatment, specifically antibiotics, should she develop a further chest infection and to complete a DNACPR form. Her husband has already registered as his wife's welfare power of attorney.

4 Fiona experiences severe low back pain due to her increasing immobility and muscle spasms. Fiona and Gary talk to their GP about travelling abroad as they are concerned that Fiona may become unwell during the flights. They are also concerned about travelling with opioids.

5 Fiona and Gino ask her GP about assisted dying after reading about it on the internet.

Key considerations

- How would you promote person-centred care within a healthcare organisation?
- How would you support Fiona if she presented with symptoms of depression?
- Gino and Fiona ask for your advice about writing an advance decision. What information would you offer the couple about an advance decision to refuse treatment?
- What legal, ethical and communication issues would you consider when assessing a person's capacity prior to discussing a treatment escalation plan, DNACPR or a Recommended Summary Plan for Emergency Care and Treatment (ReSPECT)?
- What are the legal and ethical issues raised by requests for euthanasia and physician-assisted dying, and how should the multidisciplinary team approach the situation when Fiona and Gino raise the subject of physician-assisted dying?
- What information would you give to Fiona and Gino about travelling abroad with opioids?

Person-Centred Care in Palliative Care

The importance of person-centred palliative care was emphasised by Dame Cicely Saunders (2001):

> 'The losses of parting cannot be removed but their devastating effects can be ameliorated. For this we must give attention to the whole person with all the insights the humanities can give us.'

It is generally accepted that people should be treated with dignity, compassion and respect. This is encapsulated in the ABCD approach (see 'The importance of dignity' (p. 4) in Chapter 1 – Principles of Palliative and End-of-Life Care)

There are many definitions of, and dimensions to, person-centred care (PCC). The Healthcare Quality Strategy for NHS Scotland described it as (Scottish Government, 2010):

> 'Mutually beneficial partnerships between patients, their families and those delivering healthcare services which respect individual needs and values, and which demonstrate compassion, continuity, clear communication and shared decision making.'

This could be summarised as 'What matters *to* you?' rather than 'What's the matter *with* you?'. In practice it means finding out who and what is important to the person, and working with them and their loved ones to support their wishes and care. Achieving this involves providing the information people need to be fully involved in decision making, ensuring that services are, as far as possible, organised around their needs, and enabling them to be involved in their care, at whatever level they choose. This requires a holistic approach from healthcare professionals encompassing the physical, emotional, practical, social and spiritual needs of the patient. It involves a change in practice to ask about what is important to the patient, rather than simply concentrating on their diagnosis and past medical history. The CARE approach (Connecting, Assessing, Responding, Empowering) described in Chapter 3 – Communication (p. 54) is a useful tool for assessing needs and facilitating PCC.

The Royal College of Nursing (RCN, 2021) stressed that:

> *'People have their own views on what's best for them and their own priorities in life. So as health care workers we have to be flexible to meet their needs – we have to make our system suit them, rather than the other way round.'*

If PCC is successful the patient's care is not only tailored to meet their needs, but also, with the patient's consent, the needs of their family/carers who play a crucial role in supporting patients at the end of life, enabling care at home, and preventing hospital (re)admission. Carers' needs differ from those of patients and should be assessed separately. Carers require support as 'co-workers' and it is vital to ensure that they have the information, skills and equipment they need. They may also need support as 'clients,' in their own right, to preserve their own well-being and health. Families and carers will differ in what they find helpful, and what they need is often very different to what practitioners expect (Ewing and Grande, 2018).

People living with long-term conditions value consideration of their personal circumstances, and what matters to them to enable them to live a good life, as particularly important (Chatterjee, 2016). There are, however, a number of barriers to a patient receiving PCC including individual patient and practitioner beliefs, funding and organisational structures, systems, cultures and leadership (Ewing and Grande, 2018; Byrne, Baldwin and Harvey 2020). Conversely PCC can be facilitated by staff education and self-compassion, leadership, patient-centred care champions, resource availability and organisational culture, structure and development (Burton et al., 2017; Biddy et al., 2015; Haraldsdottir et al., 2019; Byrne, Baldwin and Harvey, 2020). A number of models and techniques have been shown to help provide PCC (see Table 2.1).

Table 2.1   Initiatives that promote Person-centred Care.

Initiative	Model	Outcomes
Schwartz round (The Point of Care Foundation, 2021)	A structured forum where all staff, clinical and non-clinical, come together regularly to discuss the emotional and social aspects of working in healthcare. The purpose is to understand the challenges and rewards that are intrinsic to providing care. The underlying premise is that the compassion shown by staff can make all the difference to a patient's experience of care, but that in order to provide compassionate care staff must, in turn, feel supported in their work.	Helps staff feel more supported in their jobs, allowing them the time and space to reflect on their roles. Staff feel less stressed and isolated, with increased insight and appreciation for each other's roles. Also helps to reduce hierarchies between staff and to focus attention on relational aspects of care. Staff have confidence in their ability to attend to the emotional aspects of patient care.
House of Care (The Health Foundation, 2016)	A model that draws on international evidence and best practice to show that effective care planning relies on four key elements in the local healthcare system. Patients feeling engaged in decisions about their treatment and care and able to act on these decisions. Professionals being committed to working in partnership with patients. Systems being in place to organise resources effectively. Having a whole-system approach to commissioning health and care services.	The House of Care illustrates the importance and interdependence of each element of holistic care. The model can act as a checklist highlighting what needs to be in place, a metaphor emphasising that care and support planning is complex and that all the components need to be in place to make it a success, and a flexible framework guiding each local community to build a stable house designed round the needs of local people.
'What matters to me' boards (The Health Foundation, 2016)	An information board placed by beds to make sure everyone can see what is most important to each patient. They are used to write down the patient's preferences and priorities, such as whether they want friends and family close by, or preferences about pain relief, sleep or treatment options.	The boards help share information about what matters to the patient, and encourage PCC.
Hello my name is ... (2021)	A national campaign founded by Kate Granger, a doctor living with terminal cancer, to encourage all staff to introduce themselves by name and profession when meeting a new patient. This includes wearing 'Hello my name is ...' badges to start the conversation.	Kate said, 'In my mind it (introducing yourself properly) is the first rung on the ladder to providing compassionate care.'

Do Not Attempt Cardiopulmonary Resuscitation (DNACPR)

It is important to consider CPR in the context of anticipatory care planning discussions and future care for patients. CPR was first described by Kouwenhoven et al. in 1960 as a method of restarting the heart in the event of a sudden cardiac arrest, where the envisioned recipients were otherwise well individuals who were expected to make a good recovery from the episode and its treatment.

The cessation of the heartbeat and/or breathing occurs as part of the natural process of dying from any cause. The average survival discharge rate for people who survive a hospital cardiorespiratory arrest and CPR is 15–20%, whereas following an arrest in the community, where CPR is attempted, the average survival rate is 5–10% (BMA et al., 2016). Survival depends on many things, including the cause and circumstances of the cardiorespiratory arrest, comorbidities, how soon CPR is started and the availability of resuscitation equipment and trained staff (BMA et al., 2016). Figures do vary, due to a variety of factors. In a meta-analysis study, Ebell and Afonso (2011) found that 3.1% of 'dependent' patients survived to discharge following in-hospital CPR, and only 1.9% of patients with a metastatic malignancy survived. CPR in these and similar circumstances is likely to either subject patients to traumatic physical treatment at the end of their life and deprive them of a dignified death, or restart their heart for a brief period of time and potentially prolong their suffering from their underlying illness. In other words, the burdens of CPR can outweigh the benefits in some situations, for example when attempts are made to prevent a natural and inevitable death. Chan et al. (2013) found, in a study of patients aged 65 years and over, that old age was associated with poorer survival following hospital CPR. However, in patients who were 85 years or older and discharged from hospital following CPR, half were still alive after a year, prompting the suggestion that discussions about advance directives should be individualised and informed by patients' preferences and health status.

Ideally the appropriateness of CPR should be considered in advance when there is an identifiable risk of cardiac or respiratory arrest, either due to a terminal illness, a significant co-morbidity or an acute, severe event, to avoid the need for assessments in crisis situations (BMA et al., 2016). There is generally an initial presumption that CPR should be attempted when a person dies or suffers a sudden cardiac arrest unless a decision to the contrary is formally recorded (BMA et al., 2016), and anticipatory care planning has therefore emerged as a method of minimising the improper use of CPR. Standardised 'do not attempt' CPR (DNACPR) forms are available for the purposes of clear documentation and communication, and guidance published jointly by the British Medical Association (BMA), Resuscitation Council (UK) and Royal College of Nursing (BMA et al., 2016) is available to assist healthcare professionals in making these often difficult judgements. Importantly, a DNACPR decision refers only to CPR (BMA, 2007) and does not preclude other forms of active treatment such as chemotherapy, non-invasive ventilation or intravenous antibiotics; it must not compromise the high-quality delivery of any other aspects of care.

Who can make DNACPR decisions?

There must be a presumption of involvement of the patient unless there is reason to believe that it will cause them significant physical or psychological harm (*Tracey v Cambridge University Hospitals NHS Foundation Trust*, 2014).

Decisions regarding CPR are complex and sensitive and should be made by healthcare professionals with the necessary training and expertise, which includes suitably skilled nurses (BMA et al., 2016). There should be discussions with the wider multidisciplinary team to ensure their agreement, but the ultimate responsibility lies with the most senior clinician in charge of the patient's care (BMA et al., 2016).

Making DNACPR decisions

As a result of differences in clinical and personal circumstances, it is essential that CPR decisions are made on an individual patient basis following a careful assessment and not as part of 'blanket' policies (BMA et al., 2016). However, key ethical and legal principles apply in all cases.

Ethical considerations

The four principles of biomedical ethics (Beauchamp and Childress, 2013) are particularly relevant to CPR decisions. They are beneficence, non-maleficence, autonomy and justice. The ethical principle of beneficence refers to acting in a way that promotes the well-being of others, for example administering CPR when it is likely to be successful. Non-maleficence refers to avoiding the causation of harm to a person. If a patient clearly has deteriorating health and CPR would not restart the heart and breathing for a sustained period, it should not be offered or attempted (BMA et al., 2016). The principle of autonomy refers to respecting the choices that a person makes about their own life, for example, respecting a competent patient's choice to refuse CPR when the healthcare team believe CPR is likely to be successful. Justice refers to treating other people fairly, this might be ensuring that all staff CPR training is up to date. Whilst ethical principles may guide the decision-making process, they may also at times conflict, for example beneficence and autonomy may conflict if a patient in whom CPR would not be successful expresses a wish to be resuscitated. In these circumstances a second opinion should be offered, although this may be avoided if all members of a multidisciplinary team agree with the DNACPR decision (BMA et al., 2016).

Legal considerations

Human Rights Act

The Human Rights Act 1998 is the principal law that protects human rights in the UK. It covers sixteen human rights or 'Articles'. Several of its articles are relevant to resuscitation decisions, such as the right to life (Article 2), the right to be free from inhuman or degrading treatment (Article 3) and the right to hold opinions and to receive information (Article 10) and the right to be free from discriminatory practice with respect to these rights (Article 14). Healthcare professionals must be able to demonstrate that the spirit of the Act is reflected in their practice. A helpful learning resource is available through the British Institute for Human Rights and Sue Ryder (2016).

Withholding treatment

Withholding and withdrawing treatment are both considered to be acts of omission. Acts of omission that intentionally result in death, such as withholding CPR, are permissible when it is not in the patient's best interests to continue treatment (*Aintree University Hospitals NHS Foundation Trust v James, 2013*).

Capacity and DNACPR

If a patient with capacity, discussed fully later in the chapter, refuses CPR and is free from coercion, this must be respected, even if CPR may be successful in that individual and the healthcare team disagrees with the decision. The patient is an autonomous adult, and CPR in these circumstances would amount to battery. If CPR may be successful in a patient who lacks capacity, attempts should be made to understand their previously expressed wishes, beliefs and values by contacting those close to them, although it is important for relatives/carers to be aware that they are not responsible for making the final decision; instead, they have a role in helping the healthcare team to act in the patient's best interests (BMA et al., 2016). If CPR would not be successful in a patient who lacks capacity, it cannot be demanded by those close to them; should relatives/carers express a wish for the patient to be resuscitated, it may be necessary to offer a second opinion unless all members of the multidisciplinary team agree with the DNACPR decision (BMA et al., 2016).

The role of a power of attorney and the use of an advance decision are discussed later in this chapter. If a person in England and Wales lacks capacity and has no appropriate relatives/carers with whom to discuss 'serious medical treatment', an independent mental capacity advocate (IMCA) must be consulted in accordance with the *Mental Capacity Act 2005*. An IMCA does not have the authority to make decisions regarding CPR but is involved in determining the course of action that would ultimately be in the patient's best interests. While the *Adults with Incapacity (Scotland) Act* has no such stipulation, consideration should be given in these circumstances to involving an appropriate advocacy service (BMA et al., 2016).

Communication and DNACPR

Discussing CPR with a patient and those close to them may, at times, be challenging. Current guidelines (BMA et al., 2016) state that it is necessary either to encourage shared decision making when appropriate or to explain a medical decision and the reasons for it. This advice was issued following a Court of Appeal judgment in the case of *Tracey v Cambridge University Hospitals NHS Foundation Trust*. Doctors at Addenbrooke's Hospital deemed Janet Tracey to be an unsuitable candidate for CPR but failed to discuss this with her prior to completion of the relevant paperwork. Learning about it at a later date caused the patient and her family considerable distress which prompted her widower to bring a judicial review claim seeking a declaration that her right to a private life under Article 8 of the European Convention of Human Rights had not been respected. The court ruled in his favour, and while it was acknowledged that decisions regarding CPR are ultimately made at the discretion of medical staff, it was declared that there must be a presumption of involvement of the patient unless there is reason to believe that it will cause them significant physical or psychological harm.

Some patients strongly decline to discuss dying or end-of-life care, including decisions regarding CPR. In such cases, the patient's wishes should be respected; it is poor practice to inflict conversations about DNACPR on those who have clearly stated that they do not want to have them (BMA et al., 2016).

Documentation

Decisions regarding CPR and details of the accompanying discussions should be documented clearly and comprehensively in the case notes in addition to full completion of the DNACPR form if appropriate (BMA et al., 2016). The use of standardised forms that are recognised and accepted across geographical and organisational boundaries is recommended, and the form should accompany a patient when they transfer from one healthcare setting to another (BMA et al., 2016). Whenever discussions do not take place, this should be documented with a suitable explanation.

Review

A DNACPR decision should be subject to review according to the patient's individual circumstances. In the context of an acute illness, it should be reviewed in response to a patient's clinical progress or deterioration; in the context of end-of-life care for those with progressive irreversible conditions, there may be little or no need for review (BMA et al., 2016). It may be appropriate to suspend a DNACPR decision temporarily during an operation or procedure, particularly if prompt treatment of the arrest is likely to be successful, and a review should therefore take place ahead of the intervention (BMA et al., 2016). Finally, a DNACPR decision does not take precedence over professional judgement should cardiac or respiratory arrest occur due to an unforeseen and reversible event – for instance choking – as it is not in itself legally binding (BMA et al., 2016).

Wider anticipatory care planning

For many patients, decisions regarding CPR are best made in the wider context of anticipatory care planning, which allows other treatment options to be considered and a record to be made of those that are likely to be acceptable to the patient and those that are not (BMA et al., 2016). This generally results in a more positive discussion than focusing solely on whether or not CPR should be withheld in the event of cardiorespiratory arrest. Tools for anticipatory care planning are outlined in Chapter 1 – Principles of Palliative and End-of-Life Care (p. 10).

Further information

- Decisions relating to cardiopulmonary resuscitation: Guidance from the British Medical Association BMA, the Resuscitation Council (UK) and the Royal College of Nursing. 3rd edition (1st revision), 2016
- General Medical Council (GMC)
- Joint NMC/RCN statement regarding Decisions Relating to Cardiopulmonary Resuscitation (CPR). Available at: https://www.nmc.org.uk/news/news-and-updates/joint-nmc-rcn-statement-cpr/
- Local and regional policies may offer more detailed guidance
- Defence unions will be able to assist with enquiries regarding specific cases.

Capacity

Introduction

A proportion of patients receiving palliative care experience either a fluctuating or an irreversible decline in their ability to make decisions for themselves. This is more likely in the advanced stages of a long-term condition. It is the practitioner's responsibility to assess the patient's capacity in such circumstances, and to provide sufficient support to enable the patient to make appropriate decisions (NICE, 2018).

Circumstances where capacity decisions may be required

Capacity can be compromised in a patient with palliative care needs for a number of reasons. The person may already have impaired capacity, for instance due to a learning disability, a mental health condition, a brain injury or dementia (NHS, 2021). There may also be loss of capacity due to a deteriorating long-term condition, declining consciousness, an acute event or the development of delirium (National Council for Palliative Care and NHS Improving Quality, 2013).

Types of decisions that might have to be made

Diminished capacity at the end of life is a significant problem because of the important decisions which may have to be made at this time concerning treatment and care (GMC, 2010). These include how nutrition and hydration needs are to be met, whether cardiopulmonary resuscitation should be attempted, whether to consent to further treatment or investigations and the choice of place of care.

Assessment of capacity

The Mental Capacity Act 2005 and the *Adults with Incapacity (Scotland) Act 2000* specify that capacity should be assumed unless loss of capacity is formally established. Except in emergency situations, the assessment of capacity should be carried out by a practitioner who is familiar with the person being assessed. The assessment should be based on the person's condition and on the decisions which are to be made. Repeated assessments may therefore be required if the person's condition fluctuates or new decision challenges arise. The practitioner should gather insights from those known to the person, for example family or professional carers, and may consult more experienced or specialist colleagues, such as mental health practitioners or speech and learning therapists, where doubt exists. Assessment tools, for example the Mini-Mental State Examination, may also be used if appropriate (NICE, 2018).

Lack of capacity requires a demonstration of both an impairment of, or a disturbance in, functioning of a person's mind or brain (cognitive impairment, mental disorder, delirium, intoxication) and an inability to do any of the following (Nicholson et al., 2008):

- Understand information relevant to the decision in question
- Retain relevant information for long enough to use it to inform decision making
- Use or weigh up information
- Communicate the decision.

Putting in place mechanisms for decision making

Where it has been deemed that a patient's capacity is limited or absent, alternative processes must be implemented to support decision making to serve their best interests (NICE, 2018). The practitioner should take into account any documented wishes of the patient, such as anticipatory care plans, advance statements or advance decisions to refuse treatment (ADRT). Documents including DNACPR and ReSPECT should also be considered (Resuscitation Council UK, 2021; Fritz et al., 2017). Any individual(s) formally appointed to make decisions on behalf of the person who is lacking capacity should be involved in the decision-making process. Power of attorney is discussed later in the chapter.

Regardless of local and national practices, the same, broad model is used to guide decision making in these circumstances. The doctor will attempt to maximise the patient's capacity to make decisions. Where this has been assessed as inadequate, an assessment will be made of the patient's condition, their stated wishes, any advance statements, the potential benefits and disadvantages of any treatments and investigations, and the opinions of family, informal carers and other members of the multidisciplinary team. Where a legal proxy has been identified, the options for proceeding will be presented to him or her and the appropriate course of action agreed. Where there is no legal proxy, a decision will be made on the basis of the assessment just completed. In cases where 'serious medical treatment' is being considered, external advocacy should be sought via an independent mental capacity advocate in England and Wales, or an independent court ruling in Scotland (GMC, 2010). Please see *Adults with Incapacity (Scotland) Act 2000* documentation and flowchart in Appendix 2.1 at the end of this chapter. Each health board has their own variation.

Advance Directives, Advance Decisions and Power of Attorney

Advance directives, advance decisions and power of attorney can all assist in realistic discussions, and support the patient in being clear about their wishes for future care and treatments. There is more information regarding the differences between these across the UK in Tables 2.2 and 2.3.

Valid and applicable

Detailed guidance about how to assess the validity and applicability of an advance decision or an advance directive is provided by the GMC (2010) and the BMA (2019).

Advance decision, advance directive, and advance decision to refuse treatment forms

- My Advance Decision to Refuse Treatment document. Available at: https://www.macmillan.org.uk/_images/ADRTDocument_20170505_JS_tcm9-311758.pdf
- Advance Decisions Assistance. Available at: http://adassistance.org.uk/
- Compassion in Dying (Scotland). Available at: https://compassionindying.org.uk/making-decisions-and-planning-your-care/scotland/advance-directives/
- My Living Will. Available at: https://www.mylivingwill.org.uk/home

---

Table 2.2   UK advance directives, advance decisions and advance decisions to refuse treatment.

Country	Scotland	England and Wales	Northern Ireland
Legal term used	Advance directive. (Scottish Government)	Advance decision. Advance decision to refuse life-sustaining treatment. (UK Government)	Advance decision. Advance decision to refuse treatment. (Northern Ireland Assembly)
Definition and purpose	A document or a verbal statement that enables an adult, aged 16 years or over, to refuse any treatment, including life-sustaining treatment, in advance of a time where they do not have capacity to make that decision or to communicate their wishes. An advance directive only comes into effect when either of these situations occurs. The document should be signed and dated. (Healthcare Improvement Scotland and Scottish Government, 2017)	A written or verbal statement that enables a person with capacity, aged 18 or over, to refuse specified medical treatment in the future should they lack capacity to consent to, or refuse, that treatment. An advance decision refusing life-sustaining treatment must: • Be written • Be signed and witnessed • Clearly state that even if the person's life is at risk the decision applies • State what specific treatment is being refused. *Mental Capacity Act 2005.*	An advance decision to refuse treatment is valid and effective when there is proof that: • The decision exists • The decision applies to the existing circumstances • The person had capacity when the decision was made • The person who made the decision understood the consequences of refusing treatment • The person who made the decision was not unduly influenced by a third party. *Mental Capacity Act (Northern Ireland) 2016.* Review of the law relating to advance decisions to refuse treatment. (Northern Ireland Government Department of Health, 2019).

Table 2.2   (*Continued*).

Country	Scotland	England and Wales	Northern Ireland
Legal status	No specific legislation or case law. The principles of the *Adults with Incapacity (Scotland) Act 2000* should mean that a doctor is bound to consider an advance directive as evidence of the person's wishes and feelings. (Scottish Government, 2018a) In Scotland, valid and applicable advance refusals are potentially binding although there has not yet been a test case in court. (GMC, 2010)	Legally binding if written by an adult, and is valid and applicable to the treatment circumstances. *Mental Capacity Act 2005*. Healthcare professionals must follow a valid, applicable, advance decision or may risk criminal prosecution. (Department of Constitutional Affairs, 2007).	No specific legislation or case law. Under current common law ADRTs are legally recognised. Failure to respect an advance decision can result in legal action against the medical practitioner. The law relating to advance decisions will be reviewed by 2022. *Mental Capacity Act (Northern Ireland) 2016*. Review of the Law relating to advance decisions to refuse treatment. (Northern Ireland Government Department of Health, 2019).
Code of practice or guidance	Anticipatory Care Planning: Guidance for Health and Care Professionals. (Healthcare Improvement Scotland and Scottish Government, 2017)	*Mental Capacity Act 2005:* Code of Practice. (Department of Constitutional Affairs, 2007)	Forthcoming 'Code of Practice' will expand on advance decisions. *Mental Capacity Act (Northern Ireland) 2016*.

Table 2.3   UK Power of attorney.

Country	Scotland	England and Wales	Northern Ireland
Power of attorney	Types of power of attorney (POA) are: 1. Welfare (WPOA) 2. Continuing (financial) POA. 3. Combined POA A WPOA is a legal document that enables the 'granter' to appoint an 'attorney' or 'attorneys' to make health and welfare decisions for the granter. The granter must have capacity and be aged 16 or over to write a WPOA. WPOA only comes into effect at the onset of incapacity related to the powers granted, and can consent to or withhold consent for medical treatment, except where excluded from doing so by the Act. WPOA must be registered at Office of the Public Guardian (Scotland). (Scottish Government, 2018b)	Types of lasting power of attorney (LPA) are: 1. Personal welfare LPA 2. Property and financial LPA. A personal welfare LPA is a legal document that enables the 'donor' to appoint one or more 'attorneys' to make, personal welfare decisions for the donor. The donor must have capacity and be aged 18 or over to write an LPA. A personal welfare LPA: ● Must be registered with the Office of the Public Guardian. ● Can only be used when the donor lacks capacity to make a specific welfare decision. ● Can only consent to or refuse life-sustaining treatment for the donor if the donor has specified, in the LPA, that the attorney is given this power. (UK Government, 2021)	Types of power of attorney (POA) 1. General (GPOA) 2. Enduring (EPOA). A power of attorney (POA) is a legal document made by a 'donor' that gives authority to an 'attorney' to make decisions about the donor's property and affairs. Decisions about the donor's medical treatment and care are not the remit of the attorney. Whereas a GPOA ceases if the donor becomes mentally incapable of managing their affairs, an EPOA continues. The donor must be aged 18 or over and have capacity to sign an EPOA. An EPOA must be registered at the High Court (Office of Care & Protection). (Northern Ireland Government, 2021; *Mental Capacity (Northern Ireland) Act 2016* (c. 18)).

Table 2.3   (*Continued*).

Country	Scotland	England and Wales	Northern Ireland
Relationship between advance decision and power of attorney	If there is doubt about what the person who made the advance decision and appointed the welfare power of attorney wanted, the Court of Session can clarify the situation. (BMA, 2018)	An LPA cannot override an advance decision to refuse treatment unless it was made after the advance decision and the donor specified that the attorney has the power to do so. (Department of Constitutional Affairs, 2007)	There is no power of attorney for health and welfare legislation in Northern Ireland.

Mental Health Problems in Patients with Palliative Care Needs

There is no clear agreement on the prevalence of mood disorders in palliative care settings, as the way in which depression is defined and identified varies (Hotopf et al., 2002; Ly, Chidgey and Hotopf, 2002; Mitchell et al., 2011; Wasteson et al., 2009) but there is universal recognition of its impact on people's quality of life and functioning and the impact on families and carers (Hotopf et al., 2002; Wasteson et al., 2009). Prevalence of depression in palliative care has been quoted as between 5 and 30 percent of patients (Ly, Chidgey and Hotopf, 2002; Mitchell et al., 2011). Doctors' and patients' perspectives also differ in the interpretation of depression (Hotopf et al., 2002). All patients with palliative care needs should be screened for depression (Scottish Palliative Care Guidelines, 2020).

Depression and mood problems are common in patients with a life-limiting illness, yet often remain unrecognised and overlooked as they can be challenging to diagnose and classify (Mitchell et al., 2011; Noorani and Montagnini, 2007; Hotopf et al., 2002; Rosenstein, 2011; Moussavi et al., 2007). This, in part, is due to the complexity of overlapping physical symptoms such as insomnia, fatigue and changes in appetite and also the difficulty in differentiating between depression and anxiety symptoms in patients with life-limiting illness (Hotopf et al., 2002; Hugel et al., 2004). Insomnia specifically can be multifactorial in hospice inpatients (Hugel et al., 2004). Be alert to dysphoric mood, feelings of guilt, worthlessness and hopelessness, as well as social withdrawal in patients with palliative care needs (Scottish Palliative Care Guidelines, 2020). See Figure 2.1 for risk factors associated with depression in palliative care.

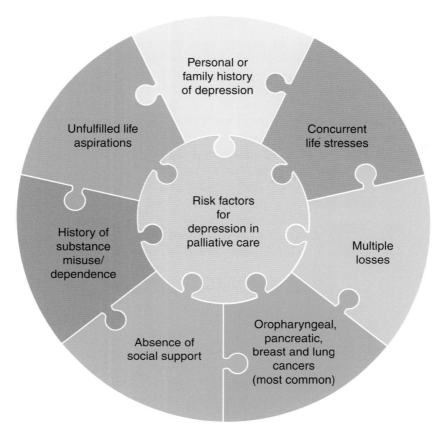

Figure 2.1 Risk factors for depression in palliative care.

Source: Based on information from the Scottish Palliative Care Guidelines, 2020.

There is a lack of consensus on which screening tool or assessment method should be used for depression in palliative care (Hayes et al., 2017 Lloyd-Williams et al., 2003; Warmenhoven et al., 2012; Wasteson et al., 2009). A healthcare professional's ability to recognise any suicidal thoughts that the patient may have is crucial and if identified should prompt further assessment and support (Rosenstein, 2011). If a patient is at risk of suicide, their care plan should include an immediate safety plan co-produced with the patient (Royal College of Psychiatrists, 2020). Downloadable safety plan templates are available at stayingsafe.net. Thoughts of self-harm and suicidal ideation are independent predictors for depression in palliative care patients (Lloyd-Williams et al., 2003). The Hospital Anxiety and Depression Scale (HADS) is easily available but focuses on physical symptoms, so its use can be limited (Scottish Palliative Care Guidelines, 2020). There is some discussion, however, as to whether the HADS could be used as a screening tool for earlier detection of symptoms (Holtom and Barraclough, 2000). The Brief Edinburgh Depression Scale is suitable for us in patients with palliative care needs and the PHQ-9 can be used as a screening tool for community patients (Scottish Palliative Care Guidelines, 2020).

Other depression assessment tools have been used in palliative care studies, but were validated with physically unwell patients (Lloyd-Williams et al., 2003; Hotopf et al., 2002). A screening question, 'Are you depressed?', can also be particularly useful (Lloyd-Williams et al., 2003). Diagnostic interviewing can be used but is time-consuming and burdensome for frail patients (Hotopf et al., 2002). For more information on this topic please see 'Further Reading' at the end of this chapter. See Figure 2.2 for potential barriers to the diagnosis of depression in palliative care.

Treatment of depression can significantly improve quality of life and is as effective in palliative care as in other situations (Scottish Palliative Care Guidelines, 2020). The *European Clinical Guidelines for the Management of Depression in Palliative Care* (Rayner et al., 2010) recommend that clinicians should consider psychological therapy and antidepressants for the treatment of depression in palliative care, based on evidence gathered from randomised controlled trials and expert clinical opinion. Pharmacological management should be tailored to the individual patient with consideration of side effects, contraindications and interactions. Pain control should be optimised and use of non-pharmacological approaches and referral to psychiatric services should be considered on an individual basis (Scottish Palliative Care Guidelines, 2020).

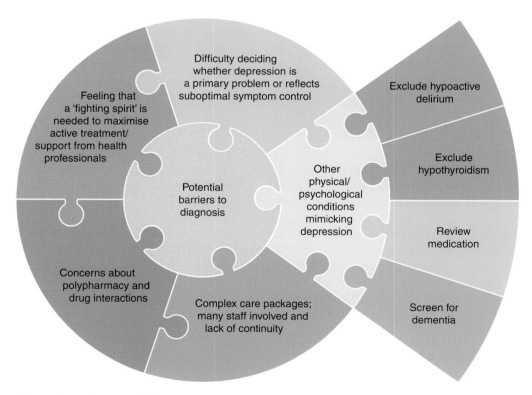

Figure 2.2 Potential barriers to diagnosis of depression in palliative care.

Source: Based on information from the Scottish Palliative Care Guidelines, 2020.

Controlled Drugs

The *Misuse of Drugs Act 1971* discusses the manufacture, supply and possession of controlled drugs (except where permitted by the 2001 Regulations or under licence from the Secretary of State). *The Misuse of Drugs (Safe Custody) Regulations 1973* discuss the storage and safe custody requirements for controlled drugs.

The Misuse of Drugs Regulations 2001 (and subsequent amendments) define those who are authorised to supply and possess controlled drugs (British National Formulary (BNF), 2020; NICE, 2020). Drugs are divided into five schedules, each specifying issues including: import, export, production, supply, possession, prescribing and record keeping (NICE, 2020). The Home Office controlled drugs list (2019) details which drugs are included in each schedule (BNF, 2020; NICE, 2020):

- *Schedule 1* includes drugs not used medicinally, for example ecstasy-type substances, raw opium, and cannabis.
- *Schedule 2* includes opioids, major stimulants, ketamine, cannabis based products. Schedule 2 controlled drugs (except for some liquid preparations) are subject to the full controlled drug requirements relating to prescriptions, safe custody, and the need to keep a controlled drug register.
- *Schedule 3* includes barbiturates, buprenorphine, gabapentin, midazolam, pregabalin, temazepam, and tramadol hydrochloride that are all subject to the special prescription requirements.
- *Schedule 4* includes, in Part I, drugs that are subject to minimal control, such as benzodiazepines (except temazepam and midazolam, which are in Schedule 3), non-benzodiazepine hypnotics and Sativex®. Part II examples include androgenic and anabolic steroids and clenbuterol.
- *Schedule 5* includes preparations of certain controlled drugs such as codeine, pholcodine or morphine, which due to their low strength are exempt from virtually all controlled drug requirements other than retention of invoices for two years. Schedule 5 prescriptions are valid for 6 months from issue (NICE, 2020).

The Health Act 2006 introduced the 'accountable officer' with responsibility for the management of controlled drugs and related governance. In 2013 The Controlled Drugs (Supervision of Management and Use) Regulations were published to ensure good governance (NICE, 2020).

Controlled drug prescription requirements

Prescribing

Prescriptions for controlled drugs can be electronic but must have a handwritten signature, be dated by the prescriber and include the patient's name and UK address. Full prescription writing requirements:

- Name, the drug form, for example capsules or tablets and strength of drug.
- Total quantity in words and figures: State total number of dosage units in words and figures or total volume in millilitres for liquids in words and figures,

- Prescription(s) valid for 28 days.
- Only 30 days' supply on prescription
- Instalment amount and interval of supply to be stated

When prescribing liquids write the total volume in millilitres (words and also in figures) and for dosage units (tablets, capsules, ampoules) write the total number (in words and also in figures) of drug to be supplied (NICE, 2020).

Travelling abroad

Travelling abroad with prescribed controlled drugs raises a number of issues. A patient going in or out of the UK needs to prove that medicine is prescribed for them if it contains a controlled drug. A letter will be required from the person who prescribed the controlled drug which includes the prescriber's signature, the patient's name, address and date of birth, the destination and travel intinerary and the names, forms, strengths, doses and total amounts of drug being carried (PCF 7). Patients should check restrictions within the country they are travelling to and should contact the embassy or high commission (Macmillan Cancer Support, 2020a; Wilcock et al., 2020). If travelling for more than three months a Home Office licence may be required (NICE, 2020; Macmillan Cancer Support, 2020a; Wilcock et al., 2020). If travelling for more than three months patients should approach clinicians to prescribe medication prescribed in that country (NICE, 2020; BNF, 2020). A licence can take ten working days to issue. Applications for obtaining a licence must be supported by a prescriber's covering letter as discussed above (Wilcock et al., 2020; Macmillan Cancer Support, 2020a).

Patients cannot travel with schedule 1 controlled drugs. If the drug is schedule 2, 3 or 4 on the controlled drugs list, and the patient will be travelling with a 3-month supply of medication, the patient will need to apply for a licence from the Home Office. A licence can take 10 working days to issue. Applications for obtaining a licence must be supported by a covering letter signed by the prescribing doctor or drug worker, which must confirm (Macmillan Cancer Support, 2020):

- The patient's name and address
- The travel itinerary
- The names of the prescribed controlled drug(s), doses and total amounts to be carried.

Applications for licences should be sent to the Home Office, Drugs and Firearms Licensing Unit, Fry Building, 2 Marsham Street, London, SW1P 4DF (dflu.ie@homeoffice.gov.uk). Telephone: 020 7035 6330, 9am to 5pm, Monday to Friday (UK Government, 2020).

The Macmillan Cancer Support website has a wide range of advice and support for people with health problems travelling abroad, including information about travelling with medications, travelling with oxygen and accessing health insurance and services abroad (Macmillan Cancer Support, 2020b). There may also be flight restrictions to be considered (Macmillan Cancer Support, 2020c; Fit for Travel, 2019).

Unlicensed medications

A marketing authorisation or product licence defines a medication's characteristics, the indications, recommended doses, contraindications, and special warnings and precautions for use (Medicines and Healthcare products Regulatory Agency, MHRA, 2014). The individual circumstances for prescribing unlicenced medications should be assessed by the prescriber. The prescriber should be satisfied there is sufficient evidence or that they have the experience to justify their decision and should also be satisfied with the safety and efficacy of their decision. They should arrange a follow-up and make clear records. Patients and relatives should have adequate information and be supported to make an informed decision (GMC Online).

Physician-Assisted Dying

Physician-assisted dying and euthanasia are illegal in the United Kingdom, but this is something that patients, and their families, do sometimes want to discuss. Parliamentary bills attempting to change this have been brought to governments both in Scotland and Westminster. Professional bodies in the UK including the BMA, Royal College of General Practitioners and the Association of Palliative Medicine are against legalisation of physician-assisted dying (Association of Palliative Medicine (APM), 2018). The Royal College of Physicians recently changed their position on the issue to neutral (Royal College of Physicians (RCP), 2019a) and the Royal College of Nursing have adopted a neutral stance on assisted dying (Royal College of Nursing (RCN), 2014).

Definitions

There are no universal definitions of physician-assisted dying or euthanasia, however the definitions used by the Royal College of Physicians (RCP, 2019b) are:

- Physician-Assisted Dying: A physician intentionally supplies a patient who has capacity with the means to self-administer a lethal dose of a medicine.
- Voluntary Euthanasia: A physician intentionally administers a lethal dose of a medicine to a patient who has capacity and who has expressed a wish to die.
- Involuntary Euthanasia: A physician intentionally administers a lethal dose of a medicine to a patient without capacity, whether or not that patient has expressed a wish to die, but with the intention of acting in the best interests of the patient.

Physician-assisted dying covers not only the prescription of a lethal dose of medication but also advising on lethal doses of medications that could be used (NHS, 2017).

History in the United Kingdom

In Scotland the *Assisted Suicide (Scotland) Bill* was debated in 2015 and defeated. The bill included a number of criteria that would need to be met before completing assisted dying, including the patient being 16 years or over, having a terminal condition and having capacity. The bill proposed that a series of formal requests supported by two medical practitioners would be required before physician-assisted death could occur.

In England and Wales, bills proposing the legalisation of physician-assisted dying have been brought to Westminster. The most recent bill, defeated in 2015, stated that the patient must be at least 18 years of age, have a terminal condition, capacity, and not have been coerced. Terminal conditions covered progressive irreversible conditions and a prognosis of less than 6 months (*Assisted Dying Bill*, 2015).

Current law

It is not a specific crime to assist someone to die in Scotland. However, assisted dying could result in conviction of a number of crimes under Scottish law such as murder, culpable homicide or reckless endangerment (Robson and Harvie-Clark, 2015).

Under English law it is illegal to assist someone to complete suicide under the *Suicide Act 1961* and can result in a 14 year prison sentence (NHS, 2017). In addition, carrying out euthanasia or physician-assisted dying could result in life imprisonment by conviction of manslaughter or murder (NHS, 2017).

Global examples

Currently, physician-assisted dying and euthanasia are legal in the Netherlands, Belgium, Luxembourg, Colombia and Canada (Emanuel et al., 2016).

Physician-assisted dying is legal in Switzerland and some American states such as Oregon, Washington, Montana, Vermont and California (Emanuel et al., 2016). In Victoria, Australia the *Voluntary Assisted Dying Act 2017*, including physician-assisted dying, came into effect in 2019 (Victoria State Government, 2021) and more recently, in July 2021, Western Australia legalised physician-assisted dying through the implementation of the *Voluntary Assisted Dying Act 2019* (Government of Western Australia, 2021).

Arguments for and against physician-assisted dying

For physician-assisted dying

- It relieves patient's physical and/or mental suffering as palliative care cannot relieve all suffering (Brock, 1992).
- Even with universal access to specialist palliative care, some dying people will still experience severe, unbearable physical or emotional distress that cannot be relieved. Forcing dying people to suffer against their wishes is incompatible with the values of twenty-first-century medicine (BMA, 2020).
- It respects patient autonomy (Steinbock, 2005). Doctors should not be able to impose their personal beliefs on competent, informed adults who wish to exercise this voluntary choice (BMA, 2020).
- There is no significant difference in the morality of withholding/withdrawing life-sustaining treatment and physician-assisted dying (RCP, 2019b).
- It is possible to distinguish between physician-assisted dying in those with capacity and voluntary/involuntary euthanasia (RCP, 2019b).

- In countries where physician-assisted dying is legal there has been no reported increase in deaths of patients not expressing a wish to die (RCP, 2019b).
- Physician-assisted dying is a legal option for over 150 million people around the world. In jurisdictions where it is lawful, there are eligibility criteria, safeguards and regulation in place to protect patients (BMA 2020).
- Guidance in the UK for end-of-life practices, such as the withdrawal of life-sustaining treatment, contains safeguards to ensure decisions are made voluntarily and that potentially vulnerable people are protected. These safeguards could be used effectively in assisted dying legislation. (BMA, 2020).
- Legalisation of physician-assisted dying would be reassuring to patients and the general population as they would know that the option of physician-assisted dying exists for them (Brock, 1992; BMA, 2020).
- The current law is not working. UK citizens travel abroad to avail themselves of physician-assisted dying, but this option is only available to those who have the funds to do so. There is no oversight under UK law about who travels abroad for an assisted death; anyone who provides assistance is breaking the law, which can lead to criminal investigations (BMA, 2020).
- If death is inevitable then why not have the option of a controlled death? (Brock, 1992).
- Safeguards can be put in place to protect vulnerable people (RCP, 2019b).

Against physician-assisted dying

- Non-maleficence is a key ethical value of medicine and physician-assisted dying would go against this (Miller and Brody, 1995).
- Allowing physician-assisted death would decrease the general population's trust in doctors (Brock, 1992).
- Allowing physician-assisted death would devalue the lives of disabled people (RCP, 2019b).
- There is a moral difference between withdrawal or withholding of life-prolonging treatment and physician-assisted death (RCP, 2019b).
- Palliative care can relieve almost all patient suffering and legalisation of physician-assisted dying could result in reduced efforts towards good palliative care (BMA, 2020).
- Legalising physician-assisted dying would lead to a 'slippery slope', resulting in legalisation of involuntary euthanasia (Brock, 1992).
- It is impossible to guarantee the safety of vulnerable people and to ensure that decisions are truly voluntary with safeguards (BMA, 2020).
- In countries where physician-assisted dying is legal there have been cases of patients who are not in the original categories stated being helped to die (RCP, 2019b).
- An assisted dying law would alter society's attitude towards elderly, seriously ill, and disabled people and send the subliminal message that assisted dying is an option they 'ought' to consider (BMA, 2020).

- Some seriously ill patients might fear that healthcare professionals will give up trying to relieve their distress, seeing death as an easy option (BMA, 2020).
- Factors behind a request for assisted dying are predominantly personal or social rather than clinical. Assisted dying is not a role for hard-pressed doctors (BMA 2020).

Summary

Internationally the debate surrounding physician-assisted dying and euthanasia is ongoing. It remains illegal to provide physician-assisted dying in the United Kingdom. Public and professional opinion is divided over this highly emotive and challenging ethical issue reflected in the results of the recent survey of BMA members on the topic (BMA, 2020).

Scenario Recap

Fiona's disease journey and the issues she faces are complex. It is clear that in order to focus on the needs of Fiona and her husband the multidisciplinary team needs to take a person-centred approach to empower and support them both while also supporting Gino within his co-worker role. Decision making may be challenging for Fiona given her complex issues, including fluctuating capacity and likely communication difficulties. Fiona's individual experiences and health beliefs will also influence her choices and the team's subsequent approach. A number of strategies, underpinned with staff education and support, could be employed to facilitate a person-centred approach to Fiona's care. A person-centred multidisciplinary care approach, including early planning and discussions, active listening, empathy and honesty, will enable Fiona to have more control over her care. The multidisciplinary team involved in Fiona's care will need to have an understanding of any complex legal and ethical issues that may arise.

Further Reading

Ahmedzai S et al. (2011) Managing passengers with stable respiratory disease planning air travel: British Thoracic Society recommendations. *Thorax*, 66(Suppl 1): 1–30.

British Lung Foundation (2018) Going on holiday. Available at: https://www.blf.org.uk/support-for-you/going-on-holiday

General Medical Council (2012) Protecting children and young people: the responsibilities of all doctors. Available at: https://www.gmc-uk.org/ethical-guidance/ethical-guidance-for-doctors/protecting-children-and-young-people/about-this-guidance

Macmillan Cancer Support (2019) Travel insurance. Available at: https://www.macmillan.org.uk/cancer-information-and-support/impacts-of-cancer/travel/buying-travel-insurance

Marie Curie (2019) Mental capacity and making decisions. Available at: https://www.mariecurie.org.uk/help/support/terminal-illness/rights/mental-capacity#meaning

NHS (2014) Improving quality capacity, care planning and advance care planning in life limiting illness. Available at: https://www.england.nhs.uk/improvement-hub/wp-content/uploads/sites/44/2017/11/ACP_Booklet_2014.pdf

Office of Care and Protection – Northern Ireland Courts and Tribunals Service (2021) Information on Enduring Powers of Attorney. Available at: https://www.justice-ni.gov.uk/articles/information-enduring-powers-attorney-epa

Office of the Public Guardian in Scotland (2015) What is a power of attorney? Available at: https://www.publicguardian-scotland.gov.uk/power-of-attorney#:~:text=PoA%20is%20a%20written%20document,holds%20a%20licence%20to%20practise

The Enduring Powers of Attorney (Northern Ireland) Order 1987. Available at: https://www.legislation.gov.uk/nisi/1987/1627

Queensland University of Technology (2019) End of life law in Australia: euthanasia and assisted dying. Available at: https://end-of-life.qut.edu.au/euthanasia

Victoria State Government (2021) Voluntary Assisted Dying. Available at: https://www2.health.vic.gov.au/hospitals-and-health-services/patient-care/end-of-life-care/voluntary-assisted-dying

Wilcock A, Howard P and Charlesworth S (2020) Palliative Care formulary (PCF7). 7th edn. London: Pharmaceutical Press.

References

Adults with Incapacity (Scotland) Act (2000) (c.1). Available at: https://www.legislation.gov.uk/asp/2000/4/contents

Aintree University Hospitals NHS Foundation Trust v James [2013] EWCA Civ 65. Available at: https://www.bailii.org/uk/cases/UKSC/2013/67.html

Assisted Dying Bill (2015) Parliament: House of Lords. Bill no.6 Available at: https://publications.parliament.uk/pa/bills/lbill/2014-2015/0006/lbill_2014-20150006_en_2.htm

Assisted Suicide (Scotland) Bill (2013). Parliament: Scottish Parliament, Bill no. 40. Available at: https://archive2021.parliament.scot/parliamentarybusiness/bills/69604.aspx

Association of Palliative Medicine (2018) APM physician assisted dying web materials. Available at: https://apmonline.org/news-events/apm-physician-assisted-dying-web-materials/

Beauchamp TL and Childress JF (2013) Principles of Biomedical Ethics. 7th ed. New York: Open University Press.

Biddy R et al. (2015) *A Quality Initiative Endorsed by Cancer Care Ontario in Partnership with the Program in Evidence-Based Care (PEBC)*. Ontario: Ontario Cancer Care.

British Institute of Human Rights and Sue Ryder (2016) *End of Life Care and Human Rights: a practitioner's guide*. Available at: https://www.sueryder.org/for-healthcare-professionals/education-and-training/human-rights-end-of-life-care/download

British Medical Association (2007) *Withholding or Withdrawing Life-Prolonging Medical Treatment*, 3rd edition. London: Blackwell Publishing.

British Medical Association (2018) Consent toolkit. Card 9: Advance decisions. Available at: https://www.bma.org.uk/advice/employment/ethics/consent/consent-tool-kit/9-advance-decisions

British Medical Association, Resuscitation Council (UK) and Royal College of Nursing (2016) Decisions relating to cardiopulmonary resuscitation: guidance from The British Medical Association, The Resuscitation Council (UK) and The Royal College of Nursing, 3rd edition, 1st revision. Available at: www.resus.org.uk/dnacpr/decisions-relating-to-cpr

British Medical Association (2019) Consent and refusal by adults with decision making capacity: a toolkit for doctors. Available at: https://www.bma.org.uk/media/2481/bma-consent-toolkit-september-2019.pdf

British Medical Association (2020) Physician-assisted dying survey and briefing pack. Available at: https://www.bma.org.uk/advice-and-support/ethics/end-of-life/physician-assisted-dying-survey

British National Formulary (2020) Controlled drugs and drug dependence. Available at: https://bnf.nice.org.uk/guidance/controlled-drugs-and-drug-dependence.html

Brock DW (1992) Voluntary active euthanasia. *The Hastings Center Report*, 22(2): 10–22.

Burton C et al. (2017) The value of different aspects of person-centred care: a series of discrete choice experiments in people with long-term conditions. *BMJ*, 7: e015689.

Byrne A-L, Baldwin A and Harvey C (2020) Whose centre is it anyway? Defining person-centred care in nursing: an integrative review. *PLoS ONE*, 15(3): 1-21. Available at: https://journals.plos.org/plosone/article?id=10.1371/journal.pone.0229923

Chan P et al. (2013) Long-Term Outcomes in Elderly Survivors of In-Hospital Cardiac Arrest. *New England Journal of Medicine*, 368(11): 1019–1026.

Chatterjee J (2016) Improving person-centred care for hospice patients who have difficulty expressing their needs. Leeds: St Gemma's Hospice.

Department of Constitutional Affairs (2007) *Mental Capacity Act 2005*: Code of Practice. Available at: https://assets.publishing.service.gov.uk/government/uploads/system/uploads/attachment_data/file/497253/Mental-capacity-act-code-of-practice.pdf

Ebell MH and Afonso AM (2011) Pre-arrest predictors of failure to survive after in-hospital cardiopulmonary resuscitation: a meta-analysis. *Family Practice*, 28(5): 505–515.

Emanuel EJ et al. (2016) Attitudes and practices of euthanasia and physician-assisted suicide in the United States, Canada and Europe. *The Journal of the American Medical Association*, 316(1): 79-90.

Ewing G and Grande GE (2018) *Providing Comprehensive, Person-Centred Assessment and Support for Family Carers Towards the End of Life: 10 Recommendations for Achieving Organisational Change*. London: Hospice UK.

Fit for Travel (2019) Air travel – health issues. Available at: https://www.fitfortravel.nhs.uk/advice/general-travel-health-advice/air-travel

Fritz Z, Slowther A M and Perkins GD (2017) Resuscitation policy should focus on the patient, not the decision. *BMJ*, 356: j813.

General Medical Council (2010) Treatment and care towards the end of life: good practice in decision making. Available at: https://www.gmc-uk.org/ethical-guidance/ethical-guidance-for-doctors/treatment-and-care-towards-the-end-of-life

Government of Western Australia (2021) Voluntary assisted dying. Available at: https://ww2.health.wa.gov.au/voluntaryassisteddying

Haraldsdottir E et al. (2019) Person centred culture in a hospice: myth or reality. Available at: https://eresearch.qmu.ac.uk/bitstream/handle/20.500.12289/5357/5357aam.pdf?sequence=1&isAllowed=y

Hayes J, Hart B, and Phillips J (2017) Specialist palliative care nurses' management of the needs of patients with depression. *International Journal of Palliative Nursing*, 23(6): 298–305.

Health Foundation (2016) *Person-Centred Care Made Simple: What Everyone Should Know about Person-Centred Care*. London: The Health Foundation.

Healthcare Improvement Scotland and Scottish Government (2017) Anticipatory care planning: guidance for health care professionals. Available at: https://ihub.scot/project-toolkits/anticipatory-care-planning-toolkit/anticipatory-care-planning-toolkit/

Hello My Name Is ... (2021) A campaign for more compassionate care. Available at: https://www.hellomynameis.org.uk/

Holtom N and Barraclough J (2000) Is the Hospital Anxiety and Depression Scale (HADS) useful in assessing depression in palliative care? *Palliative Medicine*, 14(3): 219–220.

Home Office (2019) Controlled drugs list. Available at: https://www.gov.uk/government/publications/controlled-drugs-list--2

Hotopf M et al. (2002) Depression in advanced disease: a systematic review. Part 1. Prevalence and case finding. *Palliative Medicine*, 16(2): 81–97.

Hugel H et al. (2004) The prevalence, key causes and management of insomnia in palliative care patients. *Journal of Pain and Symptom Management*, 2(4): 316–321.

Human Rights Act 1998 (c. 42) Available at: www.legislation.gov.uk/ukpga/1998/42

Kouwenhoven WB, Jude JR and Knickerbocker GG (1960) Closed-chest cardiac massage. *JAMA*, 173(10): 1064–1067.

Lloyd-Williams M, Spiller J and Ward J (2003) Which depression screening tools should be used in palliative care? *Palliative Medicine*, 17(1): 40–43.

Ly KL, Chidgey J and Hotopf M (2002) Depression in palliative care: a systematic review. Part 2. Treatment. *Palliative Medicine*, 16(4): 279–284.

Macmillan Cancer Support (2020a) Travel and cancer. Available at: https://www.macmillan.org.uk/cancer-information-and-support/stories-and-media/booklets/travel-and-cancer

Macmillan Cancer Support (2020b) Taking medication abroad. Available at: https://www.macmillan.org.uk/cancer-information-and-support/impacts-of-cancer/travel/taking-medication-abroad

Macmillan Cancer Support (2020c) Planning for your trip checklist. Available at: https://www.macmillan.org.uk/cancer-information-and-support/impacts-of-cancer/travel/planning-for-your-trip-checklist

Medicines and Healthcare products Regulatory Agency (2014) Off-label or unlicensed use of medicines: prescribers' responsibilities. Available at: https://www.gov.uk/drug-safety-update/off-label-or-unlicensed-use-of-medicines-prescribers-responsibilities

Mental Capacity Act 2005 (c.9). Available at: https://www.legislation.gov.uk/ukpga/2005/9/

Mental Capacity Act (Northern Ireland) 2016 (c.18). Available at: http://www.legislation.gov.uk/nia/2016/18/contents/enacted

Miller FG and Brody H (1995) Professional integrity and physician-assisted death. *The Hastings Center Report*, 25(3): 8–17.

Misuse of Drugs Act 1971 (c. 38). Available at: https://www.legislation.gov.uk/ukpga/1971/38/contents

Misuse of Drugs (Safe Custody) Regulations 1973 (no. 798). Available at: https://www.legislation.gov.uk/uksi/1973/798/contents/made

Mitchell AJ et al. (2011) Prevalence of depression, anxiety, and adjustment disorder in oncological, haematological, and palliative-care settings: a meta-analysis of 94 interview-based studies. *Lancet Oncology*, 12(2): 160–174.

Moussavi S et al. (2007) Depression, chronic diseases, and decrements in health: results from the World Health Surveys. *Lancet*, 370(9590): 851–858.

National Council for Palliative Care and NHS Improving Quality (2013) Advance decisions to refuse treatment: a guide for health and social care professionals. Available at: https://www.england.nhs.uk/improvement-hub/wp-content/uploads/sites/44/2017/11/Advance-Decisions-to-Refuse-Treatment-Guide.pdf

NHS (2017) Euthanasia and assisted suicide. Available at: https://www.nhs.uk/conditions/euthanasia-and-assisted-suicide/

NHS (2021) Mental Capacity Act. Available at: https://www.nhs.uk/conditions/social-care-and-support-guide/making-decisions-for-someone-else/mental-capacity-act/

NICE (2018) NICE Guideline NG108: decision-making and mental capacity. Available at: https://www.nice.org.uk/guidance/ng108/evidence/full-guideline-pdf-6542486605

NICE (2020) Controlled drugs and drug dependence. Available at: https://bnf.nice.org.uk/guidance/controlled-drugs-and-drug-dependence.html

Communication

Kirsty J Boyd with Claire Clark
and Elaine Stevens

Learning Objectives

This chapter will help you to:

- Have sensitive and effective discussions about deteriorating health, death and dying with people who have life-limiting illnesses and their families
- Describe and apply person-centred communication in the context of palliative care
- Use effective approaches to communication in specific situations including sharing bad news, shared decision making about treatment and care, care planning, and care when a person is dying
- Ensure there is effective communication when a person lacks capacity
- Communicate with parents, children and young people
- Communicate with people who have disabilities or communication difficulties
- Take account of culture, religion and beliefs in communication about palliative and end-of-life care.

Scenario

Background

Pete is a 56-year-old engineer with metastatic bowel cancer. He lives with his partner, Sarah, and their two children Asha (7) and Kelly (12). Pete has an adult son, Mark, from a previous marriage. Mark has Down's syndrome and lives in supported accommodation.

Pete's greatest worry is how his family will cope as he deteriorates and dies.

Key points

- Throughout a person's illness journey, effective communication with them and their family is a core aspect of care.
- Many professionals are involved and can offer person-centred information and support.
- Evidence-based approaches to good communication with people receiving palliative care are well-established best practice.

Timeline

Pete had surgery and chemotherapy 7 years ago for sigmoid colon cancer. Last year, Pete visited his GP with tiredness and a persistent cough.

(1)

(2) GP shares abnormal test results with Pete and Sarah clearly and sensitively.

Tests at oncology confirm multiple liver and lung metastases. Pete chooses a clinical trial but after 4 months has signs of progressive lung disease. A recent scan shows multiple brain metastases. Pete struggles with having to stop the trial treatment so it is difficult to talk about the future and care planning.

(3)

(4) District nurse asks what Pete understands about his cancer while checking his bloods and this helps him share his worries about talking with their children; Pete and Sarah are supported to be more open with the girls.

Mark's key worker tells Pete that his son has been quite upset recently and they agree that it is time for the staff to start preparing Mark for what is going to happen.

(5)

(6) Pete is less well and may die in the next few weeks. He becomes acutely unwell with breathlessness, a temperature and a swollen, painful leg. Sarah and Pete choose admission as it might give him more time with his family. Pete is treated with antibiotics but continues to deteriorate. Sarah opts for care on the medical ward where Pete dies peacefully the following day.

Key considerations

- Why is it important to involve everyone close to the person who is deteriorating and dying by sharing information adapted to their individual needs and concerns?
- Think about why open and effective communication is vital for people who are deteriorating and the people who are close to them.
- How could you put some of these communication behaviours and approaches into practice yourself?
- Why is it important to use language that is clear, unbiased and realistic when sharing bad news and planning care with people and their family?

Introduction

Effective communication is an essential component of palliative care as conversations can often be complex and emotionally charged. People with advanced illness and their families require a sensitive, empathetic approach, with careful use of language in order to balance hope and realism (Clayton et al., 2008). Our ability to communicate and listen well are often the most valuable attributes we can offer. Colleagues from different settings and professional backgrounds deliver palliative care together so effective teamwork supported by good communication is essential.

All staff caring for people with advanced illness and providing palliative care benefit from high quality communication training (NHS Education for Scotland, 2017). A combination of clear information about effective approaches, opportunities to take part in experiential learning, and self-reflection are the best ways to improve.

This chapter covers the principles of person-centred communication, effective communication approaches, and topics relevant to palliative care, such as care planning and care around death. This is applicable not just to patients but also their families. We use the term 'family' to mean anyone who is important to the person and involved in their life and care. It is also relevant to people of any age, illness or culture and in all care settings.

Person-Centred Communication in Palliative Care

Person-centred care means treating people as individuals, prioritising their thoughts, feelings and concerns. It builds therapeutic relationships based on trust and understanding (McCormack et al., 2010).

Person-centred communication is the use of established principles and behaviours in clinician–patient or family discussions that facilitate person-centred care (Figure 3.1).

Connecting	**Assessing**
Engaging to build rapport Letting the person tell their 'story' Using effective non-verbal communication	Active listening Picking up on cues Understanding the person's feelings and concerns
Responding	**Empowering**
Showing understanding/reflecting back Showing care and compassion Responding with clear explanations	Confirming the person understands you Helping the person take control Action planning

Figure 3.1   The 'CARE' approach.

Source: Mercer SW et al., 2004.

It is a broad approach, rather than being a specific interview structure or model, although these can also be helpful. Effective person-centred communication has multiple benefits, such as:

- It improves patient, family and professional well-being
- Results in emotional and care needs being met
- Promotes patient independence and 'life near the end of life'
- Is central to effective shared decision making
- Reduces later regrets and complaints.

There are core interview steps in person-centred communication that will be familiar to most professionals, and some potential problems in the context of palliative care.

Build a relationship

- Listen without interruption, and allow silences; they give people time to reflect and volunteer more information
- Comments intended to be empathetic can in fact cause distress
  - ✗ *I know/understand how you feel.*
  - ✓ *It makes sense that you feel that way.*
- Introducing a serious topic using informal language underplays its importance
  - ✗ *Can we have 'a chat' about resuscitation?*
  - ✓ *There is something important about your treatment for us to discuss, is this a good time?*

Gather information

- Ask about the person's ideas, concerns and expectations. What is important for them, and their beliefs and values?
  - ✓ *What matters most for you in this situation?*
  - ✓ *What are you expecting might happen?*
  - ✓ *What would they say about this if we could ask them?*
  - ✓ *What do we need to know about you to care for you as well as possible?*

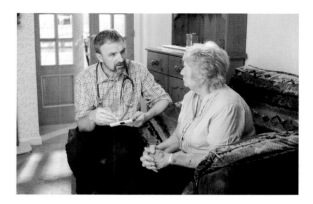

Figure 3.2 Person-centred care.

Source: © sutrti/iStock.

- Clarify the person's understanding or emotions by asking questions
  - ✓ *What do you know about your illness now?*
  - ✓ *How are you feeling about that?*
- Leading questions or questions that are too broad hinder effective communication
  - ✗ *You don't have any problems with your bowels, do you?*
  - ✗ *So how are things these days?*

Respond

- Pick up cues you hear from the person to explore feelings, concerns, and questions
  - ✓ *You said 'worried' about your husband … what is it that worries you most?*
- Keep sentences short, and check for mutual understanding
  - ✓ *What have you understood from what we talked about so far?*
- Be honest and clear but soften the impact with effective non-verbal communication: tone, posture, eye contact, gentle touch of the hand or arm
- Summarise sections of a discussion, and pause to let the person respond
- Signpost a change of topic after a summary and checking understanding.

Plan together

- Find out what the person can do for themselves: their strengths and interests
- Support self-efficacy as much as is realistic

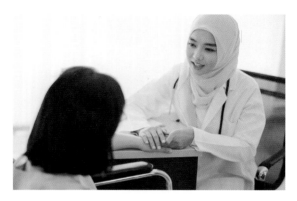

Figure 3.3 Treating people as individuals.
Source: © CMYK/Shutterstock.

- Discuss what is important and what people want to aim for: a functional goal, a family or home-related matter, legacy work, preferred place of care, plans for a pet.
- Emphasise that treatments are available for pain and other symptoms.
- Identify areas where some control and hope are possible. This could be thinking and planning ahead in the short or medium term.
- Acknowledge uncertainty and talk about ways to manage it.

Common Reactions to Life-Threatening Illness, Death and Dying

In advanced illness or frailty, there are topics which patients and professionals can find challenging to discuss because they connect with deteriorating health, loss and dying. These reactions often change and vary over time. People may have different responses within a family so it is important to explore these individually as well as together.

As a general guide to addressing these responses, *acknowledge* the emotions, *explore* the reasons behind them, *check* the person's perspective of the situation and that we have enough understanding of the reason for their response, and *summarise* what has been discussed before giving information or suggesting any actions. Agreeing some next steps is important, including offering help if this is within your role, or enabling the person to make contact with another colleague or service.

Seek advice and support early if emotional responses are strong or complicated.

Tips for responding to distress/grief

'They are crying all the time. It's too upsetting to talk about.'

- Listen and respond in an empathetic way, before moving on sensitively so that the person and the professional avoid 'emotional fatigue'
  - ✓ *You seem very upset at that …*
  - ✓ *What worries you the most about …?*
- Try to move on to identifying the main concerns and priorities, then an action plan
  - ✓ *What is the most important thing for us to do?*
  - ✓ *Who do you know that could help and support you right now?*
  - ✓ *What do you think could help with that?*

- Reassure the person that help and support are available but don't offer premature or false reassurance

    ✗ *Don't worry, it will be ok. We can look at other treatments.*

Tips for addressing anger/blame

'It is that doctor's fault. If they had treated them properly ...'

Common causes are:

- Expectations of people/services not being met
- Loss of control in the face of deteriorating health or treatment not working
- Conflicting information from different professionals and/or specialties
- Disagreement on care arrangements or place of care for the patient
- Experiencing or witnessing uncontrolled pain or other symptoms
- Unrelated issues such as family problems or conflicts; mental health problems
- Guilt about responsibility in some way for the situation.

How to handle anger:

- Remain calm – try to get everyone to sit down; maintain eye contact
- Listen without interruption. Allowing people to express anger often reduces it
- Use effective non-verbal communication; speak slower, fewer words, even tone of voice, open body posture with unfolded arms
- Acknowledge the anger

    ✓ *I can see why that would make you angry.*

    ✓ *I agree that not getting an answer to that question would be frustrating.*
- Apologise for the distress caused and any errors made. Take responsibility for addressing adverse events, and act to prevent future harm
- Try to negotiate a way forward that would help the person who is dying and/or the situation of the person who is complaining, now or in future
- Keep yourself and others safe if anger/aggression is severe or escalating.

Tips for responding to bargaining

'You might have made a mistake.' 'They were seen by the wrong doctor!'

This needs to be distinguished from anger and blame. This person is not making a complaint but is struggling to come to terms with the situation.

- Acknowledge the person's reasons for wishing things were different
- Explore the person's understanding of what we do know about the situation
- Talk about ways to move forward that the person can cope with. This could be finding one thing that is important to focus on.

Tips for dealing with guilt

'If only I had got them to see the GP ...'

Guilt can come across as anger or complaints about care. It may happen if the person has not been able to support the patient well or their relationship is complex. Listen in a non-judgemental way; negotiate looking at the things we can do for the person now.

Tips for handling denial

'It can't be true ... I don't want to believe it ...'

Denial is a coping mechanism to manage internal distress. Although denial may enable a person to cope for a time, it can have a negative impact on communication within a family including with children. It hinders shared decision making and care planning. At different times in an illness trajectory, people tend to be more or less open about what is happening. A diagnosis of cancer brings initial fears about dying, but the person may then move on to talking solely of active treatment or 'fighting' the illness ('dual narrative') (Kendall et al., 2015). Some people try to appear positive and want to avoid disappointing or letting down family members or professionals. Complete denial is uncommon but many people choose to focus on 'living in the present'. They take life 'a day at a time', while also knowing things will change at some point, and cope well in this way. It can be harmful for clinicians to challenge an effective coping strategy, but a time will come when helping the person be more open is important. Do this gradually.

- Acknowledge how hard it is to think about what is happening and the future
- Explore the person's understanding of their current situation gently
- Listen for any 'window of doubt' that could be a way into a conversation
- Gently challenge inconsistencies in their account, if present
- Discuss the benefits of talking about the future more openly
- Go slow and do not 'push' further than what is comfortable for the person
- Talk about 'hoping for the best' and focusing on the present while also making some plans 'just in case'.

Tips for managing withdrawal

'What's the point? Just leave me alone.'

A withdrawn mental state – non-engagement or silence – might be a conscious response, or caused by medical conditions such as depression or hypoactive delirium (screen and treat).

- Listen, offer support and make a commitment to try to help the person
- Acknowledge the difficulty of the person's situation
- Invite the person to explain why talking is difficult
- Explain the benefits of starting a conversation: it helps the clinicians to help the person and their family more effectively
- Invite the person to talk about what matters to them.

Tips for addressing collusion

'Don't tell them, it will be too distressing … they will give up …'

It is common in the context of palliative care for people to want to protect those they see as vulnerable from the truth to avoid distressing them. However, denying people the truth about a serious illness in a family can be more distressing in the long run (Fallowfield and Jenkins, 2002). Sharing information clearly and sensitively allows the dying person and their family to talk about their situation, express feelings and make plans for the future (Stevens, 2018).

Collusion can be the result of a well-intentioned agreement between one or more family members to deliberately withhold information from a patient. A person may choose not to be open with family or close friends about their illness and prognosis and has a right to confidentiality. However, the benefits of involving the people who are close to them are such that professionals should seek to explore why the person does not want to share information. Occasionally a patient and family conceal information from professionals, or a patient may appear overly positive as they try to avoid disappointing or letting down family members or professionals. Collusion commonly involves a *'don't tell me/him/her/them'* request. Having the knowledge and skills to deal effectively with a collusive situation is important for all professionals providing palliative care. Strategies to help manage this situation are:

- Acknowledge and explore the underlying reasons behind the *'don't tell'* request; this can help dispel fears or misconceptions
- Check current understanding of the situation with the person requesting secrecy
- Explore the possible impact of continued collusion on the person and/or family
- Explore the benefits and potential disadvantages of being more open about what is happening
- Negotiate finding out what the other person or people actually know
- Offer reassurance that sensitive information will not be given but only shared gently and honestly in response to the person's questions
- If the patient is blocking information, gently check what they want to know, without giving unwanted or unnecessary information. These people may cope with talking about hoping for something positive while also suggesting that it can be a good idea to talk a little about what might happen just in case things turn out less well
- Try to bring everyone together and offer or plan extra support if collusion has caused ongoing damage to relationships.

Barriers to Effective Communication

Clinicians may feel uncomfortable when sharing bad news and discussing prognosis, deteriorating health and death (Baile et al. 2000). When this happens, professionals can consciously, or unconsciously, hinder person-centred communication with the use of 'blocking' behaviours. These close down further exploration and discussion of a person's feeling and concerns. Box 3.1 lists some of these behaviours and the reasons professionals may use them.

Through reflective learning and training, self-awareness and competence can improve. Professionals need to recognise how their own emotions, values and beliefs might affect their practice. Sometimes seeking support from a colleague or sharing care in a particularly challenging situation helps. The vast majority of patients and families want open, honest communication tailored to them as individuals (Fallowfield and Jenkins, 2002). The rest of this chapter looks at evidence-based approaches to good communication in palliative care.

Box 3.1 Communication barriers

Some less helpful communication behaviours are:

- Quickly changing the topic of conversation
- Use of too many closed questions or questions that are too vague
- Use of medical jargon or complex words and concepts
- Interrupting someone expressing strong emotions
- Dominating the conversation with long or overly detailed explanations
- Asking leading questions which hint at a desired response
- 'Jollying along' and not exploring the impact of distressing information
- Premature reassurance that everything will be fine or problems can be treated
- Use of negative language that causes people to feel abandoned or denied care when talking about the limitations of treatment or limited options.

Some reasons why blocking may happen are:

- Fear of upsetting the person or causing more distress
- Fear of destroying hope, for example when discussing prognosis
- Fear of 'unleashing a can of worms': emotions or a level of distress which the professional feels unable to deal with
- Fear of being asked a difficult or unanswerable question
- Lack of confidence/skills in dealing with emotions
- Poor time management due to lack of structure in conversations
- Fatigue or burnout
- Brings up personal experiences or those of someone close to the professional
- Professional pressure to make a plan for ending or avoiding treatment.

Source: Adapted from de Caestecker, 2012.

Using helpful language

There are evidence-based approaches to talking about deteriorating health and dying that allow people to adjust to potentially distressing information (Box 3.2). Some people choose to be very open and clear about the future from the start, but many opt for living more 'day to day' and prefer a less direct conversation that allows them to hope and cope (Jackson et al., 2013).

> ## Box 3.2   Helpful ways to talk about deteriorating health and dying
>
> ### Generalisation
>
> ✓ '**Sometimes people** choose family members or close friends to help make decisions for them if they get less well in the future. Have you thought about that?'
>
> ### Hypothetical questions
>
> ✓ '**If** you were less well like this in the future, what do you think we should do?'
>
> ### Sharing decisions
>
> ✓ 'Can we talk about what is **important** for you? That will let us make good decisions together.'
>
> ✓ 'How would **you like** to be cared for in that situation?'
>
> ### Hope linked with concern
>
> ✓ 'We **hope** the (treatment) will help, but I am **worried** that at some stage, maybe even soon, you will not get better ... what do you think?'
>
> ✓ 'I **wish** we could give you more treatment ... could we talk about **what we can do** if that is not possible?'

Sharing Bad News

Bad news is any information that has a negative effect on a person's future life (Pereira et al., 2013). This suggests that it is not only the 'big' news such as diagnosis and prognosis that may affect the well-being of the person and their family but other issues such as no longer being able to work, having to take on new roles in the family or not being able to be cared for in a preferred place. Bad news can be shared in a sensitive and empathetic way so that it does not cause additional distress (Monden et al., 2016). It is important to prepare for the discussion if at all possible and to start by finding out how big the gap is between what the person already knows or suspects and the reality of their situation. The SPIKES model of sharing bad news is recommended (Baile et al., 2000). Using the six steps can allow clinicians to share bad news in a way that lessens distress (see Table 3.1).

Table 3.1   The SPIKES model.

SPIKES stages	What to consider when sharing bad news
Before the interview takes place	
Setting and setting up	Suitable private place. All the relevant information. An understanding of the relationships of the people who are at the interview. Preparation can include suggesting a family member or friend is present.
During the interview	
Perceptions	Begin by asking everyone what they already know about the current situation. This allows the professional to tailor the information given to these people.
Invitation	Allow each person to decide how much they wish to hear, and how much information they need just now.
Knowledge	This may begin with a 'warning shot' to prepare people for bad news. Share information in a clear and simple way to allow people to understand and respond. 'Chunks and checks' or 'Ask-talk-ask' are used. Avoid 'jargon' and complicated clinical details or long sections with no pauses.
Emotions	Bad news is likely to cause emotional distress that needs to be expressed before anything further can be discussed. It is usually helpful to stay close at this time but some people choose to be alone for a while. The interview proceeds once everyone feels able to move on with discussing people's main concerns and the way forward.
Strategy and summary	Begin to plan a way forward for the future. If people remain very emotional, only one or two concerns can be addressed and other problems may need to be postponed until later. End the interview with details of who to contact should they have any further questions or need more support.

Source: Adapted from Baile et al., 2000.

Shared Decision Making and Capacity

Sharing decisions is a key requirement of person-centred care, informed consent and realistic medicine. It increases satisfaction with care and people's confidence in treatment and care decisions while reducing complaints and regrets.

Shared decision making involves:

- Shared responsibility, using evidence well and thinking together about the available options tailored to the person's situation and wishes

- Making sure the person **understands** they have a choice to make, what might happen, and they can **remember** and **use** the information we have given them to reach a decision and **communicate** it
- Talking about any **risks** or harms that could be considered important by a person in this situation as well as the benefits of an option.

Patients and family members cannot demand a treatment or intervention that is contraindicated or illegal, or one that would definitely not have a clinically successful outcome. Professionals explain why some treatments will not work, or are unavailable, or why outcomes are poor for a person like this. If a decision cannot be reached, another clinician, specialist or team is asked to offer an opinion and additional support.

Only the patient or a legally-appointed, proxy decision-maker (a welfare attorney) can consent to a treatment. If the person lacks capacity to make decisions, has not made a valid advance directive, and has no proxy, the professionals responsible for the person's care need to make decisions that are of overall benefit to the person, taking account of any available information about the person's likely views.

Shared decision-making discussions

It is helpful to have a clear framework for these discussions and explore the balance of responsibility for the final decision in line with patient wishes and realistic, available options. Some people need factual information to enable them to choose the best option for them. Others prefer a dialogue with the professional, supported by evidence-based decision aids where appropriate, to help them find the best way forward. Another group look to the professional to suggest a recommended course of action or the best available option. Table 3.2 gives a stepwise approach that can be applied to many shared decision-making discussions. This is called the DECIDE model. The key elements of a shared decision-making model are below. DECIDE gives the steps and language to use.

- Build a relationship of trust and encourage participation and partnership
- Clarify the roles and responsibilities of the person, family or close friends (including any welfare attorney/proxy decision-maker) and the professionals
- Find out how much information is needed and think about how best to present it
- Check what everyone knows and understands about the situation and any decisions to be made
- Provide tailored information and evidence that is person-centred
- Find out what is most important for this person at this time and in the future
- Discuss what we can do and the options available, including not having more tests or treatments, or making a decision later
- Discuss the benefits and risks or harms of the options and how likely they are
- Check everyone has understood and address any further questions or concerns

Table 3.2   DECIDE model for shared decision making.

Shared decision making using DECIDE	
Define decision	*'We are making a decision with you about X.'* *'Is this a good time to do that? Should anyone else be involved?'*
Explain situation	*'Can we start by talking about your health problems and situation?'* *'Can you tell me what you know already?'* Share relevant, individualised information (in chunks with checks). *'Do you have any thoughts, questions or worries I can help with?'*
Consider options	*'Let's talk about available options and the likely benefits, risks or harms.'* *'We need to work out what option is the best one for you.'* *'Each of them has pros and cons.'* *'You might choose to wait and see what happens.'*
Invite views	*'I would like to hear about what matters to you (your relative) in this situation.'* *'That is important in helping us make good decisions together.'*
Decide together	*'Given what we can do and what you said matters, let's find the right option for you'* *'What do you think the best option might be?'* *'What do you think they would say, if we could ask them?'* *'Would it help if I suggest a way forward and explain what might happen?'*
Evaluate decision	*'You think the best option is Y, because ... Is that right?'* *'Are you clear about what that means for you?'* *'Do you want to think about it, and we can talk again later?'*

Source: Developed by Kirsty Boyd with NHS Education for Scotland education lead (September 2021 version: used with permission from Dr Boyd, Macmillan Reader in Palliative Care, The University of Edinburgh).

- Agree a decision and a clear action plan; offer further resources/information
- Before closing, summarise the discussion and plans, check people's understanding of what the decision will mean for the person and if there are more questions or worries; make follow-up arrangements.

Anticipatory Care Planning

Care planning conversations are part of good care for any person whose health is declining and should start early (Box 3.3). These discussions are about thinking ahead and making plans for what a person would like to happen, anything they do not want and how best to care for them if their health, care or personal situation changes. Care planning can also include an emergency or urgent care plan to help guide treatment and care if a person's health changes rapidly. Although 1–2% of people living at home, and up to 30% of those admitted to hospital as an emergency, will deteriorate and die in the next year, it is impossible to predict accurately what will happen to an individual person (Clark et al., 2014). That means accepting inherent uncertainty and planning ahead to reduce the risk of an acute crisis due to a complication or new life-threatening illness (Kimbell et al., 2016).

Box 3.3   Care planning

- Identify the right people
- Find out what matters
- Talk about what we can do
- Explain what will not help
- Plan care together.

People close to the person are involved in these discussions as is anyone with a power of attorney for them. NHS Inform/ NHS Direct, Healthcare Improvement Scotland, NHS Education for Scotland and other national organisations offer information for people, their families and friends, and professionals to support care planning.

It can be helpful to think of care planning as three overlapping phases to guide conversations with patients and families (Figure 3.4). If loss of decision-making capacity is likely, planning ahead is particularly important; for example, with people who have dementia, Parkinson's disease, or motor neurone disease.

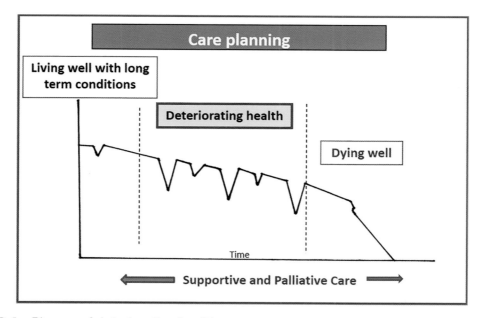

Figure 3.4   Phases of deteriorating health.

Source: Used with permission of Dr Kirsty Boyd, Macmillan Reader, The University of Edinburgh.

Table 3.3   Care planning discussions using RED-MAP.

Talking about care planning with RED–MAP	
Ready	*Can we talk about your health and care?* *Who should be involved?*
Expect	*'What do you **know**?'* *'Do you want to **tell/ask** me about anything?'* *'What has changed?'* *'Some people think about what might happen if …'*
Diagnosis	*'What we **know** is … We **don't know** … We are **not sure** about …'* *'Do you have questions or worries we can talk about?'*
Matters	*'What is **important** to you and your family?'* *'What would you like to **be able to do**?'* *'How **would you like** to be cared for?'* *'Is there anything you **do not want**?'* *'What would (name) say about this situation, if we could ask them?'*
Actions	*'What we **can do** is … Options that **can help** are …'* *'This **will not help** because … That **does not work** when …'*
Plan	*'Let's **plan ahead** for when/if …'* *'Making plans in advance helps people get better care.'*

Source: Developed by Kirsty Boyd for Building on the Best (September 2021 version: published with permission from Dr Boyd, Macmillan Reader in Palliative Care, The University of Edinburgh; Scottish Partnership for Palliative Care and Macmillan Cancer Support).

General triggers or indicators of poorer health due to one or more advanced conditions are used to identify people; for example, Supportive and Palliative Care Indicators Tool (SPICT™) (2021). Frailty tools for older people can be helpful too. Sometimes people have noticed these changes themselves. If not, the professional can refer to them as a way of opening a discussion and starting a care planning conversation. Some examples of these indicators are:

- A new diagnosis of a serious illness
- An unplanned hospital admission
- A call to out-of-hours or unscheduled care services
- Persistent symptoms despite optimal treatment of underlying conditions
- A general decline in performance status and ability to function day to day
- Increasingly dependent on others for care due to physical and/or mental illness
- Low weight or loss of muscle mass (for example advanced heart failure with oedema)
- Moving into supported accommodation or a care home.

A six-step approach to care planning conversations (RED-MAP) helps professionals find out what matters to the person, share information about the situation and available options to agree a person-centred care plan (Table 3.3).

Words and phrases known to be helpful when talking about planning future care are part of the RED-MAP model. We can start to open these conversations when people are still well but at risk of deteriorating health (Figure 3.5).

Care planning discussions continue when a person is deteriorating with progressive illness, a new complication of an underlying condition or general frailty. That may include an infection not responding to treatment, or when further antibiotics are not of benefit. Sometimes a new life-threatening illness such as a major cardiovascular event or stroke, or the complications of trauma/falls mean care planning only happens when the person is closer to dying. Any wishes a person has expressed to those close to them or recorded in an advance directive or plan should inform care planning (Figure 3.6). It is also important for different professionals and teams in primary and secondary care or specialist palliative care services to share information about care planning, and ensure plans are reviewed and updated.

Starting care planning conversations

- *Can we talk about what is happening with your health and care in case things change?*

- *When would be a good time to talk? Should anyone else be involved?*

- *Can we talk about how you are doing? Has anything changed recently? Have you talked about care planning before?*

- *How do you see things going in the next weeks/months/years?*

- *What do you like doing/would you like to be able to do?*

- *Can we talk about what is important if you (or your carer) get less well in the future?*

- *Do you have questions or worries you'd like to talk about?*

- *Let's start making a plan with you.*

| Clear language | Short sentences | Pauses |

Figure 3.5 Starting care planning.

Source: Reproduced with the kind permission of Dr Kirsty Boyd, Macmillan Reader, The University of Edinburgh; Scottish Partnership for Palliative Care and Macmillan Cancer Support.

Talking about getting less well

- *Start or continue conversations about care planning (Figure 3.5).*
- *How have you been doing recently? What has changed?*
- *Is there anything you would like to tell/ask me?*
- *What **we know** is ... We do **not know** ...*
- *We **hope** you will stay well/improve ... but I **am worried** that/about ...*
- *It **is possible** you will not get back to how things were because ...*
- *What is important to you that we should know about?*
- *Are there things **you would like** to happen or **do not want**?*
- *What we **can do** is ... This does not work well/help people with ...*
- *We don't know exactly what will happen, but planning ahead helps people get better care.*

| Clear language | Short sentences | Pauses |

Figure 3.6   Care planning when someone is getting less well.

Source: Reproduced with the permission of Dr Kirsty Boyd, Macmillan Reader, The University of Edinburgh; Scottish Partnership for Palliative Care and Macmillan Cancer Support.

Communication with Families

Families are diverse and include the biological family, the family of acquisition (through marriage and adoption for example) and family of choice through friendship. The best way to identify family members is to acknowledge that 'family is who the patient says it is' (Irish Hospice Foundation, 2021). Illness in the family often has severe and wide-ranging impacts. Interpersonal stresses or tensions can arise due to the illness or may pre-date a diagnosis of serious illness. 'Communication breakdowns' are an added source of family suffering, and should be a focus of the team's intervention. Effective family assessment and person-centred communication, in particular active listening, helps family members continue to function and prevents worsening of mental health when a person is dying and on into bereavement.

General approaches to communicating with families

- Try to understand the family structure first; a genogram is useful
- Try not to make assumptions about how a family functions – find out by asking them
- Try to understand the family dynamics and usual functioning
  - ✓ *Who in your family is closest to you? What are the strongest relationships?*

✓ *How is your family coping with your illness and treatment?*

✓ *How do people in your family usually communicate with each other?*

✓ *How has your family coped in the past with stress or illness?*

- Remember that family members' main needs are *information* (with consent from the patient to share this) and *emotional support*

Conflict and complex relationships

Family functioning is not either 'good' or 'bad' but varies along a spectrum (Steele et al., 2014). In different cultures families may interact in very unique ways. Features of families with poorer functioning include:

- High levels of conflict
- Low expression of emotions
- Lack of cohesiveness and teamwork
- Low ability to cope with change, or to accept outside help
- 'Estranged' members of families who may live at a distance
- Ongoing problematic substance use
- Existing psychiatric illness such as severe depression or personality disorder.

Such families are likely to require more psychosocial support in the form of group meetings (see below), individual updates with clinicians and involvement of the wider multidisciplinary team, including chaplaincy and social work. Increased support aims to improve, or contain, rather than alter family dysfunction.

In the most severe cases, family dysfunction may impede care provision for the ill person, or cause or worsen psychiatric illness. Referral to psychology or liaison psychiatry services is an option but may not be widely available.

Family meetings

Meetings between professionals and family (involving the patient or with their consent) are a frequently used way to:

- Share information openly with several family members, therefore saving time compared with individual updates and avoiding confusion or misinformation
- Observe interactions and functioning within the family
- Acknowledge and legitimise the stresses/emotions/challenges of the situation
- Focus on family strengths and resources
- Provide a forum in which to problem-solve for the patient and agree shared goals, even when tension or conflict may exist.

Communication with Parents, Children and Young People

When a parent has a terminal illness, communication between parents and with their children is stressful. Parents want support from healthcare professionals to guide them on how to talk to their children and what to say (Fearnley et al., 2017). However, professionals can find this very difficult and fear upsetting those involved or making things worse.

Bereaved children are statistically at risk of numerous adverse outcomes later in life such as psychiatric problems, early school leaving and offending. It is therefore crucial that children are well informed and prepared, as their age allows, regarding death and bereavement. Often parents tell children about a terminal illness late in the disease due to the pursuit of life-prolonging treatments, reluctance to engage with care planning and uncertainty about what to say (Chowns, 2009). A parent may be struggling with their illness, the need to care for their child, and how to ensure appropriate arrangements are in place for the child following their death. Parents often underestimate children's information needs and their awareness that things are very different in the family.

Specialist palliative care services may have a staff member trained in providing children and family support. However, all staff providing generalist palliative care should have basic knowledge and skills in this area. Good communication is the key to supporting families with children. Clinicians involved with the family can offer information in the form of online or print resources and provide support or 'coaching' of parents or guardians on how to share bad news with children and young people and involve them in what is happening. Children of all ages and young people need to be prepared in advance for the death of someone close to them (Warnick, 2019). There are many benefits including the following:

- It creates an environment of open and honest communication
- Allows children to get accurate, factual information from appropriate care providers

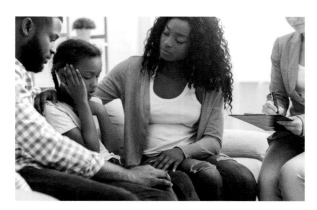

Figure 3.7 Communicating with children about death.

Source: prostock-studio/Shutterstock.

- Helps children make sense of the physical changes they see in the person who is seriously ill
- Involves the person who is ill in preparing children for the possibility of his/her/their death
- Gives time to put additional support in place, such as school counsellors and bereavement support, where available
- Enables children to grieve with the adults in their lives, instead of alone and from the periphery
- Helps children understand that their emotions and those of others around them are healthy and natural

- Gives opportunities to say goodbye in a way that feels appropriate for them or to just be with the person
- Enhances the trust between children, their primary caregivers and healthcare personnel.

What children understand about death

Children's understanding of death varies according to age, or cognitive maturity, so it is vital to bear this in mind when working with a family and speaking with children. Table 3.4 is an outline of this but children's charities offer more detailed information – see Resources.

Table 3.4   Children's understanding of death at different ages.

Age	Understanding	Actions
0–2 Years	Are aware of changes in routine and the people looking after them. Babies may become withdrawn or display loud outbursts of crying and angry tears.	Maintain the child's usual routine.
2–5 Years	Do not understand the finality of death. React to emotions and physical changes in close adults. Around age 5, begin to understand what illness is. Developmental regressions such as being clingy or having tantrums.	Explain dead people cannot return to life. Provide opportunities for the child to ask questions and answer simply and honestly. Maintain usual routines.
5–8 Years	Children accept that death is final and affects all living beings. Anxiety about the imminent death of other significant people in their lives. Fears or misconceptions that the illness is somehow their fault or is contagious.	Provide reassurance and opportunities to talk about their feelings. Explain that their words or actions did not cause the illness/death.
8–12 Years	Children understand that death is irreversible, inevitable and universal. Changes in behaviour, concentration, schoolwork and friendships. Distress expressed as physical symptoms.	Provide reassurance and honest communication about what is happening including any changes such as place of residence and school.
Teenagers	Usually understand the illness/death but may be reluctant to talk about it. Variable emotional maturity. May express feelings and emotions through art or music. May be more comfortable talking to others rather than parents. May want to help but also have their independence, leading to mixed emotions.	Provide reassurance, opportunities to ask for support and do not burden the child with adult responsibilities.

Source: Adapted from Macmillan Cancer Support, 2016, and Irish Hospice Foundation guidance, 2021.

Caring for a family with children

Assessment: taking a family history, the child as part of a family group

- What is the family structure and ages of children? A genogram can be useful here.
- What does each child or teenager know already, and how have they coped so far? The child's understanding may be different from their biological age.
- What is the relationship with the parents or guardians? This may affect how the child copes with the parent's illness and in bereavement.
- What support is available from extended family? For example help with childcare/other people the child trusts or has a close relationship with.
- What are the parents' or guardians' views on the level of openness and involvement in the family when a parent is dying and after their death?
- What are the expectations and fears of what will happen to their parent?

Supporting adults to communicate with children

- Take an individualised, holistic approach with every family.
- Encourage/facilitate open discussion between parents and children, allowing children to ask questions and finding out what they know already.
- Adults can provide reassurance that even though they do not have all the answers it is still important to talk about these difficult things together.
- Adults can encourage children to share their feelings safely and without judgement. Allowing children to see adults show and talk about feelings helps children express their own.
- Provide information to children as soon as possible. It is better to share information as the situation evolves. Developmentally appropriate books and leaflets can be helpful.
- Giving facts and concrete explanations can help them focus on things that are within their control and avoid misunderstandings. Knowing what to expect can help them let go of things beyond their control. Help the whole family to cope with uncertainty.
- Teenagers may want medical and prognostic information, and can prefer talking to someone other than a parent.
- Prepare children for what may happen to their parent next, for example becoming more tired and weak, not eating as much, and not waking up anymore. Explain what to expect when they are visiting.
- Give reassurance to younger children that they have not caused the illness in any way.
- Be prepared for children moving quickly in and out of talking about death, dying and grief.
- Explaining what is happening in stages can be useful.
  - Mum is ill
  - Mum is very ill/may not get better
  - Mum won't get better/is getting worse
  - Mum is dying/will die

- Use age appropriate, clear, simple language.
  - Dead means the body doesn't work anymore/can't come alive again
  - Do not talk about the patient 'going to sleep'
  - Avoid euphemisms like 'lost', 'gone', 'passed' and use words like 'death' and 'dead'

Other support and advice for parents

- Continue doing ordinary family routines and activities together.
- Engage in memory work e.g. memory boxes, card writing, special family nights.
- Older children/teenagers commonly need 'time out' and support from their peers.
- Agree on consistent parenting and boundaries for children.
- Provide information to other carers of their children, including the school/teachers.
- Support from local community networks, social work or other family support workers may be helpful.

Communication in Specific Circumstances

People with dementia

Due to the nature of dementia, no two people have the same impairments and subsequently have a range of communication difficulties needing an individual approach. Identifying how much a person with dementia understands can be challenging as they may use other methods such as behaviours rather than words to express themselves (James, 2011). It is important to identify how the person with dementia communicates problems such as distress, pain, fear and anxiety and how this information can be used in a person-centred approach to improve communication and ultimately their well-being (James, 2011).

The Canadian Virtual Hospice website and the Irish Hospice Foundation (2015) have provided guidance on how to communicate information when a person with dementia or someone close to them is dying. This approach can be helpful in sharing other types of news about a serious illness in the person themselves or a close relative or friend.

1. One person shares information or bad news to avoid overwhelming the person with a group of people.
2. Find a quiet, comfortable place, and choose a time of the day when the person is not tired.
3. Use clear, simple sentences and avoid ambiguous phrases. This improves the chances of the person understanding what they are being told.
4. See how the person reacts to the news. This may indicate how much of the information has been understood.

People with a learning disability

It is often difficult to share information about a serious illness with family members who have a learning disability as they may have a limited understanding of what is going on. However, as in other situations it is better to be open with the person. The level of disability of the person needs to be taken into consideration, and people require information in different forms. The person may not understand the meaning of words fully, be able to read, or be able to process more complex information (Mencap, 2019). It is good practice for a professional who knows the person well to communicate important information. Sometimes having a close family member offer support is helpful too. The key worker should use their knowledge of how to communicate most effectively as well as how the person is likely to react when they understand the information and when they are upset (National Institute for Health and Care Excellence, NICE, 2018). The use of aids such as photographs, pictures and symbols may be helpful to allow the person to understand what they are being told and specific communication tools such as 'Talking Mats' may allow them to communicate their views and concerns to others in a person-centred way (Cameron et al., 2017).

A specific model can be used to share information about a significant diagnosis with a person who has learning disability. It centres on 'Building a foundation of knowledge' to allow the person to understand fully and cope with change over a period of time. The model uses a series of guiding questions to allow the professional to plan their communication and is applicable to all people with learning disability. The questions (adapted from Tuffrey-Winje, 2012) are:

- Does the person have capacity?
- What knowledge does the person have already?
- What size of knowledge chunks can the person cope with?
- Is the person able to understand this chunk of information at this point in time?
- How many more chunks of knowledge can the person be helped to understand?
- Is it important that the person understands this specific information now?
- What is the best way/place/time to give the person the best chance of understanding?
- Who can help the person to understand the best?
- Can the person be harmed by receiving this chunk of knowledge at this point in time?

Following careful consideration of all these questions, the professional can begin with giving the first chunk of information. The setting of the meeting should be comfortable and supportive, as is the case when sharing bad news more generally (Baile et al., 2000). Using the knowledge the person has already, information should be given in a format they understand and that has meaning for them. This will allow the person to work out what this news means for them now and in the future (Tuffrey-Winje, 2012). The time taken to develop an understanding of what the information means will vary depending on the level of disability. Sharing further chunks of information is paced accordingly. A personal learning disability 'passport' helps record information about how to communicate well with this individual and improves communication with the person when they are moving between care settings.

Sensory impairment

There are a substantial number of people who have one or more sensory impairments that impact on their ability to communicate effectively (Think Local Act Personal Partnership, 2012). NICE (2013) recognised that sensory impairment, if not identified and managed appropriately, leads to poor communication. That affects confidence and independence and ultimately quality of life. It is always important to check whether patients and family members have any sensory impairments and develop a plan to ensure their preferred method of communication is available at all times (Think Local Act Personal Partnership, 2012). This information should be clearly documented in the person's care plan to enable other team members to use the preferred communication method effectively (NICE, 2013).

Culture and language

Culture is broadly defined as 'that complex whole which includes knowledge, beliefs, arts, morals, laws, customs, and any other capabilities and habits acquired by [a human] as a member of society' (Tyler, 1871). A society may include members from many different cultures, including some of whom are minority or marginalised groups. Such groups may include people from ethnic minorities, the homeless, and people with drug dependency, those with disabilities and those with diverse sexuality and/or gender identities.

Regardless of the makeup of a society, each person's culture is moulded by the history and tradition of their 'group' and is central to their human existence (Cain et al., 2018). An individual's healthcare experience may be affected negatively by culturally insensitive healthcare practices (Long, 2011). Cain et al. (2018) highlight that cultural diversity means that people with advanced illness will vary and particularly in terms of:

- The meaning they attach to suffering
- Their preferences for treatments and care provision
- How they make decisions
- The verbal and non-verbal communication they use to express their needs
- What they wish to happen when a person is dying or has died.

Culturally sensitive communication that meets the needs of all members of society is essential (NHS Education Scotland, 2010). There are a number of ways in which individual professionals and care teams can ensure they communicate with people and their families in a culturally sensitive way (adapted from Brooks et al., 2019). These include the following:

1. Acquire a good insight into one's own culture and that of others and how this can affect the care experience
2. Respect cultural preferences and adapt communication to meet people's needs
3. Ask people to say how they would prefer to be cared for and how they would like staff to support them and those close to them

4. Enable patients and families to understand how the care environment operates and involve the members of the team who can support them best

5. Use culturally appropriate verbal and non-verbal communication to develop a therapeutic relationship.

Where a patient or family member communicates in a language not understood by the care team, the use of a professional interpreter is essential to support informed decisions and improve the overall patient experience (Schouler-Ocak et al., 2015). Best practice guidance suggests that interpreters should be qualified and come from within the health or social care organisation as this ensures that unbiased information is passed to the patient and family and any questions can be answered accurately (NHS Scotland, 2011).

In 2011, NHS Scotland developed a competency framework to enable professionals to work effectively with people where spoken English is not their preferred way to communicate (NHS Scotland, 2011). It can be readily adapted for other organisations to allow people to receive information in an understandable way.

Talking about Dying

Even when people know their health is deteriorating and that they will die at some point, facing the reality of dying is often difficult. For others who have lived with a very long and disabling illness, reaching the last phase of life can bring a mixture of emotions, sometimes including relief. It is best to avoid making any assumptions about how people view the approaching death of a family member or close friend. Be open and explore their thoughts and feelings by listening as they share some of their life story. Exploring what people understand and expect before sharing information about being seriously ill, having a final illness and dying enables the professional to adapt their approach depending on how the person is coping with their situation.

Choosing language carefully is particularly important when treatment is no longer working or further treatment is not a realistic option, and can avoid distress and misunderstanding for patients and families (Table 3.5) (Australian and New Zealand Intensive Care Society (ANZICS), 2014). Even talking about 'goals of care' can seem like jargon for some people. Simple, clear language is especially important when people are tired and under emotional strain. Often non-verbal communication is what makes the greatest impression; kindness, empathetic tone and posture, appropriate touch.

Some people have prolongation of life and survival as their main priority. In this situation, it is best to avoid focusing on the 'futility' of a treatment or how unpleasant/harmful it might be as this is seen as reluctance to help or denial of a person's rights. Do try to 'reach common ground' by finding out about their reasons, priorities, beliefs, concerns and fears. Ask what is important to them in this situation, and then look for an agreed 'best way

Table 3.5 Using helpful language in conversations about death and dying.

Poor word choice	Possible interpretation	Do say
What do you want us to do next?	Professional focus is on treatment not what matters to the person; the family is responsible for making all the decisions.	*'What would be important for them?'* *'What would they say if we could ask them?'* *'How would they like to be cared for?'*
There is nothing more we can do. They are is being 'made palliative'. Treatment is 'futile'.	Patient and family are being abandoned. Person is not valued.	*'We will do everything we can to make sure they are cared for well, and is as comfortable as possible.'*
We are going to 'withdraw' treatment.	The professionals will give less care and attention to the person.	*'We are continuing to care for them while stopping treatments that are not working and may do harm.'*
The doctor makes decisions about their treatment.	The person and those close to them have no role in sharing decisions about treatment and care.	*'We look at the options and ask what you think they might say so our team can make decisions about what will help them most.'*
'Ceiling' of treatment or care.	People think they are being denied treatment that could help.	*'There are things we can do, but some treatments do not work or help when a person is dying/has a final illness.'*

forward'. Seek a second opinion (for example, from a senior colleague and/or a palliative care specialist) to support shared decision making.

Talking about dying using RED-MAP

The RED-MAP steps for care planning conversations can also be used when talking with people who are approaching the last days of life and their families (Table 3.6). Find out what people know and expect and then share information about what happens when someone is dying. Go on to talk about what matters to this person and what we can do to care for them as they are dying and offer support to their family.

Discussing uncertainty and responding to 'difficult' questions

Find out what the person already knows, what they want to know now, and why they are asking a question before responding. A pause and 'reflecting back' the question softens the response and helps us answer clearly but gently. Acknowledge uncertainty and talk about how we can hope and plan at the same time.

Table 3.6   Talking about care in the last days of life using RED-MAP.

RED-MAP: Care planning in the last days of life	
Ready	'Can we talk about what is happening with your health and care?' 'Who else should be involved? Is there someone we should talk to?'
Expect	'How have you been recently?' 'What has changed?' 'What do you **know** about your health problems?' 'What do you think is happening/might happen?' 'Do you want to **tell/ask** me about anything?'
Diagnosis	'We **know** you are less well because ...' 'We **hope** you will improve, but I **am worried** that ...' 'It **is possible** you will not get better ... I'm afraid (name) is seriously ill.' 'I'm sorry but you **could die soon** with this illness' 'Do you have questions or worries we can talk about?'
Matters	'What is **important** to you and your family?' 'How would **you like** to be cared for?' 'Is there anything you would **not want**?' 'What would **(name) say** about this situation, if we could ask them?'
Actions	'What we **can do** is ... Things that **can help** are ...' 'This **will not help** because ... That **does not work** when ...' 'I **wish** that was possible ... let's talk about what **we can do**.'
Plan	'Can we talk about how we care for someone who is dying?' 'We are **not sure** how quickly things will change.' 'We can make a care plan for you (name) and your family.'

Source: Developed by Dr Kirsty Boyd, Macmillan Reader in Palliative Care, The University of Edinburgh and reproduced with her permission.

'What are the "chances" of the treatment working?'

    ✓ *I'm not sure if the (treatment) will help ... we'll have a better idea in ...*

    ✓ *We are as certain as we can be that your (condition) means that ...*

    ✓ *I think you might not get better this time ... Can we talk about that?*

'How long have I got?'

    ✓ *No one can tell you for certain how much time you have, but I am worried that you are much less well than you were when/because ... I think we are probably looking at days to weeks/weeks to months. We are likely to have a better idea as time goes on and we see how you are.*

    ✓ *Can we talk about what is most important for you now, and how we might cope with not knowing exactly what will happen or when?*

'Am I going to die? Should we call the family?'

- ✓ *Can I ask what makes you think that you might be dying ...?*
- ✓ *I am not expecting you to die in the next few days, but you are very ill. It is possible you could get more unwell at any time. If time is short, what would be important for you?*
- ✓ *We are looking at a short time ... I think that they are is likely to die quite soon ...*

Talking about cardiopulmonary resuscitation (CPR) as part of care planning

Shared decision making with people who are seriously ill needs to take account of capacity. People may be able to make choices about some things while lacking capacity for more complex decisions including CPR (see 'Capacity' (p. 30) in Chapter 2 – Ethical and Legal Considerations). 'Do not attempt cardiopulmonary resuscitation' (DNACPR) discussions should never happen in isolation. They form part of wider care planning conversations that start with what the person understands of their current condition and what is likely to happen as they get less well.

People say they prefer a series of conversations about CPR, being prepared for decisions in advance, avoiding discussions in a 'crisis', conversations involving family members, and discussions with a trusted professional (Hall, 2019). In the acute hospital setting, focussing on a DNACPR decision and documentation of this without a wider discussion leading to agreement about a treatment escalation plan was much less effective (Lightbody, 2018). We always start by exploring what the person knows about their health problems, and what matters to them before explaining how CPR relates to that (see: Figure 3.5 and 3.6). Finding out what people know about CPR, and if it has been discussed previously can reduce distress and avoid giving information that is not relevant. The ReSPECT process supports these conversations (Resuscitation Council UK, 2021).

There are four situations when discussions about CPR happen as part of a wider care planning review. The approach to each of these is different and needs to take account of the person's current health status including decision-making capacity, the care setting, and a clinical assessment of the likely outcome of CPR. The person's wishes are respected where CPR is a realistic treatment option but a person (or a proxy decision-maker) cannot request a treatment that will not work. (Box 3.4) Always make it clear that DNACPR decisions only apply to CPR (Resuscitation Council UK, 2021). A few people do want more information about the process of dying, what CPR treatment means and the likely outcomes in their situation, but many do not. It is better to have a general discussion using clear and straightforward language first and offer more detailed information to those who want it. Occasionally a person or family refuse to have a DNACPR record in their home. The reasons for this are recorded in their GP practice health record and electronic care summary along with a clinical assessment stating why CPR would not have a successful outcome. An experienced clinician can decide not to start CPR or to stop it without a DNACPR record being in place.

Box 3.4 Talking about cardiopulmonary resuscitation during care planning discussions.

Ways to talk about a CPR decision

- *'Can we talk about what might happen if your health gets worse?'*
- *'Something we talk about these days is resuscitation or CPR. Do you know anything about CPR? Have you talked about it before?'*
- *'CPR is treatment to restart the heart and breathing after they have stopped. It can help some people. For others it doesn't work or leaves them in very poor health.'*
- *'It is better for us to make a plan about CPR in advance if it will not work, and then we make sure everyone knows about it. A DNACPR record is used to do this.'*
- *'Making a decision that CPR would not work does not change anything else. All other treatments and care that might help treat your illness and keep you comfortable are still given.'*

Talking about cardiopulmonary resuscitation in five clinical situations

I. A person makes a decision in advance not to have CPR.

'Yes, you can choose not to have CPR even if it could work. Can you tell me why you think that is the right decision for you? Do you know what it means?'

II. A person is dying so CPR is contraindicated.

'When someone is dying, they become unconscious and their heart and breathing stop, so we make a plan to care for them as well as possible at that time.'

III. A person has advanced illness such that CPR will not work.

'I'm afraid your health problems mean that treatment to restart your heart and breathing would not work. Making a decision that CPR will not be given does not change what we do about other treatment and care. We will continue to give you all the treatments that can help you.'

IV. CPR is a treatment option with an uncertain or poor outcome.

'CPR means treatment to restart the heart and breathing. It can work for some people but we know that when a person has health problems like these, they either do not recover or are often left in much poorer health.'

V. Discussions when the person lacks decision-making capacity.

'We need to make some decisions about treatments that are going help and those that would not work. Can you tell us if (name) has said anything about what they think is important or how they would like to be cared for when they are very ill and may die soon?

Communication and COVID-19

The COVID-19 pandemic has focused attention on communication in new ways. Staff, patients and families have had to adapt to remote consultations by telephone or video call and use of masks for all face-to-face discussions. Challenging conversations will remain so regardless of the circumstances. The principles of effective communication still apply and following them leads to better outcomes. In the future, continued use of remote consultations is likely and they have benefits as well as disadvantages when used appropriately in line with UK and WHO guidance (Sutherland et al., 2020).

Telephone conversations should have a clear introduction including checking you are speaking with the right person and they are able to have an effective consultation this way. Pace the conversation using short sentences and clear language, and signpost topics. Summarising and checking for understanding and emotional reactions is even more important. Non-verbal communication such as tone of voice matters too. A structured ending ensures the person is safe and that there is a clear plan to follow up any outstanding issues. Similar principles apply to video calls (See Table 3.7).

Face coverings pose additional problems for many people including those with hearing impairment, learning disabilities, cognitive impairment or mental illness. Existing language barriers increase. Clinicians have found a range of ways to overcome these challenges and developed resources to support effective communication including digital flash cards (Mheidly et al., 2020). CardMedic core resources are available free of charge at https://www.cardmedic.com/.

Table 3.7 Talking with people by phone.

Prepare	**Right place:** Quiet, no interruptions.
	Right information: Name of patient and relative; information to be shared; paper and pen.
	Right time: For you, for the person, for the situation.
	Right words: Think about what you'll say.
Opening	'Hello, my name is … I am calling from … about (*patient name*). I'm the (*role*) in the team.'
	'Please can I speak' to (*name*)? Is this a good time for you or would later on be better?
	'I'm sorry we are having to speak on the phone and not in person.'

Table 3.7 (*Continued*).

Tips for talking on the phone	Imagine the person is sitting opposite you as you speak. Use clear, simple terms; no jargon/abbreviations. Talk slowly in short sentences. Use: *ask-talk-ask.* Pause often and check how the person is. Tone (kind), pitch (even) and pace (slower) really matter on the phone. Listen for changes in tone, breathing, pitch or pace from the other person. This helps you judge how they are reacting. If things are not going so well, pause and restart. Apologise if they seem upset or confused. Ask them to tell you what they really mean or if there's anything either of you have not understood. Say how much it matters to you to help them as best you can.
Ending	**Manage:** If you have talked for long enough, signpost ending: *'We have a few minutes left ...'* **Summary:** *'So, what we've talked about is ...' 'I'm so sorry to have had to tell you this (sad) news ...'* **Check:** *'As we are talking by phone, it's important for me to check what you've understood about what we've been saying ... Is there anything else important you'd like to tell me just now ...'* **Plan:** *'I wish we could have met face to face to talk about this ...' 'So, what we've agreed is ...'* **Safety net:** *'Please call us back at this number and ask for x, if you have any questions or worries or if you change your mind about any of the plans we've made just now/what I have told you ...'*
Finish	**Record** discussion in patient record; share plans with team. **Remember** follow-up actions and plan for them. **Refresh:** Take time to debrief; seek support if needed.

Scenario Recap

Pete struggled to come to terms with his progressive cancer. Good support, based around sensitive and effective communication from many professionals, helped Pete and his family be open with each other and make decisions about what mattered to them. After Pete died bereavement counselling was offered to members of his family.

Resources

DNACPR

- Scottish Government (2010) Do Not Attempt Cardiopulmonary Resuscitation (DNACPR) – integrated adult policy: guidance. Available at: https://https://ihub.scot/acp

ACP

- Healthcare Improvement Scotland: Improvement hub. Anticipatory care planning. Available at: https://ihub.scot/project-toolkits/anticipatory-care-planning-toolkit/anticipatory-care-planning-toolkit/

Child bereavement

- Childhood Bereavement Network. Available at: https://childhoodbereavementnetwork.org.uk/
- Cruse Bereavement Care: Hope again. Available at: https://www.hopeagain.org.uk/
- Winston's Wish: Giving hope to grieving children. Available at: https://www.winstonswish.org/

Palliative care for people with learning disabilities

- PCPLD Network: Palliative care for people with learning disabilities. Available at: https://www.pcpld.org/
- St Oswald's Hospice and Northumberland, Tyne and Wear NHS Trust: The Disability Distress Assessment Tool. Available at: http://www.aettraininghubs.org.uk/wp-content/uploads/2016/02/DisDAT_Howtoguide.pdf

Palliative care for people with dementia

- Canadian Virtual Hospice: Dementia and Palliative Care. Available at: https://www.virtualhospice.ca/en_US/Main+Site+Navigation/Home/Support/Support/The+Video+Gallery/For+Professionals/Advanced+dementia+and+palliative+care.aspx

Spiritual care

- NHS Education for Scotland Spiritual Care resources. Available at: https://www.nes.scot.nhs.uk/our-work/spiritual-care/
- Spiritual Care Matters: an introductory resource for all NHS Scotland staff (Revised 2021). Available at: https://www.nes.scot.nhs.uk/media/xzadagnc/spiritual-care-matters-an-introductory-resource-for-all-nhsscotland-staff.pdf

References

Australian and New Zealand Intensive Care Society (2014) ANZICS statement on care and decision-making at the end of life for the critically Ill (Edition 1.0). Available at: https://intensivecareathome.com/wp-content/uploads/2015/05/ANZICS-Statement-on-Care-and-Decision-Making-at-the-End-of-Life.pdf

Baile WF et al. (2000) SPIKES – a six-step protocol for delivering bad news: application to the patient with cancer. *The Oncologist*, 5(4): 302–311.

Bikker AP, Cotton P and Mercer SW (2014) *Embracing Empathy in Healthcare: A Universal Approach to Person-Centred, Empathic Healthcare Encounters*. London and New York: Radcliffe Medical Press.

Brooks LA, Manias E and Bloomer MJ (2019) Culturally sensitive communication in healthcare: a concept analysis. *Collegia*, 26(3): 383–391.

Cain L et al. (2018) Culture in palliative care: preferences, communication, meaning and mutual decision making. *Journal of Pain and Symptom Management*, 55(5): 1408–1419.

Cameron L and Matthews R (2017) More than pictures: developing an accessible resource. *Tizzard Learning Disability Review*, 22(2): 57–65.

Chowns G (2009) Swampy ground: brief interventions with families before bereavement. In Monroe B and Kraus F (eds) *Brief Interventions with Bereaved Children*. Oxford: Oxford University Press.

Clark D et al. (2014) Imminence of death among hospital inpatients: prevalent cohort study. *Palliative Medicine* 28(6): 474–479.

Clayton JM et al. (2008) Sustaining hope when communicating with terminally ill patients and their families: a systematic review. *Psycho-Oncology*, 17(7): 641–659.

De Caestecker S (2012) Communication skills in palliative care. In Faull C, de Caestecker S, Nicholson A and Black F (eds) *Handbook of Palliative Care*, 3rd edition. Hoboken, NJ: Wiley-Blackwell, pp. 109–138.

Fallowfield L and Jenkins V (2002) The truth hurts but deceit hurts more: communication in palliative care. *Palliative Medicine*, 16(4): 297–303.

Fearnley R and Boland JW (2017) Communication and support from health-care professionals to families, with dependent children, following the diagnosis of parental life-limiting illness: a systematic review. *Palliative Medicine*, 31(3): 212–222.

Hall CC et al. (2019) CPR decision-making conversations in the UK: an integrative review. *BMJ Supportive and Palliative Care*, 9: 1–11.

Irish Hospice Foundation (2015). Guidance Document 1: Facilitating discussions on future and end-of-life care with a person with dementia. Dublin: The Irish Hospice Foundation; 2015.

Irish Hospice Foundation (2021). Children's Grief. Available at: https://hospicefoundation. ie/i-need-help/i-am-bereaved/types-of-grief/childrens-grief/

Jackson VA et al. (2013) The cultivation of prognostic awareness through the provision of early palliative care in the ambulatory setting: a communication guide. *Journal of Palliative Medicine*, 16(8): 1–7.

James IA (2011) *Understanding Behaviour in Dementia That Challenges: A Guide to Assessment and Treatment*. London: Jessica Kingsley Publishers.

Kendall M et al. (2015) Different experiences and goals in different advanced diseases: comparing serial interviews with patients with cancer, organ failure, or frailty and their family and professional carers. *Journal of Pain Symptom Management*, 50(2): 216–224.

Kimbell B et al. (2016) Embracing inherent uncertainty in advanced illness. *BMJ*, 354: i3802.

Lightbody CJ et al. (2018) Impact of a treatment escalation/limitation plan on non-beneficial interventions and harms in patients during their last admission before in-hospital death, using the Structured Judgment Review Method. *BMJ Open*, 8(10): e024264.

Long CO (2011) Cultural and spiritual consideration in palliative care. *Journal of Pediatric Haematological Oncology*, 33(Suppl 2): S96–101.

Macmillan Cancer Support (2016) *Talking to Children and Teenagers When an Adult Has Cancer*, 3rd edition. London: Macmillan Cancer Support.

McCormack B et al. (2010) Exploring person-centredness: a qualitative meta-synthesis of four studies. *Scandinavian Journal of Caring Sciences*, 24(3): 620–634.

Mencap (2019) Communicating with people with a learning disability. Available at: https://www.mencap.org.uk/sites/default/files/2016-12/Communicating%20with%20people_updated%20%281%29.pdf

Mercer SW et al. (2004) The consultation and relational empathy (CARE) measure: development and preliminary validation and reliability of an empathy-based consultation process measure. *Family Practice*, 21(6): 699–705.

Mheidly N et al. (2020) Effect of face masks on interpersonal communication during the COVID-19 pandemic. *Front Public Health*, 8: 582191.

Monden KR, Gentry L and Cox TR (2016) Delivering bad news to patients. *Baylor University Medical Centre Proceedings*, 29(1): 101–102.

National Institute for Health and Care Excellence (2013) Mental wellbeing of older people in care homes. Quality statement 4: Recognition of sensory impairment. Available at https://www.nice.org.uk/guidance/qs50/chapter/Quality-statement-4-Recognition-of-sensory-impairment#quality-statement-4

National Institute for Health and Care Excellence (2018). Care and support of people growing older with learning disabilities. Guideline NG 96. Available at: https://www.nice.org.uk/guidance/ng96

NHS Education for Scotland (2010) Spiritual care matters. Available at: https://www.nes.scot.nhs.uk/media/23nphas3/spiritualcaremattersfinal.pdf

NHS Education for Scotland (2017) *Enriching and Improving Experience. Palliative and End of Life Care: A Framework to Support the Learning and Development Needs of the Health and Social Services Workforce in Scotland*. Edinburgh: NHS Education for Scotland.

NHS Scotland (2011) NHS Scotland competency framework for interpreting. Available at: http://www.healthscotland.com/documents/5227.aspx

Pereira ATG et al. (2013) Communication of bad news: systematic literature review. *Journal of Nursing UFPE Online*, 7(1): 227–235.

Resuscitation Council UK (2021) Guidance: DNACPR and CPR decisions. Available at: https://www.resus.org.uk/library/additional-guidance/guidance-dnacpr-and-cpr-decisions

Schouler-Ocak M et al. (2015) EPA guidance on cultural competence training. *European Psychiatry*, 30, (3): 431–440.

Steele R and Davies B (2014) Supporting families in palliative care. In Ferrell BR and Coyle N (eds) *Oxford Textbook of Palliative Nursing*, 3rd edition. Oxford: Oxford University Press, pp. 500–514.

Stevens E (2018) Communication in palliative care nursing. In Walshe C, Preston N and Johnston B (eds) *Palliative Care Nursing: Principles and Evidence for Practice*, 3rd edition. London: Open University Press/McGraw-Hill, pp. 117–133.

Supportive and Palliative Care Indicators Tool (SPICT™) (2021). The University of Edinburgh. Available at: https://www.spict.org.uk/

Sutherland AE, Strickland J and Wee B (2020) Can video consultations replace face-to-face interviews? Palliative medicine and the covid-19 pandemic: rapid review. *BMJ Supportive Palliative Care*, 10(3): 271–275.

Think Local Act Personal Partnership (2012) *Making it Real for People with Sensory Impairment*. London: Think Local Act Personal Partnership.

Tuffrey-Winje I (2012) A new model for breaking bad news to people with intellectual disabilities. *Palliative Medicine*, 27(1): 5–12.

Tylor EB (1871) Primitive Culture. London: J Murray.

Warnick (2019) Supporting children grieving their own death or the death of someone close to them. Available at: https://www.virtualhospice.ca/default.aspx?goto=en_US-Main+Site+Navigation-Home-Support-Support-The+Video+Gallery-Children+and+Teens-Supporting+children+grieving+their+own+death+or+the+death+of+someone+close+to+them+with+Camara+Van+Breeman+%e2%80%93+Recorded+Webinar

Symptom Management

Marie Fallon, David Carroll, Deans Buchanan,
Paul Brown and Maire O'Riordan

Learning Objectives

This chapter is separated into five parts. The chapter will help you to understand how to manage symptoms associated with:

4.1 Pain

4.2 The gastrointestinal system

4.3 The respiratory system

4.4 Mental health

4.5 And other symptoms common to palliative patients

4.1 PAIN

Marie Fallon with Mairi Armstrong and Roger Flint

Learning Objectives

At the completion of this section, you will be able to:

- Recognise the impact of pain for palliative care patients
- Provide a comprehensive assessment of pain, recognising the different components and secondary contributing factors
- Suggest potential options for management of pain being cognisant of co-existing symptoms.

Scenario

Background

Amir is a 70-year-old retired joiner with a 3-month history of right-sided chest pain and cough. He has been receiving palliative radiotherapy for right-sided Pancoast's tumour. Amir lives with his wife; his son lives in Canada, and his daughter, who has two young children, lives 30 miles away. The bedroom and bathroom he uses is upstairs. His GP was asked to visit because of worsening pain.

Key points

- Poor pain control on simple analgesia.

Timeline

Amir was reviewed during radiotherapy because of pain in right shoulder and arm. He experiences constant severe background pain, rated as 9/10. He also experiences intermittent, excruciating shooting pain associated with pins and needles and a tight sensation, rated as 10/10.

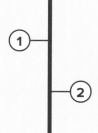

Amir is unable to sleep. He says he feels miserable and hopeless, and that he 'doesn't look forward to anything; each day is a challenge'. He has also lost weight and has a poor appetite.

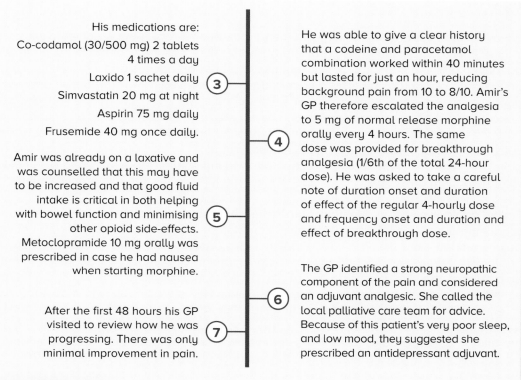

His medications are:

Co-codamol (30/500 mg) 2 tablets 4 times a day

Laxido 1 sachet daily ③

Simvastatin 20 mg at night

Aspirin 75 mg daily

Frusemide 40 mg once daily.

④

Amir was already on a laxative and was counselled that this may have to be increased and that good fluid intake is critical in both helping with bowel function and minimising ⑤ other opioid side-effects. Metoclopramide 10 mg orally was prescribed in case he had nausea when starting morphine.

⑥

After the first 48 hours his GP visited to review how he was progressing. There was only ⑦ minimal improvement in pain.

He was able to give a clear history that a codeine and paracetamol combination worked within 40 minutes but lasted for just an hour, reducing background pain from 10 to 8/10. Amir's GP therefore escalated the analgesia to 5 mg of normal release morphine orally every 4 hours. The same dose was provided for breakthrough analgesia (1/6th of the total 24-hour dose). He was asked to take a careful note of duration onset and duration of effect of the regular 4-hourly dose and frequency onset and duration and effect of breakthrough dose.

The GP identified a strong neuropathic component of the pain and considered an adjuvant analgesic. She called the local palliative care team for advice. Because of this patient's very poor sleep, and low mood, they suggested she prescribed an antidepressant adjuvant.

Key considerations

- As there was only minimal improvement in Amir's pain, what options does his GP have?
- What side-effects should the GP anticipate and how can she manage them?
- What should be considered when switching from simple analgesia to opioids?
- What should you consider for an ongoing pain review and future planning?
- What adjuvant analgesics could be considered for Amir?

Cancer Pain

Cancer pain is one of the most feared symptoms of cancer and is the commonest cause of out of hours calls (Adam et al., 2015) and one of the commonest reasons for cancer patients attending A&E (Mills et al., 2019). It is an untruth that cancer pain is well managed in western countries. There are multiple factors behind poor cancer pain management, however, a lack of a simple and consistent systematic approach to assessment and appropriate prescribing lie at the core. Numerous studies have demonstrated that cancer pain can be managed in up to 85% of cases with widely available and cheap drugs, however, as stated above, this success is not translated into clinical practice.

Opioid Analgesics

Opioid analgesics are the mainstay in the treatment of chronic pain associated with active cancer (WHO, 2019) and other chronic progressive illnesses, particularly in the context of advanced disease. Although concurrent use of other approaches and interventions may be appropriate in many patients, and necessary in some, an opioid is a preferred approach in almost every patient with moderate or severe chronic pain. The safe and effective use of opioid drugs is a key competency in palliative care and is predicated on a continual effort to balance expected benefits against the potential for harm. The common side-effects of opioids cause the barrier in pain control in most cases, rather than any inherent inability to control pain. The care taken with preventing and attenuating opioid side-effects and communication with the patient and carers about side-effects is key in successful pain management.

Opioid analgesics are conventionally distinguished from non-opioid analgesics, such as paracetamol and the non-steroidal anti-inflammatory drugs (NSAIDs), and the so-called adjuvant analgesics. The latter category includes drugs, such as the glucocorticoids, analgesic antidepressants and anticonvulsants, that have primary indications other than pain but are effective analgesics in specific circumstances. Adjuvant analgesics should be considered in all cases of neuropathic pain. Opioids have a complex pharmacology, which is reflected in great inter-individual variability in the response to different opioid compounds. Recent evidence has established the importance of genetic variability in determining not just the analgesic response to exogenous opioids but also the response to our own endogenous opioids involved in the inherent ability to attenuate pain transmission (Lee et al., 2014; De Felice et al., 2016). Concurrently, advances in neuroimaging have helped to model the long-held belief of managing 'total pain'. We now understand clearly how such problems as anxiety, depression, fear, distress, sleeplessness and hopelessness feed into the actual pain network. These common co-existing problems do not simply make the patient less able to cope with pain, rather at a central level they actually increase the severity of pain (Figure 4.1.1).

Opioids are key to the management of chronic moderate or severe pain related to active cancer or other advanced illnesses. However, the active management of any exacerbating symptoms which feed into the pain networks via emotional centres is key to the successful management of pain.

If the assessment of a patient is inadequate then pain cannot be managed appropriately.

The analgesic ladder

The 'WHO analgesic ladder' (WHO, 1996; Poulsen et al., 1996) emphasised that the severity of pain should be the prime determinant of the choice of analgesic pharmacotherapy, emphasising the importance of opioids, such as morphine, for pain that is moderate to severe. In particular:

- The intensity of pain, rather than the stage in the disease process or its specific aetiology, should be the prime consideration in analgesic selection.
- Appreciation of the underlying aetiology and pain mechanism may direct to appropriate adjuvant analgesic drugs.

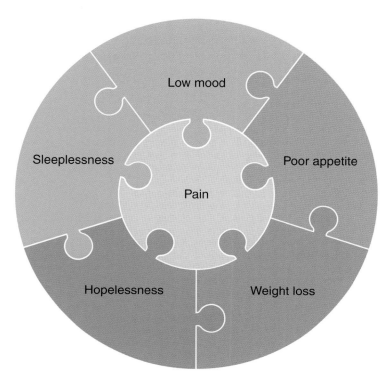

Low mood

Sleeplessness

Poor appetite

Pain

Hopelessness

Weight loss

Figure 4.1.1   Actual pain is exacerbated by non-nociceptive problems.

- Any analgesic strategy in cancer patients must be integrated with non-pharmacological methods of cancer pain control (such as radiotherapy, chemotherapy, hormone therapy, surgery, anaesthetic interventions, physiotherapy and psychological/cognitive approaches).

The analgesic ladder (Figure 4.1.2) proposes the following framework:

Step 1: Patients with mild pain should be treated with a non-opioid analgesic, which should be combined with adjuvant drugs if a specific indication for these exists.

Step 2: Patients with pain that is generally moderate, and those with generally mild pain that has not responded adequately to a trial of a non-opioid analgesic, should be treated with an opioid conventionally used for pain of this severity (WHO, 2019). This may be in the form of a combination product (for example, paracetamol plus codeine) or a low dose of a pure opioid agonist such as morphine or oxycodone. Regardless of the opioid used, a co-administered adjuvant analgesic should be considered if an indication for one exists.

Step 3: Patients with pain that is generally severe, and those with pain of lesser intensity that has not responded adequately to one or more trials of drugs conventionally used on Step 2 of the analgesic ladder, should receive an opioid conventionally used for severe pain. This group most commonly includes morphine, fentanyl, oxycodone and hydromorphone. There is no inherent superiority of one opioid over another and treatment must be individualised (Caraceni et al., 2012; WHO, 2019). It does, however, make sense to start with morphine as it is the strong opioid with which we all have most experience. Co-administration of a non-opioid analgesic or an adjuvant analgesic drug appropriate for the pain aetiology should be considered.

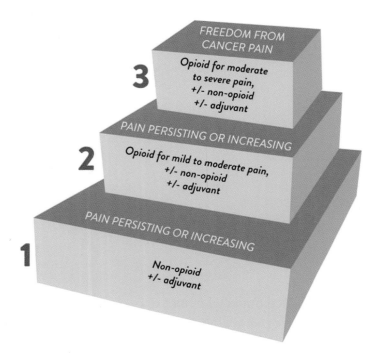

Figure 4.1.2   The WHO analgesic ladder.

Source: Reproduced from WHO, 2019.

Adjuvant therapies

It makes sense when choosing an adjuvant analgesic to think about co-existing symptoms other than pain.

- **NSAID**:
  - For bone pain, liver pain, soft tissue infiltration, or inflammatory pain
  - Side-effects: gastrointestinal ulceration or bleeding (consider proton pump inhibitor (PPI)), renal impairment, fluid retention, adverse cardiac events.
- **Antidepressant** or **anticonvulsant**:
  - For nerve pain
  - Start at low dose: titrate slowly (refer to neuropathic pain guideline)
  - No clear difference in efficacy between the two types of medicine for this indication
    - Amitriptyline (side-effects: confusion, hypotension caution in cardiovascular disease).

- Gabapentin (side-effects: sedation, tremor, confusion; reduce dose if renal impairment).
- **Corticosteroids**: dexamethasone:
  - 8–16 mg daily for raised intracranial pressure
  - 4–8 mg daily for neuropathic pain; 4–8 mg daily for liver capsule pain
  - Give in the morning; reduce to lowest effective dose. Consider PPI. Monitor blood glucose.
- **TENS, nerve block, radiotherapy, surgery, bisphosphonates, ketamine** (specialist use) and **skeletal or smooth muscle relaxants.**

(Scottish Palliative Care Guidelines, 2020b)

According to these guidelines, a trial of opioid therapy should be given to all patients with pain uncontrolled by an NSAID and/or paracetamol. The opioid chosen depends on the individual patient and drug availability. On a worldwide basis, morphine is most commonly chosen. There is increasing evidence for missing out Step 2 and moving straight to a low dose of a Step 3, a strong opioid (Bandieri et al., 2016; Fallon, 2017; Fallon et al., 2021).

Definition of Pain

International Association for the Study of Pain's definition of pain

'An unpleasant sensory and emotional experience associated with, or resembling that associated with, actual or potential tissue damage.'

(IASP, 2020)

International Classification of Diseases (ICD) definition of cancer pain

'Chronic cancer-related pain is defined as chronic pain caused by the primary cancer itself or metastases (chronic cancer pain) or its treatment (chronic post-cancer treatment pain).'

(Bennett et al., 2019)

Prevalence and Aetiology of Cancer Pain

Pain is common in cancer patients, particularly in the advanced stage of disease when the prevalence is estimated to be more than 70%, contributing to poor physical and emotional well-being. The most comprehensive systematic review indicates pain prevalence ranging from 33% in patients after curative treatment, to 59% in patients on anti-cancer treatment, and to 64% in patients with metastatic, advanced or terminal disease (Fallon et al., 2018b)

Although effective pain relief can be achieved in up to 85–90% of patients with cancer (Burton et al., 2007), numerous studies have shown that pain remains inadequately controlled in many patients (Glare et al., 2014). A lack of effective pain control can adversely affect the patient and carers in numerous domains (Brown et al., 2014).

In patients with cancer, pain may be caused by the tumour itself, treatment of the tumour, diagnostic or therapeutic procedures, or treatment-related adverse events (Breivik et al., 2009) such as acute procedural pain, iatrogenic pain, or co-morbidity-related pain. Cancer survivors often have chronic treatment-related pain; about 30% will have chemotherapy-induced peripheral neuropathy still present 6 months or later after completing chemotherapy (Ripamonti et al., 2012). Post-cancer treatment pain is generally not best managed with chronic opioid therapy. There is usually a large neuropathic pain component and adjuvant drugs along with non-pharmacological approaches remain key.

Pain Associated with Other Chronic Life-Limiting Conditions

While pain is common in other chronic life-limiting conditions, it is often less severe and less feared than cancer pain. The aetiologies are wide-ranging, such as hepatic pain in heart failure, neuropathic pain in multiple sclerosis. However, assessment and management in advanced non-malignant disease should follow the same broad principles as cancer pain.

Prevalences in chronic non-malignant life-limiting disease are as follows:

- Cardiac – 23–85% (Alemzadeh-Ansari et al., 2017)
- Respiratory – 66% (Lee et al., 2015)
- Neurological – 36% (Cragg et al., 2018)
- Renal – >60–70% (Pham et al., 2017)
- Hepatic – 30–79% (Peng et al., 2019)
- Dementia – 49.7% (Lin et al., 2018).

Much anxiety has evolved about the use of opioids in chronic non-malignant pain not associated with life-limiting disease over recent years, largely fuelled by the North American situation, which is clearly very complex. Chronic pain management teams in the UK are trying to evolve better ways of managing this otherwise-well group who are different from the patients with life-limiting chronic disease that we are referring to in this chapter.

Pathophysiology

Pain is complex. The underlying neurobiology, and the individual's unique response to that neurobiology, along with co-existing symptoms, is the cornerstone of the pathophysiology in an individual patient. We know that in cancer, bone pain and neuropathic pain are the most challenging. That said, we have evidence (see below) that human factors in poor assessment play a greater role overall in poor cancer pain control than the type of pain per se.

Assessment of Patients with Pain

We now have evidence from patients with cancer that a simple, but consistent approach using the Edinburgh Pain Assessment Tool (EPAT) can lead to improved pain relief, more individualised prescribing, faster discharge from hospital and cost savings (Fallon et al., 2018a; Diernberger et al., 2021). The principles of the assessment approach can be applied to patients with pain due to advanced life-limiting non-malignant illness, however the strong evidence for EPAT applies to cancer pain.

The key to EPAT is to use the same simple screening question, not to take a shortcut with this, and then to ask simple follow-up questions if pain falls in amber or red (Figure 4.1.3).

> 'What has been your worst pain on a scale of 0–10, with 0 none and 10 the worst imaginable?'

This is asked for the last 24 hours or, if in hospital, it is asked along with evaluating the patient's vital signs and relates to the last assessment. Move to a more detailed assessment, Step 2, if worst pain is ≥3/10 or the patient is distressed by pain. Monitor if <3/10.

The key to Step 2 (Figure 4.1.4) is the assessment of cause/s of pain/s and this is linked with management.

The key to management is the use of algorithms, which give the details on how to prescribe opioids and adjuvants, along with dose titration. These have clear advantages over broad statements of recommended drugs found in standard guidelines. Important non-pharmacological management options are also presented: please refer to Appendix 4.1.1.

No management is successful without reassessment of pain relief and of unwanted effects, especially opioid-related adverse effects. The key to preventing serious side-effects with chronic opioid use is careful monitoring of vivid dreams, hallucinations, shadows on the periphery of vision and sleepiness, as these are prodromes to frank confusion and opioid toxicity.

This approach has been proven to lead to improved, tailored prescribing and better side-effects prevention and management.

Assessment of the descriptors of pain improves the choice of therapy: pain is termed nociceptive when it is caused by ongoing tissue damage, either somatic or visceral, or neuropathic if sustained by damage or dysfunction in the nervous system (Sun et al., 2008). According to the literature, most patients with advanced cancer have at least two types of cancer-related pain which derives from a variety of aetiologies (Portenoy and Koh, 2010).

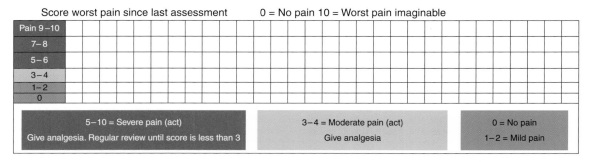

Score worst pain since last assessment   0 = No pain 10 = Worst pain imaginable

| Pain 9–10 |
| 7–8 |
| 5–6 |
| 3–4 |
| 1–2 |
| 0 |

5–10 = Severe pain (act)
Give analgesia. Regular review until score is less than 3

3–4 = Moderate pain (act)
Give analgesia

0 = No pain
1–2 = Mild pain

Figure 4.1.3   EPAT Step 1.

LOCATION
NERVE PAIN?
OVEMENT PAIN?
WIDER ISSUES
REFERRAL

Edinburgh Pain Assessment Tool (EPAT ©) –Step 2

Name: Ward: Date/Time:

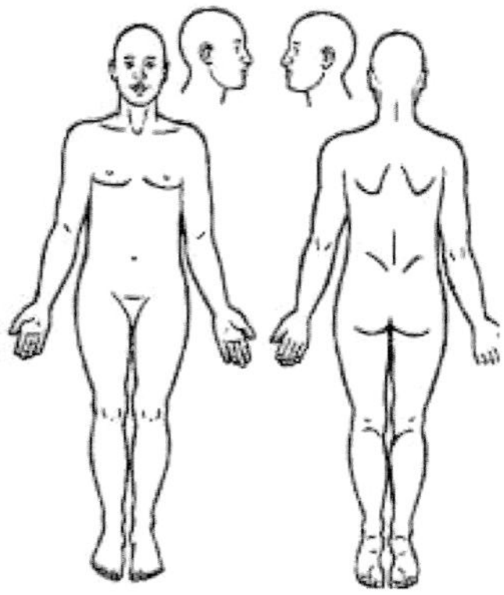

Severity Score	A Most Severe	B	C
Worst Pain in Last 24 hrs (0-10)			
Least Pain in Last 24 hrs (0-10)			

0 = No Pain 10 = Worst Pain Imaginable

On the diagram, mark the sites where you have felt worst pain (ABC)

Does your pain disturb your sleep?
Yes ☐   No☐

Is your pain…?
Shooting or Stabbing ☐   Tingling or Pricking ☐   Pins & Needles☐   Hot or burning ☐
➤

Do any areas of your skin feel numb or strange or unpleasant to touch?
Yes ☐ No ☐   Detail: _____

Does moving or any other activity make your pain worse?   Yes ☐   No☐

Does your pain come on suddenly at rest?   Yes ☐   No☐
>   **Consider** neuropathic pain. **Treat** with adjuvants
Use 'starting gabapentin/starting amitriptyline' EPAT algorithms

Does moving or any other activity make your pain worse?   Yes ☐   No☐

Does your pain come on suddenly at rest?   Yes ☐   No☐

>   Is the patient experiencing movement-related or spontaneous pain? Consider bone pain
>   **Use** WHO analgesic ladder – See EPAT algorithm. **Give** PRN analgesia before movement
>   **Consider** NSAID's / Palliative Radiotherapy / Bisphosphonates

What makes your pain better? _____

>   **Remember:** non-pharmacological interventions!
Consider: Position change / Relaxation / Physiotherapy/ Rubbing / TENS / acupuncture

☺ **Is there anything worrying or concerning you about your pain?** Discuss with patient.
>   **Remember:** ☺ anxiety/depression may co-exist with severe pain.

☎**Consider referral to your Specialist Team for patients
who have persistent pain:**
➤Patients with severe pain   ➤Patients with movement-related pain
➤Patients requiring a rapidly increasing opioid dose   ➤Pain unrelieved by initial management
➤Patients with opioid-induced drowsiness

Figure 4.1.4   EPAT Step 2.

In older age, the presence of limited communicative skills or of cognitive impairment such as during the last days of life makes self-reporting of pain more difficult, although there is no evidence of clinical reduction in pain-related suffering.

When cognitive deficits are severe, observation of pain-related behaviours and discomfort (that is facial expression, body movements, verbalisation or vocalisations, changes in interpersonal interactions, changes in routine activity) is an alternative strategy for assessing the presence of pain (but not intensity) (Van Herk et al., 2007). Observational scales are available (Van Herk et al., 2007). Sensitivity to light touch can herald neuropathic pain and is often not identified in the cognitively impaired.

Assessment and management of pain in children are not considered here but WHO guidelines on the pharmacological treatment of persisting pain in children with medical illness are available (WHO, 2012).

Psychosocial distress has to be assessed because it is strongly associated with pain (Syrjala et al., 2015). Psychological distress may amplify actual pain, and similarly, inadequately controlled pain may cause psychological distress (Tracey, 2017). As already alluded to, it is fundamentally wrong to think that a very distressed patient does not really have the pain expressed. The pain expressed is what the patient feels. The distress will impact on the central brain pain network to actually increase the severity of pain and vice versa.

Principles of Pain Management

Inform patients about possible onset of pain at any stage of disease, both during and after diagnostic interventions and as a consequence of cancer and/or anti-cancer treatments or other disease treatments. Patients must be both empowered and encouraged to communicate with the physician and/or the nurse about their suffering, the efficacy of therapy and side-effects. Patient education should include information on the appropriate use of opioids at various stages of disease and this should be set in context with other analgesic and non-pharmacological approaches (Reid et al., 2008). Patient involvement in pain management improves both communication and pain relief (De Wit et al., 1997).

It is important to prescribe a therapy that can be managed simply by patients and families themselves, especially when the patient is cared for at home. A patient-held version of EPAT has been used in rural Kenya with improved patient outcomes (Besley et al., 2014). The patient and carers are key to effective pain relief, and time invested in their education about expressing pain, management used, potential side-effects and outcomes to be expected from prescribed drugs is fundamental. The oral route, if well tolerated, should be considered the preferred route of administration (Hanks et al., 1996; WHO, 1996). Care should be given to the assessment and treatment of breakthrough pain (BTP), defined as 'a transitory flare of pain that occurs on a background of relatively well-controlled baseline pain'. Typical BTP episodes are of moderate to severe intensity, rapid in onset (minutes) and relatively short in duration (median 30 minutes) (Portenoy and Hagen, 1990).

The type and dose of analgesic drugs are influenced by the intensity of pain and have to be promptly adjusted to reach a balance between pain relief and side-effects. The rescue doses (as required) if taken by a patient for 'end of dose failure' can help with calculating the daily titration of the regular doses. An alternative to the oral route should be considered when oral intake is not possible because of severe vomiting, bowel obstruction, severe dysphagia or severe confusion, as well as in the presence of poor pain control which requires rapid dose escalation and/or in the presence of oral opioid-related adverse effects.

Clearly, analgesic drugs are only one part of cancer pain management. An integrated approach to cancer pain management should be adopted and this incorporates primary antitumour treatments, systemic analgesic therapy and other non-invasive techniques such as psychological and rehabilitative interventions (Paice and Ferrell, 2011).

Choosing an Opioid

When an individual's pain is not being managed effectively by paracetamol (with or without an adjuvant), the WHO analgesic ladder suggests moving to an opioid from Step 2 or 3. Given the heterogeneity and complexities of patients with cancer pain, choice of opioids is important and can facilitate an optimum balance between analgesia and unwanted adverse effects.

Opioids come in different dose forms: oral, transdermal, transmucosal and injectable. They also have different release characteristics: immediate release and modified release. Modified release (MR) preparations are normally used over a 24-hour period to control background pain. Immediate release (IR) preparations can be prescribed and given 'as required' for breakthrough pain.

Oral immediate release preparations, such as oral morphine, act quickly. Oral morphine will start to have an effect within 20–30 minutes of administration with peak effect at approximately 60 minutes. Titration of the background modified release opioids should be guided by how much immediate release opioids are required (Scottish Palliative Care Guidelines, 2020a).

Opioids for mild to moderate pain

Codeine

The weak opioid codeine, used in Step 2 of the analgesia ladder, has no or little analgesic effect until metabolised to morphine, mainly via CYP2D6. In poor metabolisers (about 5–10% of the population (Dean, 2017)) it is therefore essentially ineffective, while in ultra-rapid metabolisers it is potentially toxic. It has several active metabolites that are renally excreted, so should be avoided in stage 4 and 5 chronic kidney disease.

Dihydrocodeine

Dihydrocodeine is similar to codeine in structure and analgesic effect, and is also a substrate for CYP2D6. However, there is no evidence to suggest that analgesic effect is affected by an individual's ability to metabolise dihydrocodeine. It also has several active metabolites that are renally excreted, so should be avoided in stage 4 and 5 chronic kidney disease.

Tramadol

Tramadol is chemically unrelated to morphine, and has opioid and non-opioid properties. It requires the liver enzyme CYP2D6 to help with its metabolism and can therefore be poorly tolerated by some individuals. It is renally excreted so should be used with caution in stage 4 and 5 chronic kidney disease, and also severe liver failure. It should be avoided or used with caution in individuals taking selective serotonin reuptake inhibitors (SSRIs) or tricyclic antidepressants (TCAs) due to risk of serotonin syndrome and of lowered seizure threshold.

Buprenorphine patches

This is available as a 7-day, slow-release patch to treat moderate pain. It is therefore contra-indicated in patients with acute (short-term) pain and in those who need rapid dose titration for severe uncontrolled pain. It undergoes hepatic metabolism to norbuprenorphine, which has little clinical activity and does not cross the blood–brain barrier, and unchanged buprenorphine is excreted through the biliary system. It does not accumulate in renal impairment and therefore may be a good Step 2 opioid in stage 4 and 5 chronic kidney disease.

Opioids for moderate to severe pain

Morphine

As with other opioids morphine is available in immediate and modified release oral preparations, and it is essential to ensure the correct preparation is prescribed. It is renally excreted with active metabolites, so needs to be titrated slowly and monitored carefully in stage 1 to 3 chronic kidney disease. Use alternative opioids in stage 4 and 5 chronic kidney disease and patients undergoing dialysis to avoid toxicity. In liver impairment consider low doses and slow titration.

Diamorphine

Diamorphine is highly soluble opioid used both for subcutaneous (SC) injection and given via a syringe pump (CSCI). It comes in a powder preparation that is soluble in a small volume of water for injections. Because of this, it is particularly useful for high-dose SC breakthrough injections (above morphine SC bolus injections of 60 mg in 2 ml). As with morphine, it should be used cautiously in renal and liver impairment, and avoided in stage 4 and 5 chronic kidney disease.

Second-line opioids

Oxycodone

Oxycodone is used in moderate to severe pain if morphine or diamorphine are not tolerated. It also should be prescribed with caution due to the variety of preparations available. In mild to moderate renal impairment there is reduced clearance, so it needs to be titrated slowly and monitored carefully. Immediate release preparations may be used with caution for breakthrough pain in stage 4 and 5 chronic kidney disease, but modified release preparations should be avoided. It should also be avoided in moderate to severe liver impairment, where clearance is much reduced.

Transdermal fentanyl

Fentanyl is most commonly available as a transdermal patch lasting 72 hours, for use if oral and SC routes are unsuitable. It should only be used for stable pain, as the dose cannot be changed quickly. The generalist should consider seeking specialist advice before switching a patient on to it. It is a very potent opioid and can only be considered for patients who are known to be tolerant to opioids (a 12 micrograms/hour fentanyl patch is equivalent to about 30–60 mg of oral morphine in 24 hours). Inappropriate use can cause fatal overdose.

Usually there is no need for initial dose reduction in renal impairment. It may accumulate over time, as it is cleared through the kidneys. If pain is well controlled, but the patient has shown signs of mild toxicity, dose reduction should be considered, particularly if the estimated glomerular filtration rate (eGFR) is <30 ml/min. Dose reduction may also be needed in severe liver disease.

Transdermal fentanyl can be useful in patients with nausea, vomiting, problems with swallowing, constipation and poor compliance.

Fentanyl patches should not be initiated at the end of life, when the oral route is no longer available, due to the time delay for dose changes to have an effect, and it can take too long to reach a steady state.

Third-line opioids (seek specialist advice)

Alfentanil

Alfentanil is a short-acting potent opioid: 1 mg of alfentanil is roughly equivalent to 30 mg oral morphine. Due to the short half-life it is used for episodic or incident pain, and can be given by injection or sublingually (unlicensed). The dose does not need to be reduced in renal disease including stage 4 and 5 chronic kidney disease. It is the drug of choice if the eGFR is less than 30 ml/min and a syringe pump is required. Clearance may be reduced in liver impairment requiring a reduced dose and titration.

Fentanyl – sublingual/buccal/intranasal

These are potent preparations. Before rapid acting fentanyl is used, patients must have been on a stable dose of a regular opioid for approximately 7 days equivalent to a minimum of 60 mg oral morphine or 30 mg of oral oxycodone in 24 hours or a 25 micrograms/hour fentanyl patch.

In episodic or incident pain fentanyl can be given sublingually, buccally or intranasally. The effective dose of transmucosal fentanyl cannot be predicted from the background dose of opioid. Therefore it should be started at the lowest dose and titrated upwards to determine the effective dose. There are several preparations available. These products are not interchangeable due to different absorption profiles.

Fourth-line opioids (specialist use only)

Hydromorphone and methadone are both potent opiods that are available for specialist use only.

Opioid Toxicity

Many patients develop adverse effects from opioid therapy, over a wide variation in doses. These can be precipitated by several factors including rapid dose escalation, renal impairment, sepsis, electrolyte abnormalities and drug interactions. Prompt recognition and treatment are needed. There are many adverse effects. The more common include (Scottish Palliative Care Guidelines, 2020a):

- Sedation (exclude other causes)
- Nausea and vomiting
- Dry mouth
- Bowel dysfunction (constipation, incomplete evacuation, bloating, gastric reflux)
- Vivid dreams or shadows at the edge of visual field
- CNS toxicity (cognitive impairment, confusion, delirium, hallucinations)
- Muscle twitching/myoclonus/muscle jerking
- Respiratory depression (consider co-morbidities, respiratory depressive drugs)
- Abnormal skin sensitivity to touch (opioid induced hyperalgesia).

Management of opioid side-effects

The management of opioid-induced adverse effects is an important aspect of pain management because each adverse effect requires a careful assessment and treatment strategy (Benyamin et al., 2008). Opioid dose reduction can reduce the severity of adverse events. If the pain is controlled, reduce the opioid dose by a third and ensure the patient is well hydrated. If pain is uncontrolled, consider reducing opioid dose by a third, and consider adjuvant treatments, an opioid switch or both. Common adjuvant treatments include using a co-analgesic, a nerve block or radiotherapy. Since some adverse effects may be caused by accumulation of toxic metabolites, switching to another opioid and/or another route may allow titration to adequate analgesia without the same disabling effects. This is especially true for symptoms of central nervous system (CNS) toxicity such as opioid-induced hyperalgesia, allodynia or myoclonic jerks (Stone and Minton, 2011). Naloxone (in small titrated doses) is only needed for life-threatening respiratory depression, and should be used with specialist advice.

Metoclopramide and anti-dopaminergic drugs are used frequently for treatment of opioid-related nausea and vomiting, although good studies are lacking (Laugsand et al., 2011).

The most common manifestation of bowel dysfunction is opioid-induced constipation (OIC) with reduction in bowel movement frequency, increased straining, incomplete evacuation and hard stools (Larkin et al., 2018). First-line treatments for OIC typically involve laxatives, increased dietary fibre and fluid intake, along with exercise. However, more than half of patients remain constipated (Kumar et al., 2014). Methylnaltrexone administered by subcutaneous injection should be considered in the treatment of opioid-related constipation resistant to traditional laxatives (Candy et al., 2011). A newer class of agents, seeking to address the underlying pathophysiology of opioid induced bowel diseases and OIC, are called peripherally acting mu-opioid receptor antagonists (PAMORAs). Naloxegol is one and was approved for treating OIC in patients with cancer or non-cancer pain by the European Union (Chey et al., 2014).

There are no prospective randomised studies on the treatment of opioid-induced pruritus. Antihistamines and $5HT_3$ antagonists are commonly recommended. Opioid rotation may represent an additional choice (Cherny et al., 2001; Klepstad et al., 2003).

Opioid-induced hyperalgesia (OIH) can be associated with a general sensitivity to simple light touch as well as a marked increase in pre-existing pain. A high index of clinical suspicion should be present when pain becomes generalised and/or escalates rapidly in the existing location. In the past, at the end of life, we have probably misdiagnosed some patients with pain which is 'refractory' or 'total pain', when in fact it has been induced by opioids, now known as 'opioid induced hyperalgesia'. Management of OIH is based on an opioid reduction and/or opioid switch and appropriate hydration (Colvin and Fallon, 2010).

Opioid Switching

After starting the prescribed initial opioid, clinical efficacy may decrease gradually in time or even abruptly, resulting in a need for dose increase. In some cases dose increases do not provide analgesia, and further dose increments are ineffective. Alternatively, adverse effects may occur that are difficult to control with symptomatic therapies (Mercadante and Portenoy, 2001).

When an opioid fails to provide adequate analgesia or causes unmanageable adverse effects, it should be discontinued and a different opioid should be offered (Cherny et al., 2001). Opioid switching (also known as opioid rotation) is the process of substituting one opioid for another one to improve the opioid response, either improving pain relief or reducing the intensity of adverse effects (Mercandante, 1999).

There is no high-quality evidence to support this practice: no randomised controlled trials have investigated the efficacy of opioid switching. However, a switch to an alternative opioid is frequently used in clinical practice. This approach requires familiarity with equianalgesic doses of the different opioids (see Box 4.1.1).

Box 4.1.1   Guidelines for the adequate assessment of the patient with pain at any stage of the disease

1. **Assess and re-assess the pain**
   - Causes, onset, type, site, absence/presence of radiating pain, duration, intensity, relief and temporal patterns of the pain, number of breakthrough pains, pain syndrome, inferred pathophysiology, pain at rest and/or moving
   - Presence of the trigger factors and the signs and symptoms associated with the pain
   - Presence of the relieving factors
   - Use of analgesics and their efficacy and tolerability
   - Require the description of the pain quality
     - o   Aching, throbbing, pressure: often associated with somatic pain in skin, muscle and bone
     - o   Aching, cramping, gnawing, sharp: often associated with visceral pain in organs or viscera
     - o   Shooting, sharp, stabbing, tingling, ringing: often associated with neuropathic pain caused by nerve damage

2. **Assess and re-assess the patient**
   - Clinical situation by means of a complete/specific physical examination and the specific radiological and/or biochemical investigations
   - Presence of interference of pain with the patient's daily activities, work, social life, sleep patterns, appetite, sexual functioning, mood, well-being, coping
   - Impact of the pain, the disease and the therapy on the physical, psychological and social conditions
   - Presence of a caregiver, the psychological status, the degree of awareness of the disease, anxiety and depression and suicidal ideation, his/her social environment, quality of life, spiritual concerns/needs, problems in communication, personality disorders
   - Presence and intensity of signs, physical and/or emotional symptoms associated with cancer pain syndromes
   - Presence of co-morbidities (i.e. diabetic, renal and/or hepatic failure, etc.)
   - Functional status
   - Presence of opiophobia or misconception related to pain treatment
   - Alcohol and/or substance abuse

3. **Assess and re-assess your ability to inform and to communicate with the patient and the family**
   - Take time to spend with the patient and the family to understand their needs.

Source: Adapted from Ripamonti et al., 2012.

There is no evidence that one sequence is better than another one. Thus, the choice of a conversion ratio between opioids during switching should not be a mere mathematical calculation, but part of a more comprehensive assessment of opioid therapy, evaluating the underlying clinical situation, pain and adverse effect intensity, co-morbidities and concomitant drugs, and excluding any possible pharmacokinetic factor that could limit the effectiveness of certain drugs (Mercadante and Bruera, 2016). Recent evidence-based recommendations from the European Association of Palliative Care (EAPC) have been developed for conversion ratios during opioid switching (Mercadante and Caraceni, 2011).

There are various online opioid conversion tools. One example is the Safer Prescription of Opioids Tool, SPOT (Flint et al., 2019).

SPOT is a novel clinician decision support, digital health CE-marked medical device proven to significantly improve the confidence of opioid prescribing in users and adherence to best practice guidelines (Flint et al., 2019). It was created and trialled by a multidisciplinary team of experts including GPs, palliative medicine consultants, academics, independent prescribers and a clinical pharmacologist.

SPOT provides the following functionality:

- It uses a conversion algorithm based on the equianalgesic tables from best practice guidelines.
- It double-checks the prescriber's conversion of equianalgesic doses of opioids, allowing simple conversion from one opioid and route of administration to another, empowering the prescriber to independently validate their opioid conversions at the patient's bedside.
- It warns prescribers to consider their opioid choice if their patient has reduced renal function.
- All of SPOT's conversions are auditable centrally, providing a clinical governance and audit trail.

SPOT is available at www.spotopioids.co.uk and is available to download from the Android and iOS stores.

Changing opioid – seek specialist advice if uncertain

When switching from one opioid drug to another it should be remembered that conversion ratios are specific for patients in whom analgesia and side-effects from the first opioid is satisfactory. This is rarely the case and dose adjustment after conversion should be considered (Ripamonti et al., 1998; Mercadante et al., 1999; Caraceni et al., 2012).

Dose conversions

A guide to dose conversions *from* morphine *to* second-line opioid analgesics used for moderate to severe pain.

In Tables 4.1.1 and 4.1.2 the doses are approximate (≈) and not exact equivalent doses. Breakthrough opioid doses are based on a calculation of 1/6th of the daily dose –

these doses may be adjusted up or down to avoid the use of decimal points and to allow a practical dose to be administered. Some patients may require a smaller 4-hour breakthrough dose of 1/10th of the daily dose. Initiate dose with caution depending on clinical condition and judgement.

- Opioid bioavailability (particularly for oral morphine) and response are highly variable.
- It is important to exercise caution when switching opioids. Start low and titrate gradually.
- Always prescribe an appropriate drug and dose for breakthrough pain: 1/10th to 1/6th of the 24-hour regular opioid dose as required.
- Opioid conversions and ratios may vary depending on the resource used. The source for this manual is the Scottish Palliative Care Guidelines.
- Consider reducing the dose by up to 30% and re-titrating:
  - when changing opioid because of differences in pharmacokinetics and pharma-codynamics, including incomplete cross tolerance.
  - if the patient is opioid toxic, frail or elderly.
- Check the information about individual drugs if the patient has renal or liver impairment.
- Particular care is needed when changing between opioids at higher doses, or when the dose of the first opioid has been rapidly increased, as these patients are at greater risk of adverse effects.
- Morphine and oxycodone doses can be measured accurately in 1 mg dose increments. Decimal places are not recommended.
- Fentanyl and alfentanil – seek specialist advice.
- The effective sublingual/buccal dose of fentanyl cannot be reliably predicted from the background maintenance opioid dose and individual titration for a patient is required, always starting at the lowest dose.
- Monitor the patient carefully. If in doubt, seek advice.

Table 4.1.1   Conversions from weak opioids to oral morphine.

Weak opioid dose	Equivalent oral morphine dose	Conversion factor from weak oral opioid to morphine
Oral codeine or oral dihydrocodeine 240 mg/24hrs	= Oral morphine 24 mg/24hrs	Divide by 10
Tramadol 400 mg/24hrs*	= Oral morphine 40 mg/24hrs	Divide by 10
Buprenorphine 7-day patch 5 micrograms/hr**	= Oral morphine 12 mg/24hrs	

Source: Scottish Palliative Care Guidelines, 2020a.
Notes: *Not generally recommended for use in palliative care. **Buprenorphine is measured in micrograms and morphine is measured in milligrams.

Table **4.1.2**   Conversions from oral strong opioids to other strong opioids.

Oral morphine dose	Equivalent opioid dose	Conversion factor from oral morphine to other opioid
Morphine 10 mg	≑ SC morphine 5 mg	Divide by 2
Morphine 10 mg	≑ SC diamorphine 3 mg	Divide by 3
Morphine 10 mg	≑ Oral oxycodone 5 mg	Divide by 2
Morphine 10 mg	≑ SC oxycodone 2–3 mg	Divide by 4
Morphine 30–60 mg	≑ Fentanyl patch 12 micrograms/hour	Seek specialist advice
Morphine 60–90 mg	≑ Fentanyl patch 25 micrograms/hour	Seek specialist advice
Morphine 30 mg	≑ SC alfentanil 1 mg*	Seek specialist advice
Morphine 10 mg	≑ Oral hydromorphone 1.3 mg	Divide by 5 to 7.5
Morphine 15 mg	≑ SC hydromorphone 1 mg*	Divide by 10
Oral oxycodone dose	**Equivalent opioid dose**	**Conversion factor from oral to SC**
Oxycodone 5 mg	≑ SC oxycodone 2–3 mg	Divide by 2
Oxycodone 5 mg	≑ Oral morphine 10 mg	Multiply by 2
Oxycodone 5 mg	≑ SC diamorphine 3 mg	Divide by 1.5
Oxycodone 15–30 mg	≑ Fentanyl patch 12 micrograms/hour	Seek specialist advice
Oxycodone 30–45 mg	≑ Fentanyl patch 25 micrograms/hour	Seek specialist advice
Oxycodone 15 mg	≑ SC alfentanil 1 mg*	Divide by 15
Oxycodone 5 mg	≑ Oral hydromorphone 1.3 mg*	Divide by 4

Source: Scottish Palliative Care Guidelines, 2020a
Note: *Use only with specialist palliative care input.

- These doses/ratios are **approximate** (≑) and not exact equivalent doses and should be used as a **guide**.
- Dose conversions should be conservative and doses are usually rounded down. (Note – check available strengths.)
- Adjust and monitor doses closely, taking extra care with: opioid toxicity; frail and elderly patients; renal or hepatic impairment.
- Always prescribe an appropriate drug and dose for breakthrough pain: 1/6th to 1/10th of the 24-hour regular opioid dose as required.

Table 4.1.3   Indications for opioid switching and suggestions for dosing of new opioid, tendency of conversion ratios.

Reason for switch	New opioid dose
Convenience	=
Adverse effect	↓
Uncontrolled pain	=↑
Adverse effects and uncontrolled pain	↓=
Uncontrolled pain with rapid escalating doses	↓↓

Table 4.1.3 shows the suggested direction of equianalgesic dose chosen. For example, if switching because of side-effects, a lower equianalgesic dose is usually safer.

The subcutaneous route is simple and effective for the administration of morphine, diamorphine and oxycodone, and it should be the first choice alternative route for patients unable to receive opioids by oral or transdermal routes. In the UK we have largely avoided the intravenous (IV) route for opioids in palliative care. However, we should always remain open to individual patient needs and IV infusion should be considered when subcutaneous administration is not sensible, for example with significant peripheral oedema, coagulation disorders or poor peripheral circulation.

Scheduling and titration

Opioid doses should be titrated to take effect as rapidly as possible. Titration is a process in which opioid dose is modified speedily to achieve adequate relief of pain without unacceptable side-effects. The established practice with immediate-release oral morphine every 4 hours is based only on the pharmacokinetic profile of this formulation, which has a duration of effect of around 4 hours (Caraceni et al., 2012). Immediate release formulations are much more flexible than long-acting preparations. However, with patients in the community or at home, a long-acting opioid preparation can be a more practical choice. Individual titration of opioid should start dose and increase until optimum analgesia without unacceptable side-effects is reached (Klepstad et al., 2011).

All patients should receive round-the-clock dosing with provision of a 'rescue dose' to manage exacerbations of pain. The 'breakthrough dose' is usually equivalent to 1/10th to 1/6th of the total daily dose. If more than four 'rescue doses' per day are necessary, the baseline opioid treatment with a slow-release formulation should be reviewed. Usually this results in increasing the baseline 24-hour dose, but the main caveat is the case of intermittent pain associated with metastatic bone disease or neuropathic pain. These episodes, which come on quickly and resolve quickly, should not be chased with an increase in background opioid as this will only lead to opioid toxicity.

Breakthrough Pain

There is no unanimous consensus on definition and characteristics of breakthrough cancer pain (BTcP). However, the current agreement defines it as an episode of severe pain that occurs in patients receiving a stable opioid regimen for persistent pain sufficient to provide at least mild sustained analgesia. Clearly the underlying neurobiological causes of BTcP will be many.

Immediate release formulation of opioids should be used to treat breakthrough cancer pain where background cancer pain management has been optimised and where the breakthrough pain is opioid responsive. Patients on a regular opioid will require an opioid prescribed as required for breakthrough pain. An appropriate as-required dose is typically 1/10th to 1/6th of the regular 24-hour opioid dose. If the regular 24-hour dose is increased to achieve pain control, the as-required dose for breakthrough pain will usually also need to be increased.

Transmucosal fentanyl formulations (oral, buccal, sublingual and intranasal) all have a role in unpredictable and rapid onset breakthrough cancer pain. Seek specialist advice when prescribing rapid acting fentanyl preparations.

Bone Pain

Treatment of bone pain should always take into consideration the use of analgesic drugs based on the WHO ladder. In addition, external beam radiotherapy, radioisotopes and targeted therapy given in association with analgesics have an important role in bone pain management. Transcutaneus electrical nerve stimulation (TENS) machines can be very useful and are often underused (Coleman et al., 2020).

The key issue in bone pain is the rapid onset and fast resolution (within 15 minutes) in almost 50% of patients, making opioid analgesia irrelevant.

Cancer-Related Neuropathic Pain

Neuropathic cancer pain arises as a direct consequence of a cancer-induced damage to the somatosensory system. This type of neuropathic cancer pain is distinguished from other neuropathic pains due to cancer treatment (Mulvey et al., 2014). Nerve fibrosis after radiotherapy, chemotherapy-induced or postsurgical neuropathic pains are prominent examples. Always consider if there is a treatable underlying cause, such as spinal cord compression, and seek specialist advice for further management.

Pain in a dermatomal or neuro-anatomical area, *combined* with a history of a disease or a lesion that might affect the nervous system, might suggest the possibility of neuropathic pain. This should be confirmed by clinical examination or detailed imaging if appropriate. Sensory descriptors associated with neuropathic pain include burning, tingling, pins and needles, shooting and numbness. Patients often find it challenging to describe the pain as the sensations are so alien to them. Help with descriptions may be required. These symptoms by themselves are not diagnostic, however, in advanced disease they may be all that is available to assess. When examining the patient, confirm altered sensation in the area of pain by comparing responses with the non-painful contralateral or adjacent area of the body (Scottish Palliative Care Guidelines, 2021):

- Allodynia – painful response to light touch, for example stroking the skin with a finger or cotton wool
- Hypoaesthesia – an area of reduced sensation to non-painful or painful stimuli
- Hyperalgesia – an exaggerated pain response to stimulus, for example a lowered pin-prick threshold
- Altered thermal threshold to cold or hot (for example reduced or exaggerated response to a cold metal spoon, or a hot cup of tea)
- Some of the above can be assessed very well in cognitively impaired patients through observation of response

In cancer patients with neuropathic pain, non-opioid and opioid analgesics may be combined with tricyclic antidepressants or anticonvulsants. The efficacy and tolerability of the therapy have to be monitored over time. The addition of an adjuvant analgesic to an opioid regimen is very likely to cause an increase in opioid-related side-effects. It is critical to monitor for side-effects and be prepared to reduce opioid dose to allow an upward titration of the adjuvant analgesic.

Steroids should be considered in the case of nerve compression. This strategy can also buy time to allow appropriate introduction and titration of an adjuvant analgesic as while steroids can have an immediate effect, adjuvant analgesics rarely have an immediate analgesic effect, although they can have an immediate effect with improved sleep.

Invasive Management of Refractory Pain

Treatment of cancer itself by surgical or oncological treatment can be effective in controlling pain related to cancer, but can also be the cause of pain. About 10% of cancer patients have pain which is difficult to manage with oral or parenteral analgesic drugs. Interventional techniques such as peripheral nerve blocks, neurolytic blocks including spinal neurolytic blocks, cordotomy and intrathecal drug delivery (ITDD) (spinal or epidural) (Vainio et al., 1988) may allow those patients refractory to all conventional strategies and/or dose limiting analgesic-related side-effects to reach pain control when used as unique therapy or, more frequently, in combination with systemic therapy.

It is likely that rather than spinal morphine per se, it is the co-administration of local anaesthetic agents which may significantly improve the quality of spinal analgesia as compared with other routes of opioid delivery (Kalso et al., 1996).

Summary

The keystones to effective pain management are careful patient assessment and regular review, with acknowledgement of the great heterogeneity of patient phenotype related to complex disease; medical and psychiatric co-morbidities; emotional and spiritual factors; environmental dynamics; and genomic variation. We have learnt from neuroimaging studies about the complex relationship between the sensory, cognitive and emotional aspects of pain.

Yet, with all this complexity, simple approaches using combinations of non-drug management, non-opioid analgesics, opioids and adjuvant analgesics will give relief in most cases.

Distress of any aetiology will make physical pain worse. It is important to move away from dated concepts about coping less well with pain, and acknowledge that the actual pain is accentuated by distress. Always believe the patient while managing the distress exacerbating the pain.

Opioids continue to have a unique analgesic role. While the consensus that opioid-based pharmacotherapy remains the mainstay of chronic pain management it is reassuring to know that the science of opioid analgesia and optimal prescribing continues to evolve.

Scenario Recap

Pain affects, and is affected by, many other symptoms and aspects of daily living. Time spent on the initial detailed assessment of all aspects of the patient is key to successful management. For Amir quickly proposed solutions to his myriad of problems would only lead to therapeutic chaos. The key decision is what is the greatest driver of the symptoms and how does this potentially interact with other symptoms and distress.

Amir had very severe pain with a strong neuropathic component as would be expected from pressure on and/or invasion of the brachial plexus by tumour. It is not surprising that he was not sleeping because of this extremely severe pain and felt miserable and hopeless. His poor appetite and weight loss could be a result of the uncontrolled pain, however it could also be the result of the cancer process via a cachexia mechanism. It is important to recognise that neuropathic pain is particularly associated with mood disturbances.

When assessing complexities, it is important to ground decisions on information obtained directly from the patient. Amir was able to give a clear history that a codeine and paracetamol combination worked within 40 minutes but lasted for just an hour, and the clue within this is that his pain was at least partially opioid responsive. It is critical not to move sideways on an analgesic ladder and if maximum dose of codeine is not effective, the patient should move to a strong opioid such as morphine. The usual starting dose in this situation of normal renal function and such severe pain should be 5 mg of normal release morphine orally every 4 hours. If starting modified release morphine, the dose is 10–15 mg every 12 hours (Scottish Palliative Care Guidelines, 2020b). For breakthrough analgesia the dose is usually 1/6th of the total 24-hour dose, therefore 5 mg in this case. The patient should be advised that if breakthrough pain relief is required it will take 30 minutes to start having an effect. The patient should be instructed to take a careful note of duration onset and duration of effect of the regular dose, and frequency onset and duration and effect of breakthrough dose.

- Patient and family education/information is needed in respect of diet and nutrition in advancing malignancy.

Timeline

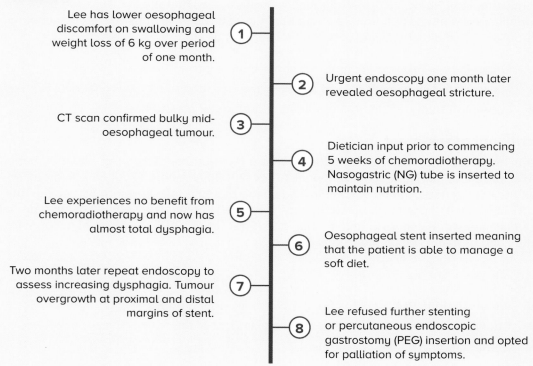

1 Lee has lower oesophageal discomfort on swallowing and weight loss of 6 kg over period of one month.

2 Urgent endoscopy one month later revealed oesophageal stricture.

3 CT scan confirmed bulky mid-oesophageal tumour.

4 Dietician input prior to commencing 5 weeks of chemoradiotherapy. Nasogastric (NG) tube is inserted to maintain nutrition.

5 Lee experiences no benefit from chemoradiotherapy and now has almost total dysphagia.

6 Oesophageal stent inserted meaning that the patient is able to manage a soft diet.

7 Two months later repeat endoscopy to assess increasing dysphagia. Tumour overgrowth at proximal and distal margins of stent.

8 Lee refused further stenting or percutaneous endoscopic gastrostomy (PEG) insertion and opted for palliation of symptoms.

Key considerations

- Nausea and vomiting, although common, are often poorly controlled. Why?
- Why is discussing the subject of nutrition and diet with patient and family important?
- Why is a team approach to patient care important at all stages of the illness?

Nutrition

Introduction

Eating and drinking has a big part to play in a person's quality of life. How a person manages with eating and drinking on a day-to-day basis has a strong relationship with how the person and their family feel about their day-to-day life. Those who are struggling with eating may experience feelings of fear and despair which may affect confidence and self-esteem and lead to social isolation and depression (Eldridge et al., 2014).

Nutrition should be considered an integral part of the assessment and management of the palliative patient (Shaw, 2011). As healthcare professionals in palliative care, we have a role to identify and address nutritional factors that impair a patient's physical and psychological well-being. The main objectives of nutritional support are to:

- Maintain or improve quality of life for the individual
- Maximise the enjoyment of food and minimise any food related discomfort (O'Hara, 2017)
- Prevent or treat avoidable malnutrition (Eldridge et al., 2014).

Nutritional assessment

Nutritional screening may identify patients who are at nutritional risk and who may benefit from appropriate nutritional intervention (BAPEN, 2003). A variety of validated screening tools are widely used, the most common being the Malnutrition Universal Screening Tool (MUST). However, these tools do not always work well in palliative settings as they do not distinguish between cachexia and malnutrition (Shaw et al., 2015) and do not account for ascites and oedema, which may skew results.

The assessment should consider:

- Weight, height, BMI, weight change over time, eating habits
- Change in appetite and the psychosocial impact of this
- Barriers to oral intake (see Table 4.2.1)
- Any need for texture modification
- Co-morbidities
- The nutritional concerns of patient, family/carers
- The nutritional goals with patients and family/carers.

Not all teams will have a dietician as a core team member, but their expertise can be valuable in addressing physical and psychological well-being when addressing difficulties with eating or drinking and weight loss (Shaw, 2011). Consider referral to a dietician if appropriate.

Social and psychological aspects

Eating habits and our food beliefs often stem from childhood. Food can be highly regarded by families as it is a time where they can socialise. A palliative patient may find mealtimes a burden if eating is difficult and can cause them to feel isolated if they cannot participate. An altered body image can affect a person's confidence and makes the thought of social gatherings/mealtimes overwhelming (Carr et al., 2013).

Some people find hope in eating as it is a fuel which provides strength in the battle against their illness whereas others may resent food as it causes discomfort or pain (Shaw et al., 2015).

Table 4.2.1   Factors affecting food intake.

Psychological	Physical
• Family worries	• Pain
• Difficulty sleeping	• Nausea and vomiting
• Anxiety	• Oral problems such as thrush/mucositis/ dry mouth
• Depression	• Taste changes
• Spiritual worries	• Diarrhoea or constipation
	• Dysphagia
	• Obstruction
	• Malabsorption

Healthcare professionals need to be aware of the tensions that often arise between patients and carers concerning a person's loss of appetite, which often becomes more significant through the palliative stages. Patients and carers may require support with adjusting and coping (Scottish Oral Nutritional Supplements Short Life Working Group (ONS SLWG), 2018). A discussion around a patient's and carer's perceptions of a decreasing oral intake can be very valuable (Raijmakers, 2013), and an emphasis should be placed on how best the patient can be supported to eat and drink when they feel able to do so, and their choices respected (O'Hara, 2017).

Nutritional management

Management should be patient centred, individualised and open to change depending on the patient's condition. Find out what is most important for the patient with regards to eating and drinking, that is, sitting down with others or eating favourite foods. Take the opportunity to discuss that loss of appetite and desire for food is part of the disease and deterioration process. The pleasure of eating and the social benefits should be emphasised, and that healthy eating is no longer a priority.

If anorexia/cachexia is present, patients and families should be counselled on what this is, and informed that increasing caloric intake does not reverse the underlying anorexia/ cachexia (Dev et al., 2017). Patients and families are often reassured when they understand what cachexia is and why it is happening.

Consider relaxing unnecessary dietary restrictions, such as those for diabetes or high cholesterol.

Treat nutrition impact symptoms – taste and smell alterations, mucositis, constipation, nausea, shortness of breath, pain, dysphagia, abdominal pain and fatigue (Omlin et al., 2013).

Practical aspects of dietary advice

- Adopt a 'little and often' approach to food consumption
- Choose energy dense foods
- Food fortification:
  - Normal foods can be 'fortified' to be made more energy dense, that is by adding butter, margarine, cheese, cream, sugar, syrup, oil, mayonnaise or dressings.
  - Fortify milk by adding 2–4 tablespoons of skimmed milk powder to 1 pint of full fat milk and use in cereal, sauces, desserts or other meals and drinks.
  - Avoid low fat/sugar products.
- Choose drinks which contain some nutrition such as milky drinks (malted drinks, hot chocolate, milky coffee, milkshake, smoothies) or sugary drinks such as fruit juice, fizzy drinks or squash. Over the counter nourishing drinks such as Meritene and Complan are available.
- Consider fresh or frozen ready meals. The local council's social care department can provide or help arrange a meal delivery service.

Guidance for carers

- Adapt meal timings depending on the patient's sleep pattern/hunger
- Smaller portion sizes may be better tolerated
- Make the table/plate/tray as attractive as possible and prepare the surroundings
- Help the patient get fresh air by taking them outside or opening a window
- Gently encourage without excessive persistence and be accepting of whatever is eaten
- Keep the patient involved in the social aspects of mealtimes.

Dietary advice for specific symptoms

Sore mouth

- Avoid spicy, salty and acidic foods
- Choose soft foods, moist foods. Consider adding extra sauce/gravy
- Avoid foods and drinks at the extremes of temperature
- Fruit juices may sting, so opt for less acidic flavours like pear/peach
- Drinking through a straw may help.

Dry mouth

- Choose soft foods, moist foods. Consider adding extra sauce/gravy
- Drink plenty fluids throughout the day
- Chewing gum can stimulate saliva
- Fizzy drinks may be more refreshing.

Taste changes

- Choose foods that the patient enjoys and avoid those that they don't
- Retry foods after several weeks as sense of taste may have changed
- Use seasonings, spices and herbs such as pepper, cumin or rosemary to flavour the food
- Try marinating meat in fruit juices or wine, or cook it in strong sauces such as curry or sweet and sour
- Sharp-tasting foods such as fresh fruit, fruit juices and sour or boiled sweets can be refreshing and leave a pleasant taste in the mouth
- Some people find that cold foods taste better than hot foods
- If the patient's sense of taste or smell has changed, it can sometimes help to serve food at room temperature
- If the patient notices a metallic taste in their mouth, try using plastic cutlery.

Nausea

- Try dry food, such as toast or crackers first thing in the morning before the patient gets up
- Avoid cooking smells
- Cold foods may be better tolerated
- Try salty foods like soup or crisps
- Fizzy drinks may be better tolerated than still
- Ice lollies can be refreshing
- Avoid foods which are fatty or fried
- Food or drinks containing ginger can help reduce feelings of sickness; try crystallised ginger, ginger tea or ginger biscuits
- Try sitting the patient by an open window while they eat, so there is plenty of fresh air in the room.

Oral nutritional supplements

Oral nutritional supplements may be helpful, particularly in early palliative care. In late palliative care they may only be of benefit to patients on psychological grounds. The focus throughout should be on choice, taste and tolerance rather than nutrient profile. A wide variety of nutritional supplements are available. A dietician is well placed to offer guidance as to whether oral nutritional supplements are appropriate.

Artificial nutrition support

The decision as to whether palliative care patients may benefit from artificial nutrition support is difficult and must be considered on an individual basis. The European Society for Clinical Nutrition and Metabolism issued guidance on the ethical aspects of artificial nutrition and hydration, stating that there is a strong consensus that artificial nutrition in palliative care has the potential to increase survival and quality of life in selected patients

(Druml et al., 2016). Each patient should be considered individually with clear goals of care and ensuring the decision made is a joint one between the patient and healthcare team. For patients for whom it is not clear whether they will benefit, it might be suitable to plan a time-limited trial with aims that can be evaluated (Shaw, 2011). Feeding regimens must be reviewed regularly and changed according to the patient's condition and circumstances (Lennard-Jones, 2000). When a patient is approaching the end of life, the volume and rate of an enteral feed often have to be reduced as tolerance decreases.

Several studies have found that in individuals with advanced dementia there is no evidence that enteral nutrition provides benefits in terms of mortality risk, survival time, physical function, incidence of pressure ulcers and quality of life (Schwartz, 2018).

Nutrition in the dying patient

Nutritional intervention in this phase of life should be considered on an individual basis. As illness develops, physiological functions such as gastric emptying, digestion, absorption and peristalsis decline. Appetite and the ability to tolerate nutrition will also decrease (Eldridge et al., 2014). Oral nutritional supplements at this stage will be of little, if any, benefit and should not be initiated (ONS SLWG, 2018).

Summary

Nutrition is an important part of the holistic management of palliative care patients. Nutrition support should be carefully considered based on a patient's wishes, prognosis and goals, with the primary nutritional objective being to maintain or improve quality of life. Healthcare professionals should acknowledge the physical and psychological impact of weight loss and changes in appetite and where appropriate be able to talk about cachexia and its impact. Open and honest communication between the patient, their family and healthcare professionals will facilitate decisions that are in the patient's best interest.

Patient literature

- The Nutrition and Diet Resources UK website offers nutrition and diet resources to purchase – ndr-uk.org
- *'Food myths'* from Macmillan Cancer Support. Available at: https://www.cancerresearchuk.org/about-cancer/causes-of-cancer/diet-and-cancer/food-controversies
- *'Eating problems'* from Macmillan Cancer Support. Available at: https://www.macmillan.org.uk/cancer-information-and-support/impacts-of-cancer/eating-problems
- *'Move More'* section of Macmillan Cancer Support, including guide, DVD and activities nearby. Available at: https://be.macmillan.org.uk/be/p-24948-move-more-your-guide-to-becoming-more-active.aspx

- Meal delivery services:
    - Wiltshire Farm Foods, www.wiltshirefarmfoods.com, Tel. 0800 773 773
    - Oakhouse Foods, www.oakhousefoods.co.uk, Tel. 0845 643 2009.

Mouth Care

Oral problems are very common in palliative care and can be the consequence of disease (particularly malignant disease), concomitant disease and recent or ongoing treatment for these conditions. Poor fluid and nutritional intake also contribute to oral problems. Prevention of oral problems is an important aspect of the palliative care of all patients and good mouth care in the form of basic oral hygiene should be encouraged at every opportunity. Potential problems should be anticipated and the appropriate treatment initiated without delay to prevent physical discomfort and associated psychosocial difficulties. Oral symptoms may lead to pain and discomfort but may also be severe enough to affect communication, oral intake and quality of life. Regular assessment is of vital importance as symptoms may not always be reported because there is often an acceptance by patients that such problems are inevitable and not worth mentioning.

Oral hygiene

The key to maintaining a healthy mouth is good, basic oral hygiene. For the majority of people this can be achieved by regular teeth cleaning, adherence to a healthy diet and regular dental check-ups. In addition to looking after teeth (if present), attention should also be paid to the gums, hard and soft palate, soft tissues, tongue and lips.

Natural teeth should be cleaned with fluoride toothpaste (1350 to 1500 ppm) after every meal, but at least twice a day if tolerated. For patients with swallowing difficulties, or who are unable to spit, non-foaming toothpastes are available.

Small-headed brushes with a soft to medium bristle are ideal for most patients. Soft or very soft toothbrushes may be required in the presence of a dry mouth or if there is pain or oral ulceration.

Dentures should be cleaned at least twice a day. They can be cleaned using a personal toothbrush with running water. Regular toothpaste should be avoided but denture cream or unperfumed soap may be used. Dentures should be rinsed thoroughly after meals and after cleaning. They should be removed at night and soaked in a suitable solution for 20 minutes, then overnight in plain water. Suitable soaking solutions are dilute sodium hypochlorite for plastic dentures or chlorhexidine gluconate 0.2% solution for dentures with metal parts.

Mouth care in the last days of life

Mouth care at the end of life should be carried out as often as necessary to maintain a clean, moist mouth with the focus on maintaining comfort. In most cases, water is sufficient and regular sips or sprays of water should be offered. Ice chips may be placed carefully in the mouth or water make be given via sponge sticks (ensuring the sponge head is secure prior to use) or other approved applicator. Attention should also be paid to the lips by applying a water-based lubricant. Loved ones may wish to be involved in this aspect of care and should be encouraged and supported to do so if they wish.

Xerostomia (dry mouth)

Dry mouth is extremely common in palliative care with prevalence reported to be between 29 and 77% (Davies et al., 2005). Effective management of dry mouth can relieve a number of associated symptoms – oral discomfort, feeling of thirst, taste disturbance, difficulty chewing, difficulty swallowing, difficulty speaking, difficulty wearing dentures and halitosis. Having a persistent dry mouth also increases susceptibility to infection, for example oral thrush. Saliva also plays an important part in maintaining dental health and referral to a dentist for assessment may be necessary.

Dry mouth may be caused by the following:

- Drugs, for example antimuscarinics, antidepressants, opioids or diuretics
- Dehydration
- Anxiety
- Mouth breathing
- Radiotherapy
- Oxygen (if non-humidified).

The management should focus on firstly identifying and treating reversible causes. The patient's medication should be reviewed and adjusted where necessary. Basic oral hygiene should be performed more frequently with the aim of keeping the mouth as moist as possible. Drinking fluids should be encouraged, especially water or sucking ice chips if preferred. Fruit juices are also useful but citrus juices are acidic and may sting. Less acidic juices include pear, peach or blackcurrant, and these may be frozen in an ice cube tray and sucked if preferred.

Very hot or very cold drinks may irritate a sore mouth, and very salty or spicy foods and foods with a dry or rough texture such as toast or pastries should be avoided. Ice cream or jellies may be more soothing and foods can be made moist by including a sauce or gravy.

Provided that there is intact salivary function, measures which stimulate saliva are preferred to saliva substitutes. Chewing sugar-free gum or sugar-free boiled sweets, pastilles or mints should be considered if the patient is able to comply. A variety of saliva substitutes are available which many patients find useful. The ideal preparation should be of neutral pH, contain electrolytes (including fluoride) and correspond closely to the composition of saliva. The selection of a product should take patient preference into account: whether they prefer a gel, spray or oral-rinse formulation. Saliva substitutes can be used as often as needed; the effects can be short lived and they may need to be used frequently throughout the day, including before and during meals.

Coated mouth

Poor oral hygiene and lack of saliva associated with a dry mouth can lead to a build up of dead cells and bacteria. Inflammation of the surface of the tongue can trap further debris resulting in a coated appearance of the tongue and other surfaces of the mouth. Smoking and alcohol intake are additional risk factors. Failure to gently remove dried secretions, debris and plaque can cause halitosis, pain, ulceration, bleeding and predisposition to infection.

Basic oral hygiene should be performed more frequently and measures to treat dry mouth implemented.

Coatings should be gently removed from soft tissues, lips and mucosa by gently soaking coated areas with wetted non-fraying gauze wrapped round a gloved finger, provided it is safe to do so.

The wetted gauze can then be used to gently remove coatings and debris. The gauze should be changed when required and several pieces of gauze used to clean the mouth. Alternatively, a moistened soft toothbrush can be used to remove coatings using gentle back to front strokes.

If sponge sticks are used, they should only be used to moisten the mouth or clean the soft tissues, not to remove plaque from tooth surfaces. Always check to ensure the sponge head is secure prior to use. Sponge sticks should be discarded after single use and must never be left to soak as this increases the risk of detachment and subsequent choking (MHRA, 2014).

If the patient is likely to bite down on the sponge stick, use a small-headed toothbrush with soft bristles or a product with a fixed cleaning head.

Painful mouth

Pain in the mouth may be a direct cause of a persistent dry mouth but may also be as a result of dental trauma such as from sharp teeth or ill-fitting dentures. Other causes include aphthous ulcers, herpes simplex infection, oral malignancy or mucositis secondary to radiotherapy or chemotherapy.

The management of a painful mouth involves identifying and targeting any underlying causes such as infection. Topically applied local anaesthetic gels such as choline salicylate (for example, Bonjela®) or benzydamine hydrochloride mouthwash or spray (for example, Difflam®) may be helpful. In some instances systemic analgesia according to the WHO analgesic ladder will also be required.

Oral mucositis should be considered as a cause of a sore mouth in patients who have received chemotherapy or radiotherapy. Follow local cancer centre guidelines or the current version of the UKOMIC (United Kingdom Oral Mucositis in Cancer Group, 2015) guidelines for recommended treatment based on the WHO assessment tool and grading scale.

Non-drug measures for a painful mouth include ensuring good basic oral hygiene and maintenance of a moist mouth with frequent sips or sprays of water. Sodium chloride mouthwashes are advised for the prevention and management of mucositis. This can be prepared at home by simply adding a teaspoon of salt to a pint of cold or warm water. Food and drinks which precipitate pain should be discouraged, for example acidic foods, citric drinks, salty and spicy food. Tobacco and alcohol should also be avoided.

Oral infections

Fungal infections

Oral candidiasis, commonly referred to as oral thrush, is the most common oral infection in palliative care with risk factors including poor dental hygiene, dry mouth, the wearing of dentures, smoking and concomitant use of antibiotics or steroids. It can present as white or yellow plaques, painful red tongue, denture stomatitis or painful cracks in the corner of the mouth (angular cheilitis). In addition to affecting the oral cavity, candidiasis may also affect the oropharynx or oesophagus.

Treatment with a topical or systemic antifungal is necessary. Nystatin mouthwash may be used four times a day, after meals and at bedtime and miconazole oral gel is useful for angular cheilitis. In patients with advanced disease or for those who are unable to comply with the instructions for applying a topical antifungal, a systemic antifungal such as fluconazole may be required. Fluconazole and even topically applied miconazole may cause significant drug interactions. Always check the BNF (British National Formulary) or seek advice from a pharmacist.

Good oral hygiene is necessary, as always, with particular attention required for dentures, ensuring they are soaked in a suitable cleaning solution.

Viral infections

Herpes simplex is the most common viral infection in palliative care, typically presenting as a cold sore but there may be more extensive oral ulceration or inflammation, particularly in immunocompromised patients. Uncomplicated infections (for example, cold sore) can be treated with a topical antiviral but more extensive infections will require a systemic antiviral such as aciclovir or related agent, with doses being doubled in immunocompromised patients.

Bacterial infections

Bacterial infections of the mouth are less common but may be present if there is poor oral hygiene, and referral to a dentist may be necessary for specific interventions. Oral cancers can become infected with anaerobic organisms requiring systemic antibiotic treatment with metronidazole to treat the infection and help with any associated odour.

Sialorrhoea (excessive drooling)

Excessive drooling of saliva is common in neurodegenerative disorders such as motor neurone disease, multiple sclerosis and Parkinson's disease and occurs usually as a result of impaired swallowing of saliva rather than excessive saliva production. Simple measures such as appropriate head positioning and a review of the patient's swallow are important.

Antimuscarinic drugs which all have the effect of reducing secretions may be tried (see Scottish Palliative Care Guidelines, 2019, for details), but these can often lead to problems of dry mouth and thickened secretions which can be even more difficult to clear.

Dysphagia

Definitions

Dysphagia is difficulty in swallowing while odynophagia is pain on swallowing. These symptoms are quite different but may co-exist in the same patient. Dysphagia may be oropharyngeal when there is difficulty initiating swallowing or oesophageal when the passage of a bolus through the oesophagus is impaired (Clark, 2015).

Physiology

Swallowing safely is a complex physiological process which involves and relies on the normal functioning of the brain stem, cranial nerves V, VII, IX, X, XII and 34 skeletal muscles (Regnard, 2005; Watson, 2005). Four distinct phases to normal swallowing have been described (Logemann, 1983):

1. Oral preparatory
2. Oral swallowing
3. Pharyngeal
4. Oesophageal.

The first two phases are under voluntary control, the others are involuntary. It has been suggested, however, that while this model is satisfactory for the swallowing of liquids, it does not entirely represent the process of eating solids (Matsuo et al., 2008).

Causes

There are many causes of dysphagia. Any structural abnormality or functional deficit involving the oral cavity, pharynx, larynx or oesophagus may impair normal swallowing (Matsuo et al., 2008). Such causes may be disease related (see Table 4.2.2) or treatment related (for example, surgery or radiotherapy), and can, in both cases, be worsened by the presence of a number of co-existing factors:

- Oral pain
- Infection e.g. *Candida*
- Dental problems
- Fatigue
- Xerostomia
- Advancing age
- Reflux oesophagitis.

Table 4.2.2   Examples of disease related causes of dysphagia.

Mechanical obstruction			Neurological/ neuromuscular defects
Malignant		Non-malignant	• Stroke
Primary	Secondary	• Oesophageal stricture	• Achalasia
• Oral cavity • Pharyngeal • Oesophageal	• Mediastinal	• Pharyngeal pouch • Reflux oesophagitis • Retro-intestinal goitre	• Cranial nerve palsy • Motor neurone disease • Multiple sclerosis • Parkinson's disease • Myasthenia Gravis • Cerebral tumour • Paraneoplastic • Dementia
Psychogenic – globus pharyngeus (hystericus) is a subjective feeling of a lump in the throat. Swallowing is normal. It is therefore not a true form of dysphagia.			

Assessment

History

In some patients, dysphagia may be a presenting or early symptom of disease, for example bulbar motor neurone disease, but in others it may develop during the course of a known progressive illness, for example oesophageal cancer. The clinical history is therefore important as the patient's description of their swallowing difficulties may help identify both the site and cause of the problem.

Timescale

Recent onset or longer?

Pattern

- Intermittent – possible oesophageal spasm
- Repeated need to swallow to clear bolus – oropharyngeal cause (Clark, 2015)
- Constant and worsening – disease progression, particularly in cancer.

Bolus consistency

Patients with oropharyngeal dysphagia frequently experience more problems swallowing fluids than solids, while the opposite is often the case for those with oesophageal dysphagia who tend to experience more problems with solids than liquids (Clark, 2015).

Site

In oesophageal obstruction a patient's subjective localisation of the obstruction can be quite accurate (Logemann, 1983; Wilcox, 1995; Ashrof et al., 2017) but the accuracy appears less precise the closer symptoms are to the epigastrium (Wright et al., 1997).

Retrosternal pain on swallowing

This may be due to malignancy, oesophagitis or spasm. If occurring after a hot drink it may indicate the presence of oesophageal candidiasis (Kaye, 1996).

Coughing/choking

Coughing or choking before, during or after swallowing is suggestive of a pharyngeal problem (Twycross et al., 2001). Coughing is typically due to aspiration (Clark, 2015).

Aspiration, however, is often 'silent' and the absence of coughing does not mean that aspiration is not occurring.

Examination

In all cases of dysphagia, evidence of weight loss should be looked for, the chest examined for features that might suggest aspiration and baseline haematological and biochemical profiles checked.

In oesophageal dysphagia the physical examination may be unhelpful. In oropharyngeal dysphagia, however, the examination may be more revealing:

- Facial asymmetry or drooling may be present
- Voice change (dysphonia) may be apparent during the consultation, for example:
  - dysarthria
  - inability to say 'pa' (impaired lip closure)
  - inability to say 'ka' (impaired tongue movement)
  - hoarseness (recurrent laryngeal nerve palsy)
- Oral cavity
- Structural abnormality, e.g. presence of malignancy, for example:
  - Abnormal tongue movements
  - Infection, e.g. *Candida*
- Cranial nerves – evidence of motor and sensory dysfunction. Simple swallow with assessment of oropharyngeal transit time (Box 4.2.1).

Box 4.2.1   How to assess oropharyngeal transit time

Place a hand over the patient's throat as they swallow and check the time between the first tongue movement and the larynx moving up and down. Times of more than 1 second are abnormal.

Multidisciplinary approach

The accurate diagnosis, evaluation and management of dysphagia require a combined specialist input (Leslie et al., 2003).

Depending on the cause/level of the problem urgent referral should be made to:

- Otolaryngology if cervical level suspected
- Gastroenterology if lower oesophageal level suspected.

In either case endoscopic examination enables visualisation of the structures and the opportunity to take biopsies. Further input may be necessary according to the nature and severity of the problem and the patient's predicted life expectancy, such as:

- NG tube (usually for short-term use only)
- Percutaneous endoscopic gastrostomy (PEG) in oropharyngeal dysphagia
- Dilatation of benign oesophageal stricture
- Brachytherapy
- Stenting of malignant oesophageal stricture.

Speech and Language Therapy (SALT)

SALT specialists have a particularly important role in oropharyngeal dysphagia. Such roles include:

- Clinical swallow assessment
- Fibre-optic endoscopy
- Video-fluoroscopy to view structures and assess coordination of swallowing
- Food texture modification
- Swallowing therapy: advice/education on manoeuvres which the patient (and family) can employ to increase the safety and effectiveness of swallowing.

Dietician

In the late stages of illness a pragmatic approach of 'a little of what you fancy' may be all that is required. For patients with a longer prognosis the input of a dietician is necessary for:

- Undertaking a nutritional assessment
- Maintaining nutritional and hydration status
- Planning nutritional support and supplementation personalised for the individual
- Enteral feeding—advice on calorie content and volume of feeds.

For more detailed information refer to the 'Nutrition' section of this chapter on page 123.

Oesophageal stents

Self-expanding metal stent insertion is a safe and effective treatment in dysphagia palliation (Yingxue et al., 2014) with successful palliation expected in up to 95% of patients (Cowling et al., 1998). As a 'stand alone' intervention for oesophageal cancer, stenting is usually considered in patients with a prognosis of 3 months or less (Clark, 2015). Although most patients experience rapid benefit, morbidity is relatively high (Twycross et al., 2002).

Possible complications:

- Immediate problems such as bleeding or perforation are very infrequent (Clark, 2015).
- Post-procedure chest pain usually settles after a few days but may require short-term analgesia (Twycross et al., 2002).
- Occlusion by food bolus.
- Gastro-oesophageal reflux, particularly if the stent is across the gastro-oesophageal junction, may necessitate the use of an antacid, proton-pump inhibitor or a prokinetic agent, such as domperidone or metoclopramide or sucralfate, for mucosal protection (Glen, 2016).
- Recurrent dysphagia secondary to stent migration or tumour overgrowth. In either situation re-stenting may be possible (Glen, 2016) and successful (Clark, 2015).

Percutaneous endoscopic gastrostomy (PEG)

Percutaneous endoscopic gastrostomy may be considered for patients with oropharyngeal dysphagia. Compared to NG tube use, PEG has been associated with a lower probability of intervention failure and may be more effective and safer with no difference in adverse events including aspiration pneumonia (Gomes et al., 2015). However, survival at 1 year from commencement of feeding is around 40–50% (Clark, 2015). Careful patient selection in respect of life expectancy is required.

Symptom control

Information and advice on the management of specific symptoms can be found in the relevant chapters of this book and the Scottish Palliative Care Guidelines.

Points of note:

- Avoid, whenever possible, medication which may cause/aggravate a dry mouth.
- Oesophageal spasm can be caused by the action of prokinetics on the lower oesophagus and may require dose reduction or cessation. Options for treatment of spasm include:
  - Glyceryl trinitrate (GTN) 400 micrograms sublingual if required (Twycross et al., 2002)
  - Nifedipine MR, for example 10–20 mg twice daily

- o   Smooth muscle relaxant, for example hyoscine butylbromide 10–20 mg four times daily
- o   Cyclizine 25–50 mg three times daily may be the anti-emetic of choice for nausea/vomiting in oral/pharyngeal disease but may, however, cause a dry mouth
- o   Dexamethasone in a daily dose of 8–12 mg (Kaye, 1996) can reduce peri-tumour oedema and allow, even if only temporarily, improved swallowing. Review response after 5–7 days.

Nausea and Vomiting

Introduction

Nausea and vomiting confers a developed survival advantage through warning of the ingestion of toxins and leads to behavioural adaptation to prevent repeating the same act.

Nausea is a profoundly unpleasant and subjective experience, the sensation projected to the epigastric region, heralding the approach of the onset of vomiting.

Nausea and vomiting can often be entirely separate entities. It is not uncommon for patients to experience constant nausea with little or no vomiting (chemotherapy/radiotherapy and pregnancy). Conversely patients with vomiting due to bowel obstruction can often experience little or no nausea, but effortless large volume vomiting (Morgan, 2010).

The nausea–vomiting relationship is not a simple continuum or one being the consequence of the other. It is almost always the case that nausea is more common, more disabling, lasts longer, and is worse than vomiting, as it is the actual act of vomiting that leads to relief in many cases. Nausea and vomiting associated with motion sickness and pregnancy can continue unabated until the causal factor is removed.

Nausea and/or vomiting occur in up to 70% of patients with advanced cancer (Harris, 2010). Nausea is an extremely unpleasant sensation with patients rating it often as bad as pain. Vomiting is the forceful expulsion of gastric contents coordinated within the medulla of the brain stem (Ganong, 1999).

As with pain control, appropriate management requires a thorough assessment so that a probable cause can be determined which then fits with the underlying neuropharmacological mechanism. A logical choice of anti-emetic can then be made (Table 4.2.3). Particular attention should be paid to the history with regards to reduced appetite, early satiety, retching and small or large volume vomiting.

Multi-level protection

The way the system has evolved confers a number of levels of protection to learn from potentially harmful and noxious stimuli with the potential harm being death.

The first level involves various cranial nerves to prevent ingestion of food stuffs which look unpleasant, smell unpleasant or have an unpleasant texture. This first level of protection

Table 4.2.3 Selection of anti-emetics.

Cause of nausea/vomiting		Anti-emetic	Class of drug	Example dose schedule	Common side-effects
Chemotherapy	Acute emesis (<24h)	Ondansetron	5HT$_3$ antagonist	8 mg twice daily orally	Constipation
		Dexamethasone	Corticosteroid	2–4 mg twice daily orally for 1–3 days	Agitation/insomnia, gastric irritant
	Delayed emesis (>24h)	Metoclopramide	Peripherally acting prokinetic and antiemetic	10–20 mg four times a day orally	Restlessness, extrapyramidal effects
		Aprepitant	NK$_1$ antagonist	3-day chemo pack or 80 mg once daily orally	GI side-effects, headache, dizziness
Anticipatory		Lorazepam	Benzodiazepine	0.5–1 mg sublingual, as required, max 4 mg/24 h	Sedation
Drugs, for example opioids, metabolic (whilst correcting the cause)		Haloperidol	Dopamine antagonist	1.5–3 mg at night orally or 0.5–1.5 mg twice daily orally	Sedation, extrapyramidal effects
		Levomepromazine	Dopamine antagonist, antimuscarinic, antihistamine and 5HT$_2$ antagonist	6–15 mg at night orally or 6 mg twice daily orally	Sedation, blurred vision, risk of urinary retention, postural hypotension
Gastric irritation including radiotherapy		Lansoprazole	Proton pump inhibitor	30 mg once to twice daily orally	
		Ondansetron	5HT$_3$ antagonist	8 mg twice daily orally	Constipation
		Cyclizine	Antihistamine and anticholinergic	25–50 mg three times a day orally/subcutaneous	Drowsiness, dry mouth, blurred vision
Raised intracranial pressure		Dexamethasone	Corticosteroid	Up to 16 mg/24 h	Agitation/insomnia, gastric irritant
		Cyclizine	Antihistamine and anticholinergic	25–50 mg three times a day orally or 150 mg/24 h/ subcutaneous	Drowsiness, dry mouth, blurred vision, risk of urinary retention

(Continued)

Table 4.2.3 (*Continued*).

Cause of nausea/vomiting	Anti-emetic	Class of drug	Example dose schedule	Common side-effects
Gastric stasis/subacute bowel obstruction	Metoclopramide	Prokinetic	10 mg four times a day orally/IV/subcutaneous	Agitation. Discontinue if colicky pain develops. Central effects less likely with domperidone
	Domperidone		10–20 mg four times a day orally or as rectal suppository	
Pharyngeal irritation, liver capsular stretch, motion sickness	Cyclizine	Antihistamine and anticholinergic	25–50 mg three times a day or 150 mg/24 h/subcutaneous	Drowsiness, dry mouth, blurred vision, risk of urinary retention
Obstruction	Cyclizine	Antihistamine and anticholinergic	25–50 mg three times a day or 150 mg/24 h/subcutaneous	Drowsiness, dry mouth, blurred vision, risk of urinary retention
	Haloperidol	Dopamine antagonist	2–3 mg twice daily or 2–5 mg/24 h/subcutaneous	Sedation, extrapyramidal effects
	Dexamethasone +/- Hyoscine butylbromide +/- Octreotide	Corticosteroid Antispasmodic antisecretory Somatostatin analogue	4–8 mg twice daily subcutaneous Up to 100 mg/24 h/subcutaneous Up to 1,000 micrograms/24 h/subcutaneous	Agitation/insomnia, gastric irritant Dry mouth, blurred vision, urinary retention
	Levomepromazine	Broad spectrum Phenothiazine anti-emetic	5–15 mg/24 h/subcutaneous	Constipation

Source: Based on Scottish Palliative Care Guidelines, 2019.

is highly evolved in animals unable to vomit, leading to avoidance behaviour as ingestion of poison would lead to certain death. If something tastes unpleasant then it can be immediately spat out without being ingested or absorbed.

The second level of protection involves the gastric and bowel mucosa as some food-poisoning toxins can be odourless and tasteless, getting past the first level of defence. Due to damage of the stomach and bowel mucosa by the toxin, there is an alteration of basal gastric motility (either slowing – bradygastria, or quickening – tachygastria). It is most often tachygastria associated with 'butterflies in the stomach' which is the precursor to nausea and vomiting, including decreasing the appetite. An example of odourless and tasteless food-poisoning toxin is bacillus cereus toxin from reheated rice. There is an immediate halt of gastric motility to prevent further absorption and dissemination of the toxin into the proximal small bowel and the expulsion of the majority of the toxin by vomiting (Stern et al., 2011; Morgan, 2010).

If some of the residual toxin does get absorbed then the third level of protection is through the detection of the toxin in the blood stream as it passes through the area postrema (AP) in the brain. This provokes further nausea and vomiting to further purge the stomach of residual food poisoning toxin (Reid, 1978).

A fourth level was postulated by Treisman in 1977 as an early warning system that all is not well through an imbalance of sensory information received by various cranial nerves (Stern et al., 2011). This is often the cause of nausea associated with travel sickness (provocative movement) when eye movements do not match the movement of the inner ear vestibular apparatus. This can be caused by reading whilst travelling in a vehicle, which causes a mismatch of vestibular and eye movement sensory information leading to sensory conflict and nausea. During movement it is imperative that eye movements are synchronised with the horizon and movement of the vehicle to prevent nausea. This type of nausea can be treated by challenge desensitisation on a regular basis until travel is possible without nausea. This is achieved using a revolving optokinetic disc or travel in the Boeing 737 KC135 zero G 'vomit comet'. This technique is used by NASA for pre-space travel training (Stern et al., 2011).

In summary, we have developed a sophisticated neuropharmacologico-psychological warning system around what and what not to eat. There is also a protective mechanism to prevent toxin ingestion, behavioural adaptation for survival combined with strong learned avoidance behaviour, which is seen in avoiding travel sickness or the continued challenge often offered by a poorly tolerated course of chemotherapy. There is a strong temporal persistence of memory even in the absence of a previously encountered cause of vomiting. This leads to conditioned anticipatory behaviour.

Mechanisms

There are many neurotransmitters, receptors and neural pathways involved in nausea and vomiting connecting the central nervous system with the periphery. The optimal choice of anti-emetic therefore requires an understanding of the potential mechanism(s) of nausea and the site(s) of action of the anti-emetic selected (Figure 4.2.1) (Reid, 1978; Ganong, 1999; Morgan, 2010).

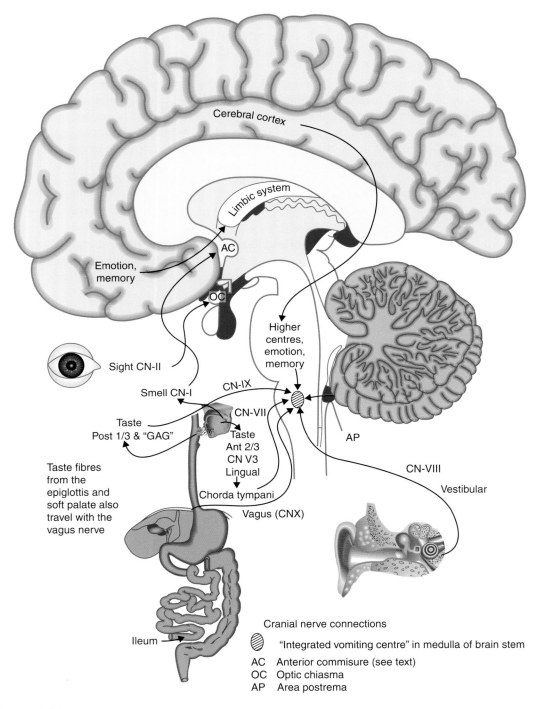

Figure 4.2.1 Neuroanatomical connections.

Neuroanatomy and description of receptors

The cerebral cortex and limbic system respond to pain and various emotional stimuli and will affect the overall threshold for nausea and vomiting within the vomiting centre (for example, low mood, depression, pain, loneliness and anxiety). The receptors of relevance within these higher neural pathways include GABA (gamma amino butyric acid) receptors, 5HT (serotonin) and the neurokinin-1 (NK_1) receptor which selectively binds the emetogenic tachykinin, substance P. The limbic system is closely associated with the olfactory pathways (smell and the memory of smell commonly evokes an emotional response) and these deep grey masses of the brain are the most primitive part of the forebrain. The limbic system is responsible for reward, memory processing and stores pleasant and unpleasant emotional responses and is responsible for aversion to previously unpleasant emetic experiences. It prevents the same mistake being repeated. An example of other primitive reflex emotional response might be 'sick at the sight of blood' (Reid, 1978; Ganong, 1999; Morgan, 2010).

Integrated vomiting centre

Over the course of the past 25 years, the area within the medulla of the brain stem concerned with the coordination of the act of vomiting and the emptying of the gastric contents has been referred to as the 'vomiting centre', 'integrated vomiting centre', or 'emetic or central pattern generator'. The most recent edition of the *Palliative Care Formulary* (PCF6) has again changed (among other things) the name of the vomiting centre to the 'nucleus of the tractus solitarius'. This goes some way to being neuro-anatomically correct but falls short of the full picture. This entirely sensory nucleus processes information received from the VIIth, IXth and Xth cranial nerves. The term 'vomiting centre' has covered both the processing of incoming afferent sensory information and the resultant output (motor efferent) resulting in the act of vomiting. The sensory afferent pathways also include information from a collection of cranial nerve nuclei including processing taste, visceral sensation and input from the vestibular apparatus which is outside the scope of the tractus solitarius. The nuclei within the brain stem are juxtaposed and connected, but the multiple sensory nuclei from the vestibular apparatus are arranged around the inferior cerebellar peduncles and are entirely separated from the tractus solitarius. It therefore makes neuro-anatomical sense that the vomiting centre relays and processes sensory input pertaining to potentially emetogenic stimuli with output to the dorsal motor nucleus of the vagus, leading to the act of vomiting. The vomiting centre therefore should be seen as a region within the medulla of the brain stem and composed of a collection of cranial nerve nuclei with both afferent and efferent components which are 'integrated' as a functional whole. The term 'integrated vomiting centre' makes neuro-anatomical and physiological sense. The most important receptors here include muscarinic acetylcholine receptors (ACh_m), histamine (H_1) receptors, $5HT_2$ serotonin receptor subtype and again, the NK_1 receptor as above (Reid, 1978; Ganong, 1999; Morgan, 2010).

Area postrema

This specialised neuro-anatomical area is located in the wall of the fourth ventricle and is an area composed of a densely vascularised sinusoidal fenestrated capillary network, which has a very high blood flow but at a uniquely slow flow rate allowing prolonged contact time of potentially emetogenic blood-borne substances with the surrounding neuronal receptors. Additionally, its location next to the cerebrospinal fluid (CSF) contained within the fourth ventricle means it is ideally placed to detect abnormalities within the CSF. The area is physiologically a chemo-receptor trigger zone and makes up part of the dorsal vagal complex along with the nucleus of the tractus solitarius and the dorsal motor nucleus of the vagus nerve. The main receptors in this area are dopamine (D_2) receptors, the $5HT_3$ serotonin subtype and the (now ubiquitous) NK_1 receptor already mentioned (Reid, 1978; Ganong, 1999; Morgan, 2010).

The connections between the vestibular apparatus (contained within the bony labyrinths) and the vomiting centre contain both ACh_m and H_1 receptors.

There are many pathways and receptors within the gastrointestinal tract, but most importantly the $5HT_3$ and $5HT_4$ serotonin receptor subtypes, ACh_m and D_2. The latter three receptors are involved in the regulation of gastrointestinal motility.

Causes

Area postrema

Drugs, biochemical derangement or blood-borne toxins will stimulate the area postrema (AP). Serum biochemistry including a corrected calcium and renal function should be checked.

Common metabolic causes are:

- Raised Ca^{2+} which may be accompanied by dehydration, constipation, abdominal pain, and confusion. Alternatively, nausea/vomiting may be the only sign
- Uraemia also causes nausea often in the absence of other clinical signs
- Hyponatraemia caused by advanced malignant disease
- Syndrome of inappropriate antidiuretic hormone secretion (SIADH)
  - Caused by specific malignancies
  - Drugs: diuretics, antidepressants
  - Chemotherapy
  - Head injury.

Opioids will cause gastric stasis and also stimulate the AP. Antibiotics, cytotoxic agents and alcohol will cause damage or irritation of the GI mucosa and stimulate the AP. Cytotoxic chemotherapy can cause acute and/or delayed emesis and anticipatory nausea and vomiting (Mannix, 1998; Regnard, 2005; Twycross et al., 2017).

Vomiting centre

Raised intracranial pressure (ICP) from brain tumours, metastatic disease or other intracranial pathology. The history may be suggestive, for example early morning headaches associated with vomiting. Fundoscopy looking for papilloedema should be performed.

Pharyngeal irritation due to, for example, a productive cough. Treat the cause if appropriate with antibiotics and aid expectoration with mucolytics such as a saline nebulizer.

Liver capsular stretch can cause nausea and vomiting as well as pain. Steroids (dexamethasone) can often help with both (Morgan, 2010).

Motion sickness

Gastrointestinal causes

(Sub)-acute obstruction: a high index of suspicion, particularly if the patient is known to have intra-abdominal malignant disease. A history detailing the timing and nature of any vomiting (for example, shortly after eating/hours after eating/unaltered food/faeculent vomitus/recent bowel habit/any flatus/associated pain, etc.) will guide in establishing the likely level of obstruction. Examination of the abdomen including a rectal examination and an abdominal X-ray (AXR) are needed. CT scan and small bowel studies may assist diagnosis of remediable causes.

Inoperable bowel obstruction: dictated by performance status, fitness for anaesthesia and the nature of the bowel obstruction. Laparotomy is not indicated in cases of widespread intraperitoneal carcinomatosis with multiple sites of obstruction (Morgan, 2010; Twycross et al., 2017; Regnard, 2005).

Squashed stomach: as above, caused by intra-abdominal pathology limiting the free and normal distension of the stomach. Significant ascites, large tumour masses or liver metastases can cause delayed gastric emptying as well as early satiety. The use of a prokinetic anti-emetic taken 20–30 minutes before mealtimes combined with an anti-flatulent antacid containing dimeticone or simethicone after meal times can be useful (Morgan, 2010; Twycross et al., 2017; Regnard, 2005).

Other causes

Pain, fear and anxiety can all precipitate nausea and vomiting and lower the threshold of the vomiting centre for emesis.

Radiotherapy may also cause sickness, particularly if the CNS or small bowel are within the radiation field.

Gastrointestinal motility and obstruction

Normal gastric motility and emptying is defined as 2.5–3.75 cycles per minute and is often demonstrated practically using an electrogastrogram (EGG). Anxiety, pain and nausea interfere with this normal basal rhythm. Bradygastria or gastroparesis (caused, for example, by opioid therapy) is defined as an EGG of 0–2.5 cycles per minute (delayed gastric emptying). Conversely, the feeling of 'butterflies in the stomach' can be caused by a tachygastria with an EGG of 3.75–10 cycles per minute, which interferes with normal stomach function and emptying reducing appetite and often a precursor to nausea and vomiting (Stern et al., 2011).

As part of a patient's ongoing management, they will probably have undergone recent imaging to identify if there is either a single level or multi-level obstruction as a cause for nausea and vomiting. Another important consideration is the patient's performance status and fitness to undergo surgical procedure.

Initial management

In all cases it may be appropriate to check urea and electrolytes and commence IV fluids, consideration being given to the use of a wide bore nasogastric tube if appropriate to relieve persistent and distressing large volume vomiting, taking the pressure off the bowel proximal to the obstructed segment. This management may allow the narrowed segment to settle spontaneously and give any peri-bowel oedema a chance to resolve. The signs of intestinal obstruction include distension, nausea and vomiting, colicky abdominal pain, constipation and an absence of the passage of flatus. Variable bowel sounds may be present, ranging from accentuated bowel sounds of normal calibre (borborygmi) to the high-pitched tinkling sounds of complete obstruction (Dicato, 1998).

Subacute obstruction

As the name suggests, the patient often cycles in and out of incomplete bowel obstruction and this may resolve spontaneously, requiring only supportive measures such as the use of intravenous fluids, hyoscine butylbromide for colic and possibly dexamethasone. A common cause may be adhesions from previous surgery rather than progressive intraperitoneal carcinomatosis. In this situation it is often worth a trial of subcutaneous metoclopramide, which may be titrated to effect, the usual dose range being 30 to 100 mg/24 hours.

Single-level obstruction

Dependent upon patient fitness, consideration may be given to a complete resection of the narrowed, stenosed, diseased segment of bowel with primary anastamosis or possibly formation of ileostomy or colostomy. There will be situations where it is impossible to resect the tumour and a decision may be made to bypass the tumour and form a gastroenterostomy or gastrojejunostomy, should the obstruction affect a more proximal part of the small bowel. If, however, the patient is unfit to undergo a surgical procedure then the help of the interventional radiologist may be sought for the consideration of using a stent.

Multi-level obstruction

Resection, bypass or stenting if appropriate may be possible proximal to the obstructed loop or multiple loops of bowel affected, but if no operative intervention is possible then the management becomes entirely dependent upon appropriate drug therapy.

Multi-level inoperable bowel obstruction

The focus in this situation is primarily to relieve distressing symptoms. The symptoms most commonly encountered are:

- Painful bowel distension
- Nausea/vomiting

- Colicky, abdominal pain
- Constipation.

This can be managed as with other pains and may require regular strong opioids, usually given by continuous subcutaneous infusion to ensure absorption.

The management of colicky, abdominal pain associated with obstruction is best managed with the use of subcutaneous anticholinergic medication such as hyoscine butylbromide (Buscopan) 20 mg by subcutaneous injection as required (De Conno et al., 1991).

Some increased comfort may be derived from emptying the lower bowel using suppositories or enemas. Other drugs include the use of dexamethasone if there is a degree of bowel oedema involved, the usual dose being 6 to 12 mg daily by subcutaneous injection. The use of a somatostatin analogue such as octreotide may have an important role to play in the management of inoperable bowel obstruction or carcinoid tumours (Fallon, 1994).

Octreotide

This analogue of growth hormone inhibiting hormone has many inhibitory hormonal actions, which reduces globally GI secretions all the way from the salivary glands through to the distal colon. It increases water and electrolyte absorption within the bowel as well as reducing all exocrine secretions from the stomach, small bowel, pancreas and biliary tract, in addition to having its own anti-neoplastic effect. The common dose range in bowel obstruction is 100 to 1,000 micrograms/24 hours by continuous subcutaneous infusion (Fallon, 1994).

Broad spectrum anti-emetic

Historically it was common practice to treat inoperable bowel obstruction with a combination of haloperidol and cyclizine. More recently, we have moved towards using a broad spectrum anti-emetic, such as levomepromazine, commonly at a dose of 6.25 to 12.5 mg/24 hours by continuous subcutaneous infusion, rarely at a dose of more than 25 mg/24 hours (Morgan, 2010; Twycross et al., 2017; Mannix, 1998; Regnard, 2005).

The above medical management seeks to address the most distressing symptoms, but in some situations the large volume vomiting persists despite all these measures and in this situation consideration is given to using a venting gastrostomy, if it is not thought appropriate or if it is too uncomfortable or distressing to use a nasogastric tube.

Treatment

A summary of treatment options in listed in Figure 4.2.2.

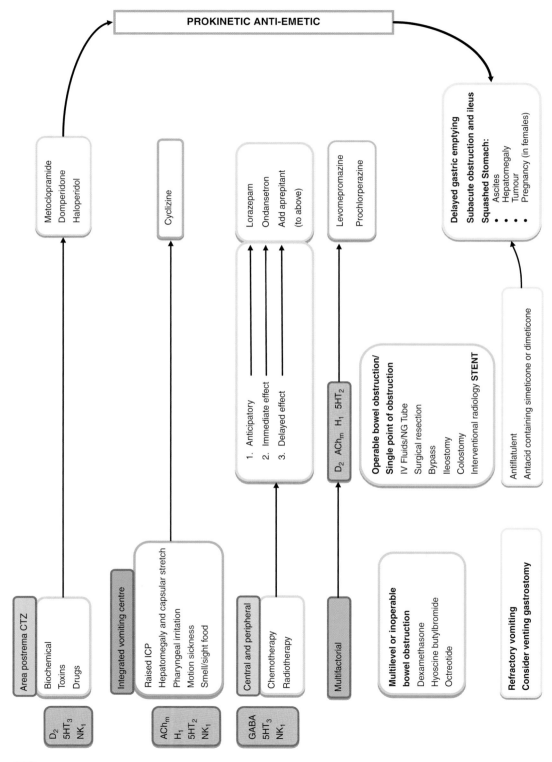

Figure 4.2.2 Summary of treatment options.

Dietary considerations/helpful strategies

Foods which should be considered to aid gastric emptying are (Stern et al., 2011):

- High protein meals and protein drinks: these reduce gastric dysrhythmias and normalise pacing
- Thin soups
- Noodles
- Rice
- Ginger.

The following foods should be avoided:

- High fat meals (fried, greasy foods), as fatty foods delay gastric emptying
- Red meat
- Sugary drinks
- All citrus fruits
- Cream and dairy-based products
- Fresh vegetables and pulpy fibrous foods, as these require more work to digest which prolongs mixing within the stomach and makes gastric emptying more difficult.

Drug profiles

Metoclopramide and domperidone: dopamine antagonists and prokinetic anti-emetics with weak central action within the AP. Not always effective for biochemical or drug-induced nausea, but especially useful to aid gastric emptying. Metoclopramide works both by countering dopamine inhibition of motility and stimulating motility as a $5HT_4$ agonist. Domperidone, however, works only by blocking the dopamine inhibition. Domperidone does not cross the blood–brain barrier and so does not cause extra-pyramidal side-effects.

Haloperidol: potent dopamine receptor antagonist useful for treating AP mediated nausea refractory to metoclopramide or domperidone. Watch for extra-pyramidal side-effects.

Cyclizine: the drug of choice for vomiting centre or vestibular apparatus mediated nausea and vomiting. Antihistamine and anticholinergic activity. First choice for nausea and vomiting caused by raised intracranial pressure, motion sickness, liver capsular stretch or pharyngeal irritation. Should not be combined with metoclopramide as its anticholinergic action will negate the pro-motility effect of the metoclopramide.

Levomepromazine: phenothiazine with useful broad spectrum anti-emetic profile. Blocks D_2, ACh_m, H_1, $5HT_2$ serotonin receptor subtype as well as α-2 receptors. This last receptor is responsible for the risk of postural hypotension at higher doses, especially when fluid intake has been marginal because of refractory nausea and vomiting.

Lorazepam: short-acting benzodiazepine, can be administered sublingually. Particularly useful as an adjuvant anti-emetic for anxiety and anticipatory nausea and vomiting.

Dexamethasone: fluorinated corticosteroid often used as part of anti-emetic regime given with chemotherapy. It acts as an adjuvant anti-emetic with other drugs. Its mechanism of action is possibly by reducing the permeability of the blood–brain barrier and the AP to emetogenic substances and by reducing GABA and leu-enkephalin release within the brain stem.

Ondansetron/granisetron: specific $5HT_3$ serotonin receptor subtype antagonists. Narrow spectrum and specifically developed to treat acute nausea and vomiting associated with both chemo- and radiotherapy. Less effective with delayed nausea and vomiting. NOT to be used as an anti-emetic when other drugs have failed. Can cause significant constipation.

Aprepitant: new NK_1 receptor antagonist developed specifically to treat the delayed emesis sometimes seen with highly emetogenic chemotherapy regimens. It is reported as having a broad spectrum of action and may have a wider role in the management of nausea and vomiting in the future (Morgan, 2010; Twycross et al., 2017).

Choice of drug

- A first-line anti-emetic is selected according to the most likely cause and is administered via a suitable route.
- If vomiting prevents oral administration other options include subcutaneous, sublingual, buccal, rectal, intravenous and intramuscular routes.
- Continuous subcutaneous administration via a syringe pump guarantees drug administration in the vomiting patient.
- Anti-emetics should be prescribed regularly.
- Second-line or combination therapy should be introduced if symptoms persist after 24 hours.
- Reversible causes of nausea and vomiting should be addressed separately, for example:

  - Correcting hypercalcaemia
  - Optimizing hydration
  - Stopping emetogenic drugs wherever possible
  - Draining ascites
  - Managing bowel obstruction appropriately.

It should be remembered that nausea and vomiting in patients with cancer is often multifactorial. If the causes are not clear, or first-line therapy has failed, then levomepromazine is an appropriate subsequent choice of anti-emetic as it acts at many different receptor sites. Its broad spectrum of activity means it is frequently effective even when combinations of specific anti-emetics have been unsuccessful. Its anxiolytic and sedative effect can also be advantageous in this group of patients, although doses above 25 mg/24 hours can frequently cause sedation and postural hypotension (Regnard, 1993).

Inoperable bowel obstruction is often treated on a surgical ward by 'drip and suck', deploying an uncomfortable NG tube and IV fluids.

A more conservative approach can be successful using a combination of broad spectrum anti-emetic such as levomepromazine and the anticholinergic (antisecretory and antimotility) drug Buscopan (De Conno et al., 1991).

Sometimes an empirical trial of subcutaneous dexamethasone can also be added to the regime.

Octreotide (a somatostatin analogue) can be useful in cases refractory to the above management.

A venting gastrostomy may have to be considered in high duodenal or jejunal obstruction. This is essentially a feeding tube used in reverse and is very effective for refractory nausea and vomiting (Morgan, 2010).

Hiccups

Pathophysiology

A hiccup is an involuntary contraction of the diaphragm and intercostal muscles immediately followed by closure of the epiglottis. The mechanism of control of hiccups is not well understood but would appear to involve a 'reflex arc'. The afferent inputs include the phrenic and vagal nerves. Central processing takes place in the brain stem and cervical spinal cord. Efferent outputs are mainly via the phrenic and accessory nerves and the recurrent laryngeal nerve (Methal et al., 2012; Steger et al., 2015).

Hiccups are usually self-limiting but can become persistent and distressing, particularly in the presence of underlying pathology (Scottish Palliative Care Guidelines, 2019). Causes can broadly be categorised as central or peripheral.

Central

- Ischaemic or haemorrhagic stroke
- Meningitis/encephalitis
- Brain injury/tumour
- Parkinson's disease
- Drugs:
  - Including anaesthetic agents, platinum-based chemotherapy
- Metabolic:
  - Hyponatraemia, hypercalcaemia, uraemia
- Excitement/stress.

Peripheral (particularly stimulation of the phrenic or vagal nerves)

- Gastric distension (probably the most common cause) (Methal et al., 2012; Steger et al., 2015; Scottish Palliative Care Guidelines, 2019)

- Gastro-oesophageal reflux
- Malignancy or inflammatory processes involving:
  - Pharynx
  - Oesophagus
  - Stomach
  - Pancreas
  - Liver
  - Lung
  - Pleura
  - Pericardium.
- Iatrogenic:
  - Pharyngeal intubation
  - Oesophageal stent placement
  - Thoracic or abdominal surgery.

Assessment

Careful assessment may identify an underlying cause. It will be important to assess the impact of the symptom on the patient, including physical and psychosocial functioning, mood and sleep. Eliciting the patient's understanding of their symptom and overall situation including their hopes and fears will put any treatment strategies in better context.

Treatment

The best symptom control is always achieved by identifying and treating the underlying cause. This is not always possible or appropriate, particularly in a palliative care scenario.

There is little robust evidence to support any individual treatment strategy (Scottish Palliative Care Guidelines, 2019). Non-drug interventions (home remedies or 'granny's cures') can be effective.

Non-drug

Most home remedies work by overloading and interrupting either the afferent or efferent arm of the reflex arc, such as (Steger et al., 2015):

- Nasopharyngeal stimulation:
  - Sipping iced water
  - Rubbing the soft palate with a swab
- Vagal stimulation:
  - Startle reflex
  - Cold key down the back
  - Cold compress to the face
- Phrenic nerve/diaphragmatic stimulation:
  - Drinking from the opposite side of a cup
  - Breath holding

- Other:
  - Digital rectal massage (Odeh et al., 1990) and orgasm (Releg et al., 2000) have both been described in the medical literature as effective in terminating intractable hiccups.

Medication (Twycross and Wilcock, 2017; Scottish Palliative Care Guidelines, 2019)

- Relief of gastric distension:
  - If possible reduce/stop medications with anticholinergic side-effects to minimise delayed gastric emptying.
  - Peppermint water acts as an antiflatulent. Avoid if gastro-oesophageal reflux. Do not co-prescribe with prokinetics.
  - Simeticone is an anti-foaming agent that facilitates belching. It is available in combination with antacids:
    - Altacite plus: 10 ml between meals and at bedtime
    - Maalox plus: 10 ml four times a day
  - Prokinetics to aid gastric emptying:
    - Metoclopramide 10 mg three times a day
    - Domperidone 10 mg three times a day
  - Treatment of gastro-oesophageal reflux:
    - Prokinetics, as above
    - Proton pump inhibitor
- In malignancy involving the liver/mediastinum/pleura/brain, reduction in peri-tumour oedema may reduce inflammation/compression
  - Dexamethasone 4–8 mg once per day in the morning. Stop after one week if no improvement. Otherwise reduce to lowest effective dose.
- Central nervous system:
  - Dopamine and GABA appear to be important in modulating the central control of hiccups (Steger et al., 2015).
    - Haloperidol 500 micrograms – 1 mg up to three times a day
    - Levomepromazine 3–6 mg at bed time
    - Benzodiazepine, for example clonazepam 500 micrograms at night, particularly if sleep disturbance
- Peripheral:
  - Relaxation of skeletal muscle
    - Baclofen 5–20 mg up to three times a day
  - Relaxation of smooth muscle (oesophagus)
    - Nifedipine MR 10 mg twice daily.

Constipation

Constipation is the passage of small, hard stools, often with difficulty. With constipation, defaecation occurs less often than is *usual* for an individual and can be associated with a sense of incomplete evacuation (NICE, 2015). The evidence base for managing constipation remains sparse in spite of the fact that its prevalence and negative impact on quality of life are well documented in palliative literature (Young, 2019). The causes can be many and concurrent, particularly in patients with advanced disease (Muldrew et al., 2018).

Causes to consider

- Medications (for example opioids, antacids, diuretics)
- Dehydration and anorexia
- Biochemical abnormalities (for example hypercalcaemia)
- Immobility
- Muscle wasting causing loss of effective peristalsis and reduced abdominal pressure during straining
- Extrinsic bowel compression
- Intrinsic bowel obstruction
- Impaired neurological control or early sign of impending spinal cord compression
- Piles or anal fissures
- Lack of privacy in hospital or with carers present.

Assessment and investigation

Objective tools and criteria to help identify constipation include the Bristol Stool Chart, Constipation Visual Analogue Scale (CVAS) and Rome II diagnostic criteria (Muldrew, 2018).

A thorough clinical assessment requires exploration of:

- Usual pattern of defaecation and stool nature
- Current laxative/dietary regimen
- Current clinical features including:
  - Pain
  - Nausea/vomiting
  - Passage of flatulence
  - Bloating
- Current medications
- An examination of the abdomen looking for tenderness, swelling, hyper-resonance, bowel sounds, evidence of ascites. Sometimes the colon may be palpable with the presence of firm, indentable faeces.

Reviewing recent imaging may be helpful to assess the potential for bowel compression or obstruction. An abdominal X-ray could be considered to identify faecal loading or dilated loops of bowel indicating obstruction.

Rectal or stoma examination may be helpful but requires sensitivity and consent.

If complete or sub-acute bowel obstruction is suspected then specialist advice should be sought.

Management

Non-pharmacological

- Encourage up to 2 litres/24 hrs or oral fluid intake where the patient is able
- Review diet (fibre, fruit, natural laxatives)
- Ensure privacy and adequate time to allow effective defaecation
- Encourage physical activity where possible.

Pharmacological

Option 1 – Stimulant and/or softner (for example senna, bisacodyl and/or docusate)

Option 2 – Osmotic laxative (for example Laxido®)

If oral interventions have not resolved the situation consider:

Option 3 – Rectal treatment

- Soft loading: bisacodyl suppository, sodium citrate or phosphate enema
- Hard loading: glycerol suppository as lubricant or stimulant; then treat as above
- Very hard loading: arachis oil enema (except in those with nut allergy) overnight followed by phosphate enema.

For details regarding dosage and further information please refer to Scottish Palliative Care Guidelines: laxative medicines information chart (Scottish Palliative Care Guidelines, 2019). It is important to prescribe a regular laxative when prescribing opioids unless there is reason not to. Any prescriptions should be reviewed over time and titrated up or down accordingly.

Specific situations

- **Opioid-induced constipation** – this should be suspected in patients on opioids for whom regular laxative use has not resolved constipation. Peripheral opioid antagonists such as methylnaltrexone or naloxegol can be considered but specialist advice is recommended (Larkin et al., 2018).
- **Paraplegic or bed-bound patients** – it may be necessary to institute an artificial bowel regimen to allow regular, effective defaecation with an element of control for the patient. Aim for a firm stool with rectal intervention every 2–3 days to prevent faecal impaction. Caution should be shown in administering rectal medications to patients with spinal cord injury to T6 or above as the stimulation can trigger autonomic dysreflexia (Young, 2019).

Diarrhoea

The WHO defines diarrhoea as the passage of more than three unformed or liquid stools in a 24-hour period. It is often associated with urgency. What patients refer to as diarrhoea varies but generally represents a pattern which is more frequent or more liquid than is usual for them. Diarrhoea is generally a less common complaint than constipation in advanced disease, with the exception of HIV AIDS (Bossi et al., 2018).

Causes to consider

- Medications (for example laxatives, antibiotics, antacids, non-steroidal anti-inflammatory drugs)
- Chemotherapy, targeted and immunotherapies
- Radiotherapy (abdominal, pelvic)
- Intestinal obstruction (including constipation) with overflow diarrhoea. This is the most common cause in elderly patients with non-malignant disease (Fallon et al., 1997)
- Malabsorption:
  o Pancreatic insufficiency
  o Post gastrectomy/ileal resection
  o Any GI surgery resulting in short bowel
- Common presenting complaint for several tumours (Bossi et al., 2018):
  o Neuroendocrine tumours
  o Colonic tumours (can alternate with constipation)
  o Pancreatic (especially islet cell tumours)
  o Phaeochromocytoma
- Patients on enteral feed regimens
- Concurrent disease (for example diabetes mellitus, inflammatory bowel disease, irritable bowel disease)
- Infection.

Assessment and investigation

A careful history should establish:

- Frequency/pattern of defaecation
- Nature of the stool (colour, consistency)
- Presence of blood or mucus in the stool
- Associated pain (nature and pattern)
- Recent oncological treatments
- Current medication (including laxative use)
- Diet/fluid intake
- Recent travel
- Past history of GI disease (for example Crohn's disease, coeliac disease)
- New incontinence which might suggest spinal cord involvement.

Symptoms and signs of a more severe situation which may require hospital admission include:

- Sepsis (with/without neutropenia)
- Peritonitis
- Delirium
- Signs of cardiovascular compromise.

Physical investigation should include observations especially lying/standing blood pressure, examination of the abdomen for tenderness, bloating and the presence or absence of bowel sounds. Rectal examination may be appropriate and should be undertaken with sensitivity and consent. Blood samples may be taken for biochemical analysis as salts may need replacing. The stool should be examined visually and sent for culture where appropriate.

Stool culture in patients with advanced cancer gives a positive yield in approximately 5% of cases. This percentage can be lower in cases of chemotherapy-associated diarrhoea (Bossi et al., 2018).

Clostridium difficile should be suspected in patients taking antibiotics – especially penicillins, clindamycin, cephalosporins – but also in patients receiving frequent enemas, prolonged nasogastric feeding or following GI surgery (Bossi et el., 2018). In cases of suspected clostridium difficile infection, Health Protection Scotland provides guidance on procedures for managing initial and subsequent infections (Health Protection Scotland, 2017). Individual health boards also publish local guidance.

Management

General management of uncomplicated diarrhoea when infective causes are excluded:

- Oral rehydration (rehydration salt preparations such as Dioralyte® can be considered)
- Review and discontinue any implicated medications where possible
- Consider the use of anti-diarrhoeal medications:
  - Loperamide – peripherally acting opioid agonist which slows gut transit time allowing fluid re-absorption, decreased faeces bulk and decreased frequency of defaecation – 2 mg after each loose stool, a maximum of 16 mg/24 hours.
  - Codeine phosphate – 30 mg as required to a maximum of 240 mg/24 hours. Can be sedating and potential for dependence should be considered. Can be used in addition to or in place of loperamide. If the patient is already established on opioids, seek specialist advice.
- Attention to peri-anal skin care, encourage hygiene, consider barrier creams.

The management of diarrhoea with specific causes is outlined in Table 4.2.4.

157

Table 4.2.4   Management of diarrhoea with specific causes.

Cause	Management
Infection	Treat underlying cause and follow general measures
Pancreatic insufficiency	Pancreatic enzyme preparations, for example CREON®
Bile acid malabsorption Short gut syndrome	Cholestyramine
Carcinoid syndrome High-output stomas	Somatostatin analogues, for example octreotide
Faecal impaction/obstruction with overflow	Investigate and manage appropriately
Chemotherapy, targeted and immunotherapy associated diarrhoea	Seek oncology advice
Radiotherapy associated diarrhoea	Seek oncology advice

Diarrhoea as a consequence of cancer treatments

Chemotherapy agents commonly causing diarrhoea include 5FU (up to 50% patients), irinotecan and capecitabine. Diarrhoea is also a common side-effect of targeted therapies and immunotherapies and can be severe where these are combined with chemotherapy (Bossi et al., 2018).

Radiotherapy can be associated with acute (<3 months) and chronic diarrhoea. The radiotherapy causes direct mucosal damage but also altered gut microflora and enzyme activity. Up to 60% of patients receiving pelvic or abdominal radiotherapy are affected (Bossi et al., 2018).

Diarrhoea in HIV AIDS

Chronic diarrhoea is common in HIV disease. Causes can differ depending on CD4 cell count, with opportunistic infections such as mycobacterium avium, cytomegalovirus and cryptosporidiosis affecting those with counts <100 cells/μl (Jacobson, 2015). The history should specifically cover travel, animal exposure, sick contacts, current medications and sexual activity. In those with CD4 counts >100 cells/μl, *C. difficile* giardia and shigella are common infective causes. Common non-infective causes include inflammatory bowel disease (can occur secondary to anti-retroviral drugs), malabsorption and endocrine abnormalities.

Ascites

Pathophysiology of ascites

Malignant

Ascites is the accumulation of excessive fluid in the abdomen. Cancer accounts for around 10% of all cases of ascites (Rosenberg, 2006). Of these, ovarian cancer has the highest incidence (30% at diagnosis, 60% in advanced disease). Other cancers include endometrial, breast, colonic, gastric, pancreatic, or unknown primary carcinoma (Keen, 2015). Malignant ascites is associated with a poor prognosis with a mean survival of around 5 months after detection. Prognosis is usually better in ovarian cancer and lymphoma, and worse in GI and unknown primary cancers (Twycross et al., 2009).

There are two main mechanisms for the development of malignant ascites:

1. Peritoneal carcinomatosis:
   o Tumour or inflammatory cell-derived cytokines increase the permeability of normal microvessels, which, along with the intrinsically leaky peritoneal neovasculature, allows extravasation of fluid (Keen, 2015; Twycross et al., 2009).
   o Obstruction of lymphatics in the peritoneum or regional lymph nodes by cancer, resulting in chylous (milky) ascites.
   o This fluid is typically an **exudate** (ascitic albumin concentration is relatively high).
2. Extensive liver metastases:
   o Increased hepatic venous pressure results in fluid leakage into the peritoneum from the sinusoids and also, via an increase in plasma rennin concentration, retention of salt and water by the kidneys. This happens as an anatomical consequence of multiple hepatic metastases, or single large (sometimes benign) tumours causing a Budd–Chiari syndrome (Keen, 2015).
   o This fluid is typically a transudate (ascitic albumin concentration is relatively low), similar to that seen as a result of hepatic cirrhosis.

Cirrhotic

Hepatic cirrhosis accounts for around 75% of all cases of ascites (Rosenberg, 2006). Cirrhotic ascites formation occurs predominantly as a result of portal hypertension and consequent splanchnic vasodilatation that results in both sodium and fluid retention and an increase in intestinal capillary pressure and permeability. This fluid is typically a transudate (ascitic albumin concentration is relatively low).

Assessment

The diagnosis of ascites relies on appropriate clinical history and examination.

Ultrasound scanning can detect as little as 100 ml of ascites and can distinguish between fluid and other causes of distension (for example cancer, organomegaly, bowel distension) (Twycross et al., 2009).

Biochemical, cytological and microbiological investigations are important to clarify the nature of the ascites:

- The serum-ascites albumin gradient (SAAG) is calculated by subtracting the albumin concentration of the ascites from the serum albumin concentration (samples taken on the same day). The gradient correlates with the portal venous pressure; a value of 11 g/L or higher is indicative of portal hypertension and indicates the fluid is a transudate. A value <11 g/L suggests the fluid is an exudate (Keen, 2015).

- Cytology is positive in up to two-thirds of malignant ascites (Twycross et al., 2009).
- In cirrhotic ascites a neutrophil count >250 cells/mm^3 usually indicates infection. These patients should be treated for spontaneous bacterial peritonitis (SBP) with intravenous antibiotics. Inoculation of ascitic fluid into blood culture bottles will identify an organism in approximately 72–90% of cases whereas sending ascitic fluid in a sterile container to the laboratory will only identify an organism in about 40% of cases of SBP (Moore and Aithal, 2006).

Management

Pharmacological management

Chemotherapy

If appropriate, some chemotherapies, either systemic or intraperitoneal, can control ascites (Twycross et al., 2009).

Diuretic therapy (transudates)

- Diuretics are the mainstay of treatment for control of non-malignant (transudative) ascites, with 90% of cirrhotic patients responding to treatment (Twycross et al., 2009).
- Spironolactone, an aldosterone antagonist, is the first-line treatment. The initial dose is 100 mg/day and can be progressively increased up to 400 mg/day. There is a lag of 3–5 days between the beginning of spironolactone treatment and the onset of the natriuretic effect.
- If spironolactone alone fails to resolve the ascites, furosemide can be added, initially at 40 mg/day, and can be increased up to 160 mg/day with careful biochemical and clinical monitoring (Moore and Aithal, 2006).
- It may be appropriate to consider a trial of diuretics in individuals with malignant ascites and a high SAAG (for example due to extensive liver metastases) (Keen, 2015).

Paracentesis

Abdominal paracentesis affords quick symptomatic relief in a population that often has a relatively short prognosis and for whom diuretic therapy may be inappropriate or ineffective (Keen, 2015). The majority of patients (90%) report symptom relief from paracentesis, even after as little as 1–2 litres of fluid (Twycross et al., 2009).

Paracentesis is appropriate for patients with:

- A tense, distended abdomen in need of rapid relief
- Ascites which is unlikely to respond, or has failed to respond, to diuretics
- Intolerance to diuretics
- An unknown diagnosis
- Possible bacterial peritonitis.

Paracentesis should ideally be done under ultrasound guidance for greater chances of success and fewer complications (Twycross et al., 2009). Ultrasound guidance is strongly recommended for patients with:

- Severe bowel distension
- Widespread intra-abdominal cancer deposits
- Previous extensive abdominal or pelvic surgery
- Difficult previous paracentesis.

Complications of paracentesis include:

- Abdominal discomfort
- Bleeding:
  - <1% of patients will bleed to the extent they need a blood transfusion.
  - The risk of bleeding is low, even in the presence of coagulopathy or thrombocytopaenia.
  - Bleeding risk increases in renal impairment (platelet dysfunction) or in the presence of varices in patients with portal hypertension.
  - Give platelet transfusion pre-procedure if platelets are $< 50 \times 10^9$/L.
  - Ideally international normalised ratio (INR) should be <1.5. Consider IV Vitamin K if INR >1.5 (The Rowans Hospice, 2011).
  - *Note*: malignant ascites may be blood-stained.
- Bowel or bladder puncture:
  - Reduce risk by using ultrasound guidance, avoid sites of old scars, and ensure bladder is empty.
- Persistent leak at puncture site:
  - <1% of patients will have a leak.
  - A colostomy bag may be needed for large volume leakage.
- Infection:
  - The risk of local infection or peritonitis is minimal with an aseptic technique.
  - Treat any local or systemic infection promptly with antibiotics.
  - Consider prophylactic antibiotics for patients at risk of SBP.
- Hypotension:
  - Large volume (>5 litres) paracentesis can lead to haemodynamic changes, for example hypotension, collapse, renal failure.
  - Consider limiting paracentesis to <5 litres in patients with cirrhosis receiving diuretics, and any patient with renal failure, hypoalbuminaemia or hyponatraemia (Twycross et al., 2009).
- Death:
  - Infection, perforation or severe bleeding can all lead to death. Even if these complications do not occur, patients with ascites and advanced disease may be very frail, and may deteriorate and die sooner than expected. Even if a patient is nearing end of life, it may still be appropriate to consider paracentesis if they are very symptomatic of

ascites, even if they may die soon after. Drainage should always be undertaken with caution to avoid the removal of excessive fluid volume at any one time.

In transudative ascites, if drainage >5 litres is required:

- Stop diuretics 48 hours before procedure
- Administer IV 100 ml 20% albumin for every 2.5 litres of fluid drained (Moore and Aithal, 2006)
- Monitor pulse and blood pressure every 30 minutes during paracentesis, then hourly for 6 hours (Twycross et al., 2009).

Indwelling tunnelled ascitic drains

For patients requiring repeated paracentesis and who have a prognosis of >1 month, an indwelling tunnelled ascitic drain can be considered. NICE have recommended the use of indwelling drains for individuals with malignant ascites likely to require repeated large volume paracentesis for palliation of symptoms (NICE, 2012). To reduce the risk of infection this drain contains a one-way valve and a polyester cuff which promotes fibrosis in the subcutaneous tissue, thus anchoring the drain in place.

Patients, carers or district nurses can drain fluid every few days at home. This reduces the frequency of hospital visits as is particularly beneficial to patients who are frail or who have to travel significant distances. The overall complication rate is similar to intermittent drainage (Twycross et al., 2009).

Scenario Recap

A major concern of Lee's family was his lack of appetite and nutritional intake. Unfortunately, the majority of patients with advancing cancer develop cachexia and anorexia is an associated symptom. It was important to acknowledge these concerns and explain that cachexia is the result of changes in one's metabolism as a result of advancing cancer and that, sadly, 'feeding' by any route would not reverse or overcome these changes and was very unlikely to make him feel better or prolong his life.

Corticosteroids may offer some temporary benefit in improving appetite and general well-being but, since dexamethasone liquid 4 mg daily had improved neither after 7 days, it was stopped.

Lee wished to be at home, cared for by his family with the support of community health and social care teams.

With time his dysphagia worsened and it became no longer possible to control his symptoms with oral medication in liquid form. A continuous subcutaneous infusion (CSCI) via a syringe pump containing morphine and metoclopramide was commenced and a 'just in case' box with appropriate medication for breakthrough (rescue) symptom control was provided. Inability to swallow saliva and the associated drooling was a source of distress for Lee but the addition of hyoscine butylbromide 80 mg to the CSCI was beneficial, as was the addition of the broad spectrum anti-emetic levomepromazine 5 mg to combat an increasing background nausea.

The importance of regular oral care, particularly when antisecretory drugs such as hyoscine are being used, was explained to family members who gladly provided this care during Lee's final days.

Further Reading

Dysphagia: Iddis.org. Available at: http://iddis.org/framework

References

Ashrof H et al. (2017) Can patients determine the level of their dysphagia? *World Journal of Gastroenterology*, 23(6): 1038–1043.

BAPEN (2003) Nutritional screening of adults: a multidisciplinary responsibility. Development and use of the 'Malnutrition Universal Screening Tool' ('MUST') for adults. Available at https://www.bapen.org.uk/screening-and-must/must/must-report

Bossi P et al. (2018) Diarrhoea in adult cancer patients: ESMO clinical practice guidelines. *Annals of Oncology*, 29(4): 126–142.

Carr B and Steel J (2013) *Psychological Aspects of Cancer.* New York: Springer.

Clark K (2015) Dysphagia, dyspepsia and hiccup. In Cherny N et al. (eds) *Oxford Textbook of Palliative Medicine*, 5th edition. Oxford: Oxford University Press, pp. 651–656.

Cowling M, Hale H and Grundy A (1998) Mangement of malignant oesophageal obstruction with self-expanding metallic stents. *British Journal of Surgery*, 85(22): 264–266.

Davies A and Finlay I (2005) *Oral Care in Advanced Disease*. Oxford: Oxford University Press.

De Conno F et al. (1991) Continuous subcutaneous infusion of Hyoscine Butylbromide reduces secretions in patients with gastrointestinal obstruction. *Journal of Pain and Symptom Management*, 6(8): 484–486.

Dev R et al. (2017) The evolving approach to management of cancer cachexia. *Oncology*, 31(1): 23–32.

Dicato MA (1998) *Medical Management of Cancer Treatment Induced Emesis*. London: Martin Dunitz Ltd.

Druml C et al. (2016) ESPEN guideline on ethical aspects of artificial nutrition and hydration. *Clinical Nutrition*, 35(3): 545–556.

Eldridge L and Power J (2014) Palliative care and terminal illness. In Gandy J (ed) *Manual of Dietetic Practice*. Chichester: John Wiley and Sons, p. 861.

Fallon MT (1994) The physiology of somatostatin and its synthetic analogue, octreotide. *European Journal of Palliative Care*, 1: 20–22.

Fallon M and O'Neill B (1997) ABC of palliative care: constipation and diarrhoea. *BMJ*, 15(315): 1993–1996.

Ganong WF (1999) *Review of Medical Physiology*, 19th edition. Stamford, CT: Appleton and Lange.

Glen P (2016) The role of stents in palliation of oesophageal cancer. *BMJ Supportive and Palliative Care*, 6(1): 135.

Gomes A et al. (2015) Percutaneous endoscopic gastrostomy versus nasogastric tube feeding for adults with swallowing disturbances. *Cochrane Database of Systematic Reviews*, 2015(5): CD008096.

Harris DG (2010) Nausea and vomiting in advanced cancer. *British Medical Bulletin*, 96(1): 175–185.

Health Protection Scotland (2017) Guidance on the prevalence and control of clostridium difficile infection in health and social care settings in Scotland. Available at: https://www.hps.scot.nhs.uk/web-resources-container/guidance-on-prevention-and-control-of-clostridium-difficile-infection-cdi-in-health-and-social-care-settings-in-scotland/

Jacobson M, Luetkemeyer A and Wlodarczyk D (2015) Managing HIV patients with prolonged diarrhoea. San Francisco: University of California.

Kaye P (1996) *A–Z Pocket Book of Symptom Control*. Northampton: EPL Publications.

Keen J (2015) Jaundice, ascites and encephalopathy. In Cherny N et al. (eds) *Oxford Textbook of Palliative Medicine*, 5th edition. Oxford: Oxford University Press.

Larkin PJ et al. (2018) Diagnosis, assessment and management of constipation in advanced cancer: ESMO clinical practice guidelines. *Annals of Oncology*, 29(4): 111–125.

Lennard-Jones JE (2000) Ethical and legal aspects of clinical hydration and nutritional support. *BJU International*, 85(4): 398–403.

Leslie P, Carding P and Wilson J (2003) Investigation and management of chronic dysphagia. *British Medical Journal*, 326(433). Available at: https://www.bmj.com/content/326/7386/433.short

Logemann J (1983) *Evaluation and Treatment of Swallowing Disorders*. San Diego: College Hill Press.

Mannix KA (1998) Palliation of nausea and vomiting. In Doyle D, Hanks GWC, MacDonald N (eds) *Oxford Textbook of Palliative Medicine*, 2nd edition. Oxford: Oxford University Press, pp. 489–499.

Matsuo K and Palmer J (2008) Anatomy and physiology of feeding and swallowing – normal and abnormal. *Physical Medical Rehabilitation Clinics of North America*, 19(4): 691–707.

Methal N, Kelt S and Jordan J (2012) Interventions for the management of persistent and intractable hiccups in adults – a systematic review. *BMJ Supportive and Palliative Care*, 2(Suppl 1): A49–50.

MHRA (Medicines and Healthcare products Regulatory Agency) (2014) Oral swabs with a foam head – heads may detach during use. Available at: https://www.gov.uk/drug-device-alerts/medical-device-alert-oral-swabs-with-a-foam-head-heads-may-detach-during-use

Moore KP and Aithal GP (2006) Guidelines on the management of ascites in cirrhosis. *Gut*, 55(Suppl 6): vi1–vi12.

Morgan TRM (2010) Symptom control in palliative care. In Cassidy J et al. (eds) *Oxford Handbook of Oncology*, 3rd edition. Oxford: Oxford University Press, pp. 134–141.

Muldrew DHL et al. (2018) Assessment and management of constipation for patients receiving palliative care in specialist palliative care settings: a systematic review of the literature. *Palliative Medicine*, 32(5): 930–938.

National Institute for Health and Clinical Excellence (2012) *The PleurX Peritoneal Catheter Drainage System for Vacuum-Assisted Drainage of Treatment-Resistant, Recurrent Malignant Ascites*. NICE Medical Technology Guidance MTG9. London: NICE.

National Institute for Health and Care Excellence (2015) Clinical knowledge summary – constipation. Available at: https://cks.nice.org.uk/constipation

Odeh M, Bassan H and Oliven A (1990) Termination of intractable hiccups with digital rectal massage. *Journal of Internal Medicine*, 227(2): 145–146.

O'Hara P (2017) The management of nutrition for palliative care patients. *Links to Health and Social Care*, 2(1): 21–38.

Omlin A et al. (2013) Nutrition impact symptoms in advanced cancer patients: frequency and specific interventions, a case-control study. *Journal of Cachexia, Sarcopenia and Muscle*, 4(1): 55–61.

Raijmakers NJH (2013) Bereaved relatives' perspectives of the patient's oral intake towards the end of life: a qualitative study. *Palliative Medicine*, 27(7): 665–672.

Regnard CFB and Tempest S (1993) *A Guide to Symptom Relief in Advanced Cancer*, 3rd edition. Manchester: Haigh and Hochland Ltd.

Regnard C (2005) Dysphagia, dyspepsian and hiccup. In Doyle D and Cherny N (eds) *Oxford Textbook of Palliative Medicine*. Oxford. Oxford University Press, pp. 468–474.

Reid C (1978) *A Primer of Human Neuroanatomy*. London: Lloyd-Luke.

Releg R and Releg A (2000) Case report: sexual intercourse as potential treatment for intractable hiccups. *Canadian Family Physician*, 46: 1631–1632.

Rosenberg SM (2006) Palliation of malignant ascites. *Gastroenterology Clinics of North America*, 35(1): 189–199.

Rowans Hospice (2011) *Policy and procedure for paracentesis*. Available at: https://www.palliativedrugs.com/download/110718_POLICY_AND_PROCEDURE_FOR_PARACENTESIS%20LOGO.pdf

Schwartz DB (2018) Nutrition support in palliative care. In Hickson M and Smith S (eds) *Advanced Nutrition and Dietetics in Nutrition Support*. Chichester: Blackwell Publishing, p.394.

Scottish Oral Nutritional Supplements Short Life Working Group (ONS SLWG) (2018) Guidelines for appropriate prescribing of oral nutritional supplements in adults (oral use). Available at: https://www.therapeutics.scot.nhs.uk/wp-content/uploads/2018/08/Gudelines-for-appropriate-prescribing-of-Oral-Nutritional-Supplements-in-adults.pdf

Scottish Palliative Care Guidelines (2019) Laxative medicines information chart. Available at: https://www.palliativecareguidelines.scot.nhs.uk/guidelines/symptom-control/constipation/Laxative-medicines-information-chart

Shaw C (2011) Nutrition and palliative care. In Shaw C (ed) *Nutrition and Cancer*. Chichester: Blackwell Publishing Ltd, 174.

Shaw C and Eldridge L (2015) Nutritional considerations for the palliative care patient. *International Journal of Nursing*, 21(1): 7–12.

Steger M, Schneemann M and Fox M (2015) Systematic review: the pathogenesis and pharmacological treatment of hiccups. *Alimentary Pharmacology and Therapeutics*, 42(9): 1037–1050.

Stern RM, Koch KL and Andrews PLR (2011) *Nausea: Mechanisms and Management*. New York: Oxford University Press.

Twycross R and Wilcock A (2001) Dysphagia. In *Symptom Management in Advanced Cancer*. Oxford: Radcliffe Medical Press, pp. 88–97.

Twycross R, Wilcock A and Stark Toller C (2009) *Symptom Management in Advanced Cancer*, 4th revised edition. Nottingham: Palliativedrugs.com Ltd.

Twycross R, Wilcock A and Howard P (eds in chief) (2017) *Palliative Care Formulary*, 6th edition. Nottingham: Palliativedrugs.com Ltd.

UK Oral Mucositis in Cancer Group (2015) Mouth care guidance and support in cancer and palliative care. Available at: http://ukomic.co.uk/documents/UK_OM_Guidelines.pdf

Watson M (2005) Palliation of head and neck. In *Oxford Handbook of Palliative Care*. Oxford: Oxford University Press, pp. 352–353.

Wilcox C (1995) Localization of an obstructing oesophageal lesion. Is the patient accurate? *Digestive Diseases and Sciences*, 40(10): 2192–2196.

Wright R and Ellis P (1997) Patient perception and localization of dysphagia – baseline study correlation. *Diseases of the Esophagus*, 10(3): 211–214.

Yingxue D et al. (2014) Interventions for dysphagia in oesophageal cancer. *Cochrane Systematic Review*, 2014(10): CD005048.

Young J (2019) An evidence review on managing constipation in palliative care. *Nursing Times*, 115(5): 28–32.

4.3   THE RESPIRATORY SYSTEM

Deans Buchanan with Alana Brown-Kerr, Emma Dymond, Lorna Frame and Fiona Reid

Learning Objectives

This section will enable you to understand:

- The epidemiology of respiratory symptoms related to palliative and end-of-life care;
- The mechanisms and palliative management of breathlessness
- The mechanisms and palliative management of cough
- The mechanisms and palliative management of respiratory secretions
- The mechanisms and palliative management of airway obstruction.

Scenario

Background

You are called to see Bilal, a 73-year-old man with metastatic lung cancer and concurrent severe chronic obstructive pulmonary disease (COPD) who has become very breathless. His wife is very distressed on the phone. She tells you that he was recently discharged from hospital to home and no oxygen was prescribed due to ongoing smoking. Full information is lacking but the hospital felt he would not benefit from further admissions should he deteriorate.

Key points

- Likely incomplete information but likely end-of-life care situation
- Need to consider place of care in context of symptoms, preferences and what support is available
- Non-pharmacological measures are useful including how you approach this situation (consider the ABCD approach, page 4),
- Medicines should be used to treat symptoms and associated distress.

Timeline

1 Upon arrival you find that Bilal feels very breathless, has had a persistent dry cough and is distressed.

2 The district nurse tells you there are subcutaneous 'just in case' medicines in the house, but they have not been used so far. He also has oramorph and lorazepam prescribed on an as-required basis, and had 5 mg oramorph 20 minutes ago. She tells you a 'Do not attempt cardiopulmonary resuscitation' (DNACPR) form is also in the house following the hospital discharge.

3 You take a brief history covering existing knowledge of condition and expectations since discharge from hospital.

4 A focused examination is carried out. His respiratory rate is 26 breaths per minute, and you measure his oxygen saturations and find them to be 84%.

5 ABCD – you ensure the patient and his wife feel you recognise the difficulty they face, that they have your full attention and that you will aim to help them at this time of distress. You are careful to find out their names and introduce yourself by name. You give reassurance that you will help settle the symptoms and distress.

Key considerations

- What are your options to palliate the distressing symptoms?
- When someone is 'sick enough to die' how do you assess when to escalate reversal interventions and when to escalate to end-of-life care approaches?

Epidemiology of Respiratory Symptoms

Respiratory symptoms are commonly experienced by those with palliative care needs and can have a significant impact on the quality of life and quality of death of those who experience them (Bausewein et al. 2013). The most common of these symptoms will be discussed in this chapter and include: breathlessness, cough, haemoptysis and respiratory secretions.

In many palliative care situations there will be more than one illness present or more than one cause of the symptom present (for example COPD is concurrent with the lung cancer in 40–70% of people (Young et al., 2009)). The causes of respiratory symptoms in those with palliative care needs can be considered in three main groups: primary lung disease (such as COPD, pulmonary fibrosis, pneumonia, lung cancers or pleural mesothelioma), secondary lung disease (such as pulmonary metastases, pleural effusion or pulmonary embolism) and extra-pulmonary diseases (such as heart failure, motor neurone disease or ascitic compression of the diaphragm) (Figure 4.3.1).

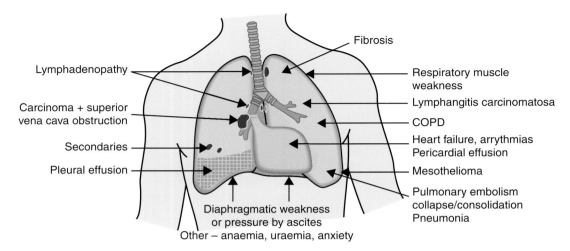

Figure 4.3.1 Common causes of respiratory symptoms in palliative care.

However, irrespective of the physical cause(s) of the respiratory symptom, managing the symptom experience can be approached through the palliative care model of 'total symptom' and a holistic approach can be taken to reduce the impact of that adverse experience. This approach includes reversing the reversible causes when wished and feasible but extends interventions beyond this on a concurrent basis when tackling the cause remains possible, or on an additive basis when maximal reversal therapies have been instituted. Framing this approach within the ABCD of Dignity ensures compassionate tone, good communication and purposeful shared decision making is promoted.

Breathlessness

Breathlessness or dyspnoea can be defined as 'a subjective experience of breathing discomfort that consists of qualitatively distinct sensations that vary in intensity', and that the 'the experience of dyspnoea derives from interactions among multiple physiological, psychological, social, and environmental factors, and may induce secondary physiological and behavioural responses' (Parshall et al., 2012). Within this definition there is a clear emphasis that breathlessness is a *subjective experience* and can only be perceived by the person experiencing it and therefore any adequate understanding of this symptom must include self-report.

There is an emerging differentiation between acute or transient breathlessness experience and the clinical syndrome of 'chronic breathlessness'. Chronic breathlessness syndrome is defined as 'breathlessness that persists despite optimal treatment of the underlying condition and that results in disability' (Johnson et al., 2017). Chronic breathlessness is highly prevalent in chronic progressive illnesses and affects >90% of people with lung cancer, COPD, interstitial lung disease and >80% of those living with heart failure (Moens et al., 2014).

An acute breathlessness crisis can occur in the context of chronic breathlessness or as a new event. When it occurs, underlying causes must be considered but it is suggested that it is most likely to occur when there are increased levels of underlying psychological, social or spiritual distress (Figure 4.3.2). If the context of this is within a setting or response that is lacking in preparation to address each of these domains then it enters a downward spiral. Acute breathlessness crisis can also occur without a readily identifiable physical change in condition, further highlighting the wider nature of the symptom experience, the role of educating those experiencing breathlessness and their carers to enable response and thinking through future events in advance (Mularski et al., 2013).

It is important to note that although reversing underlying pathology remains a key step in managing breathlessness, the experience of the symptom itself is not directly associated with severity of many conditions (for example not dependent on FEV1 in COPD). Like other symptoms, a complex array of factors can influence how breathlessness is experienced in terms of presence, severity and intensity.

Experience and impact

The language of breathing itself underlines the deep connection it has with life itself. Respiratory rate is a *vital* sign – it is essential for life. Life itself is bookmarked by the 'first breath' and the 'last breath'. The latin *'spiro' links* breath and spirit, and other cultural derivations are similar with psyche and pneuma (Greek), ruach and nedesh (Hebrew) and Qi (Chinese) all linking breath, spirit and soul (Macnaughton and Carel, 2016).

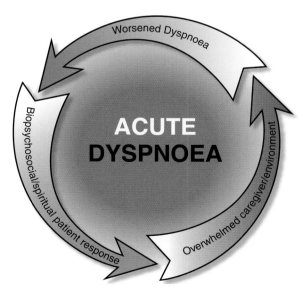

Figure 4.3.2   Dyspnoea crisis theoretical model.

Source: Reprinted with the permission of the American Thoracic Society. Copyright © 2019 American Thoracic Society. Originally published in Mularski et al. (2013).

Breathing is normally a subconscious activity. It is said when breathing is normal it is taken for granted; when breathing is not normal then nothing else matters. It is important to realise how challenging to adaptation and overwhelming a sense of breathlessness can be.

> Take a moment to think of your own breathing and bring it to attention to understand the move from subconscious to conscious experience. Then consider the presence of 'discomfort' with such breathing.

Breathlessness has a significant impact on the lives of those experiencing it, those within their social connections and those providing care to them. The impact occurs in multiple domains of life including physical, psychological, spiritual, social, practical and financial. Several studies have linked breathlessness with anxiety and depression. Carers suffer similar issues with distress, social isolation, and a feeling of helplessness. Individuals have individual experiences of the symptom and as such listening carefully to their experience will aid management (Bausewein et al., 2010).

There is evidence that although breathlessness is a core symptom experienced in several progressive conditions, there may be differences between the associated meanings which are applied. It has been reported that in cancer, breathlessness reminded people of their condition and their mortality despite any active anti-cancer treatments. In COPD an intrinsic feeling of guilt and the thought that it was self-inflicted was present and in motor neurone disease, breathlessness signalled life-threatening change (Gysels et al., 2011).

Within the definition of breathlessness, it is acknowledged that there are qualitatively distinct sensations that can be described. The increasing evidence around this area connects the descriptive words used against different causes of breathlessness. Examples include: a sense of 'air hunger' generated through raised CO_2, the 'work' or 'labour' of a rapid respiratory pattern, 'tightness' in the chest and not being able to get 'air in' or 'air out' with loss of elasticity in the respiratory response and airflow obstruction (Mahler et al., 2008). Listening carefully to the description aids assessment of the main mechanisms present and ensures the individual experience is heard, acknowledged and integrated into the therapeutic response.

Mechanisms

The neurophysiology of breathlessness is becoming clearer yet remains complex. At the heart of the experience of breathlessness is a disconnect between inspiration and expiration. The normal monitoring of effective respiration will recognise that there is a dissociation between intent (efferent signalling from respiratory centres of the brain) and results (afferent feedback). Such a mismatch can include altered mechanics of ventilation (for example emphysemic changes, extrinsic compression, muscular weakness), altered blood biochemistry (hypoxia, hypercapnia, acidosis) or other feedback processes. Neural integration of signals related to breathing experience occur in the cortico-limbic areas of the brain which are influenced by thoughts, emotions and meaning. This complexity means it is unlikely that a single intervention will be fully effective for breathlessness, instead several different interventions may be required (Fisher et al., 2009).

Assessment

Assessment approaches to breathlessness are outlined by the palliative care guidelines (Scottish Palliative Care Guidelines, 2020a):

- Undertake a holistic assessment using a multi-professional approach.
- Ask the patient to rate symptom severity and assess the level of associated distress/anxiety.
- Explore the patient's understanding of the reasons for breathlessness, fears, impact on functional abilities and quality of life.
- Clarify pattern of breathlessness, precipitating/alleviating factors and associated symptoms.
- Look for any potentially reversible causes of breathlessness, such as infection, pleural effusion, anaemia, arrhythmia, pulmonary embolism, bronchospasm or hypoxia (check oxygen saturation levels using pulse oximeter).
- Determine if treatment of the underlying disease is appropriate. Seek advice if in doubt.

It is important to understand the individual's own experience and to aim to improve the direct symptom experience. Consider the psychosocial environment and build capacity to manage it, understand the chronic breathlessness baselines and evaluate the nature of acute breathlessness crises and responses.

You should also assess for the presence and interaction of anxiety and fear associated with breathlessness. Keep in mind the breathing–thinking–functioning approach to management described below (Figure 4.3.3).

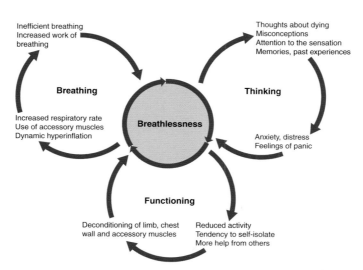

Figure 4.3.3   The breathing thinking functioning model.

Source: Spathis A (2017) The Breathing, Thinking, Functioning clinical model: a proposal to facilitate evidence-based breathlessness management in chronic respiratory disease (adapted from Booth et al., 2008).

The model is based on three predominant cognitive and behavioural reactions to breathlessness that, by causing vicious cycles, worsen and maintain the symptom. Considering each of the elements in the model allows you to tailor questions which lead to discussion of response and management.

Management

Meaningful improvement in breathlessness for the person experiencing the symptom may be a small change on a verbal rating score. Furthermore, aiming to achieve an outcome related to daily living experience may be more beneficial than a numerical gain on a symptom rating scale. This is often achieved using more than one approach to management of the symptom concurrently. Always consider non-pharmacological measures as part of the management plan and aiming for small initial incremental gain is effective. Be clear and positive about this (Kamal et al., 2012).

Non-pharmacological

Non-pharmacological intervention in a patient's breathlessness aims to reduce the work of breathing and to give patients confidence in managing periods of breathlessness.

Breathing control

For patients who are breathless, their breathing pattern sometimes alters and becomes very ineffective. This leads to muscles becoming tired, thus causing an increase in the work of breathing. Breathing control can encourage your patients to focus on how to breathe more easily, when they are relaxed but also when their breathing starts to change.

Recovery breathing: when feeling breathless, your patient should be encouraged to focus on a long breath out, instead of taking a deep breath in. This will lengthen the expiratory phase. Patients will intuitively want to breathe in more deeply to settle their breathlessness which only leads to further anxiety/panic as they are unable to achieve it. If you explain that they 'need to create space in their lungs for the air to come in' and support them to focus on the expiratory phase, you can bring significant relief. Giving patients an element of control in their breathing can help to reduce some of the anxiety around it.

Square breathing

Another technique which can be used in any setting and which can help with the concentrating on the longer expiration is square breathing or rectangular breathing. Focus on something square or rectangular in the room such as the window, TV or a picture.

Start by looking at the top left corner, breathe out as your eyes track along to the top right corner, then breathe in on the corner. Breathe out as your eyes track down to the bottom right corner, breathe in on the corner and then breathe out as you track along to the bottom left corner.

Keep continuing with this sequence around the square or rectangle until your breathlessness has eased.

Avoid attention on attempting to correct pursed lip breathing.

Fan

Handheld fans can help to reduce the sensation of breathlessness through the stimulation of the trigeminal nerve (Galbraith et al., 2010; Schwartzstein et al., 1987). There is clear evidence that air flow can offer meaningful relief of breathlessness (Swan et al., 2019).

Three-bladed fans are transportable, have no contraindications and are relatively inexpensive. From personal clinical experience and feedback from patients, handheld fans are invaluable in helping to manage breathlessness. They should ideally be held just a few inches from the face (unless the patient is claustrophobic) and may only need to be used intermittently at times when breathing is changing.

Positioning

When breathless, it can be helpful for the patient to get into a comfortable position to encourage their stomach and diaphragm to expand and encourage them to relax their chest muscles. Patients should be asked to breathe at the rate which they feel comfortable with. As they gain control of their breathlessness their breathing rate will slow. Any of the following positions can be used to ease breathlessness (Figure 4.3.4):

1. **Sitting leaning forward:** ask the patient to sit in a relaxed position with their arms resting gently on their thighs. Their knees should be shoulder width apart and they should allow their shoulders to drop downwards.
2. **Sitting with pillows**: ask the patient to sit on a chair and place a pillow on a high table in front of them. They can then lead forward and relax their head and arms on the pillow.
3. **Standing leaning back**: if your patient is standing and is unable to get to a suitable seat ask them to lean with their back against a wall and relax their neck and shoulders with their arms dropped to their side.
4. **Standing leaning forward**: the patient can stand with their arms and elbows resting on a surface such as a windowsill or kitchen worktop, so that they are supporting the weight of their upper body. Their forearms should be shoulder width apart and their chest relaxed.

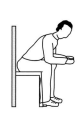
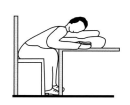
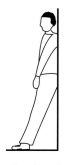
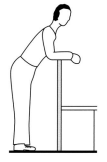

1. Sitting leaning forward
2. Sitting with pillows
3. Standing leaning back
4. Standing leaning forward

Figure 4.3.4   Positioning to relieve breathlessness.

Thinking

Breathless patients may have triggers of anxiety/panic which can themselves further trigger their breathlessness or worsen the period of breathlessness they may be experiencing.

Encouraging some form of relaxation can help. This can be through guided imagery or progressive muscular relaxation (encouraging your patient to tighten up muscles in their body and then fully relax them). There are many resources available to patients on the internet. Thinking positive statements such as 'I can manage this' or 'I have got through this before' can also be beneficial.

There may be misapprehensions about dying and some patients can be fearful about dying 'gasping for breath'. It can be useful to address such concerns with these patients.

Distraction is another technique which can aid in the 'thinking' aspect of breathlessness.

Functioning

Unassuming tasks can often become overwhelming and frightening for patients and may cause social isolation (Taylor et al., 2013). By encouraging patients to pace themselves throughout tasks, these can become more manageable:

- Eat and drink slowly with many rests – swallowing requires you to hold your breath
- Speak in small sentences
- When moving, remember about lengthening the breath out as you move
- If practical, sit down when getting dressed and undressed
- Put on a towelling robe after showering to dry yourself instead of exerting energy through using a towel
- Avoid bending
- Keep windows/vents open during tasks such as showering/washing

Pharmacological

The Scottish Palliative Care Guideline on managing breathlessness outlines pharmacological options of:

- Disease modifying therapies: identify and treat reversible causes where appropriate
- Opioids
- Steroids if breathlessness relates to lymphangitis or tumour-related airway obstruction
- Oxygen (within set criteria)
- Benzodiazepines (for treating anxiety within an anxiety–breathlessness cycle).

Opioids

Opioids, and specifically morphine, act to reduce the sense of unpleasantness associated with breathlessness. In a sense, they treat the discomfort of breathlessness. There are several meta-analyses that show benefit and a recent Cochrane Review confirms this, but with low-level evidence (Barnes et al., 2016). There is no strong evidence that nebulised opioids produce the same benefit.

Safety of the use of opioids has been confirmed in the short term (<6 weeks) in a variety of underlying conditions and up to a dose of around 30mg/day of morphine (Legrand et al., 2017).

Table 4.3.1 shows the dosing strategies for morphine that are given in the Scottish Palliative Care Guidelines.

Table 4.3.1 Pharmacological management of breathlessness with morphine.

Patient	Drug	Route	Dose	Frequency
Has not taken opioid before and is able to take oral medication	Immediate release morphine	Oral	2 mg; titrate by 30–50% if required and tolerated	Every 4 to 6 hours and/or hourly as required
Has not taken opioid before and is unable to take oral medication	Morphine sulfate	Subcutaneous	1–2 mg; titrate as above	Every 4 to 6 hours and/or 2 hourly as required
Takes an opioid regularly for pain control	<ul><li>Use existing immediate-release breakthrough analgesic dose (oral if able, or subcutaneous bolus injection equivalent) for the relief of breathlessness</li><li>A maximum of six doses can be taken in 24 hours for all indications (pain, breathlessness and cough)</li><li>Titrate both regular and breakthrough dose according to response</li></ul>			
Is frail/elderly	Immediate release morphine	Oral	1–2 mg; titrate cautiously	Every 6 to 8 hours as required; monitor closely for side-effects
Has impaired renal function	Refer to 'renal end-of-life care' guidelines (Scottish Palliative Care Guidelines, 2021a)			
Cannot tolerate morphine due to side-effects	Second-line opioids may be effective for breathlessness (refer to 'choosing and changing opioids' guidelines (Scottish Palliative Care Guidelines, 2021b)			
Has ongoing breathlessness	Try modified release (long-acting) oral morphine, plus a 4 hourly equivalent dose of immediate release oral morphine as required for additional episodes of breathlessness			

Source: Scottish Palliative Care Guidelines, 2020a.

Steroids

Steroids may be useful to treat breathlessness associated with specific issues of superior vena cava obstruction (SVCO) (see Chapter 8 – Palliative Care Emergencies), cancer-related lymphangitis, cancer-related airway obstruction and other conditions with reversible airflow obstruction. Dosing as follows:

● Trial dexamethasone 8–16 mg daily (orally or parenterally) for lymphangitis or tumour-associated airway obstruction. Consider gastric protection.

● Unless starting emergency therapy, give steroids in the morning.

● Review after 1 week, and reduce gradually to lowest effective dose where appropriate.

● If no effect, stop treatment. If continuing, ensure blood sugars are monitored to detect steroid-related hyperglycaemia.

Oxygen for management of breathlessness in palliative care

● Consider oxygen therapy for breathlessness in refractory dyspnoea (malignant or non-malignant cause) only in hypoxic patients with an oxygen saturation of less than 92% (Scottish Palliative Care Guidelines, 2020a; Hardinge et al., 2015).

● Individual patient assessment needs to be considered to assess cause of breathlessness and risk versus benefits of oxygen therapy in different environments.

● Judgement should be used by the palliative care oxygen prescriber as to the complexities of any particular patient in relation to consideration for oxygen therapy and, in complex cases, seeking specialist respiratory advice and/or discussion with oxygen services.

● Consideration of oxygen therapy should also be in conjunction with consideration of other symptomatic pharmacological and non-pharmacological treatments for breathlessness as part of a holistic approach to management.

● There is often an inconsistent relationship between oxygen therapy, dyspnoea and hypoxia which should be considered when assessing response to oxygen as a treatment (NICE, 2016a).

● There is no evidence that oxygen is beneficial in patients without hypoxia.

Benzodiazepines

There is no evidence that benzodiazepines reduce the discomfort of breathlessness itself. Benzodiazepines have a considerable place when there is a strong anxiety or panic component associated with the breathlessness, but tolerance, addiction and the increased mortality risks associated with co-prescription of benzodiazepines and opioids must be considered within the clinical context. Consider as a third line option when symptoms are unresponsive to non-drug measures and opioids. Dosing as per the palliative care guidelines:

- Lorazepam (scored tablet) sublingual 500 micrograms, given 4 to 6 hourly as required (the Genus, PVL and TEVA brands are all blue, oblong, scored tablets and are suitable for sublingual use).
- Diazepam orally 2–5 mg at night, if there is continuous distressing anxiety.
- If oral or sublingual routes are not available, midazolam can be given subcutaneously at a dose of 2–5 mg, 4 to 6 hourly as required.

Cough

Experience and impact

Cough is a very common symptom reported in patients with lung cancer, affecting 70–80% of patients (Ahmedzai, 2004). Patients with non-lung cancer diagnosis also report cough as a troublesome symptom; in one study breathlessness issues were reported by 22% of patients with colon cancer, 26% with prostate cancer, 28% with ovarian cancer and 37% with breast cancer (Portenoy et al., 1994).

It is also a feature of a number of non-malignant diseases. Molassiotis et al. (2010) found that cough, breathlessness and fatigue form a cluster of interacting respiratory distress symptoms. Cough can have distressing effects on quality of life including sleep, continence, social functioning and depression and anxiety (Molassiotis et al., 2011). It may be an under-reported symptom in the presence of other symptoms including pain. In cases of lung cancer, chronic cough may be the presenting symptom and a daily reminder of the illness.

Mechanisms

Cough is a forced expulsive manoeuvre, usually against a closed glottis, which is associated with a characteristic sound (Morice et al., 2006). A cough is thought to be a protective manoeuvre to maintain airway cleanliness and patency, protecting the airways from entry of foreign material and removing debris and secretions.

The mechanism of cough involves three phases:

1. Inspiratory: inhalation of a large volume of air to lengthen the expiratory muscles.
2. Compression: simultaneous closure of the glottis and contraction of the expiratory muscles.
3. Expiratory: opening of the glottis, accompanied by a loud sound 'cough'.

The mechanism of cough is triggered by mechanical and chemical receptors, as well as inflammatory stimuli. The sound of a cough is a result of turbulent airflow in the airways and larynx during the expiratory phase. The sound of a cough is often further described as 'wet' or 'dry'. A wet cough describes a cough with associated respiratory secretions, and a dry cough is defined by the absence of secretions.

Assessment

Assessment of cough in a palliative care patient should include the following (Scottish Palliative Care Guidelines, 2020b; NICE CKS, 2015):

- Severity, frequency, timing and duration of the cough
- Pattern and character of the cough
- Precipitating or relieving factors
- Current medications
- The impact of the person's quality of life, functional abilities and their family or carers. Ask directly about fears (including the fear of choking)
- Any associated symptoms: sputum production, blood in the sputum (haemoptysis), nasal discharge, breathlessness or chest pain
- Examine for signs of stridor (suggesting SVCO or tracheal obstruction), hoarse voice (suggesting recurrent laryngeal nerve palsy), evidence of wheeze (asthma/COPD) and signs of infection
- Consider imaging (chest x-ray or CT of the thorax)
- A number of validated questionnaires exist for cough as a symptom: Leicester Cough Questionnaire (LCQ) (Birring et al., 2003) and the Cough Specific Quality of Life Questionnaire (CQLQ) (French et al., 2002). However, these are not routinely used in clinical practice.

Causes

As shown in Table 4.3.2, the causes of cough can be categorised into those unrelated to cancer, or those either directly or indirectly related to cancer. It is important to consider the cause of the cough as this will guide treatment strategy. For some patients the underlying cause of their cough is not reversible and managing expectations of the degree of symptom control that may be achieved in this context is vital.

Table 4.3.2   Causes of cough in palliative care patients.

Unrelated to cancer	Directly related to cancer	Indirectly related to cancer
- Neuromuscular disease - Heart failure - Respiratory failure - Renal failure - Asthma - COPD - Gastro-oesophageal reflux - ACE inhibitors - Autoimmune disease - Infections and post-infectious - Pulmonary endometriosis - Immunocompromise	- Pulmonary parenchymal disease - Lymphangitis - Pleural effusion - Superior vena cava obstruction - Tumour microemboli - Pulmonary leukostasis	- Anorexia-cachexia syndrome - Aspiration - Pulmonary thromboembolism - Paraneoplastic syndromes - Radiotherapy sequelae - Chemotherapy-induced fibrosis - Chemotherapy-induced myopathy

Management

After careful assessment, we must consider if treatment of the underlying cause is appropriate/will be beneficial. For patients with a lung cancer diagnosis, the opinion of an oncologist should be sought as radiotherapy or steroids may be an option. Similarly, draining a pleural effusion or steroid treatment for lymphangitis may give symptomatic relief.

A dry cough may respond to humidified room air. In cases of suspected recurrent laryngeal nerve palsy, referral to the ear, nose and throat (ENT) department should be considered for vocal cord injection. The management of SVCO is covered already in this book. Ensure optimisation of inhaled therapy for asthma or COPD if present.

Moist cough can be caused by a number of conditions and appropriate management will depend on the cause (Table 4.3.3). Table 4.3.3 is adapted from the Scottish Palliative Care Guidelines, 2020b. In motor neurone disease, a weak, ineffective cough may be associated with excessive saliva production. An antisecretory agent such as hyoscine may help reduce salivation. Suction or a cough-assist machine are further options.

Multidisciplinary team (MDT) involvement (dietician and speech and language therapy) may be required if cough occurs after eating suggesting poor swallow and risk of aspiration.

Pharmacological

The evidence base for pharmacological interventions in the treatment of cough is poor. The 2015 Cochrane Review 'Interventions for cough in cancer' found 'an urgent need to increase the number and quality of studies evaluating the effects of interventions for the management of cough in cancer' (Molassiotis et al., 2015).

Antitussive therapy for dry cough is aimed firstly at suppressing the cough reflex. Simple linctus, available over the counter, can be effective for some patients. This is usually taken as 10 ml as required, maximum 4 times a day.

Table **4.3.3**   Management options for causes of productive cough.

Cause of productive cough	Potential treatment
COPD	Optimise inhaler therapies, consider steroids. Antibiotics if infection suspected
Infection or pneumonia	Consider antibiotics (if appropriate)
Tracheo-oesophageal fistula	Refer for consideration of stenting
Aspiration of saliva	Antimuscarinics/anticholinergics
Gastro-oesophageal reflux	Proton pump inhibitors (PPI) and prokinetic anti-emetic, such as metoclopramide
Cardiac failure	Optimise medical management

Source: Adapted from Scottish Palliative Care Guidelines, 2020b.

Morphine may also be used as an antitussive. The Scottish Palliative Care Guidelines (2020b) recommended starting at 2 mg immediate release 4 to 6 hourly as required in opioid-naive patients, before careful titration. Monitoring for side-effects and opioid toxicity is important. If a patient is already on morphine, they may use their current breakthrough dose for cough suppression as required. If these strategies are unsuccessful, referral to specialist palliative care for consideration of low dose methadone linctus as an antitussive may be appropriate.

Protussive therapy (to aid expectoration) should be the first strategy with a wet cough. This will usually be in nebulised form (nebulised saline, 5 ml four times a day) (Scottish Palliative Care Guidelines, 2020b).

Non-pharmacological

If it is a wet productive cough, refer to the information in the non-pharmacological management of respiratory secretions (see p. 183).

If the patient has a dry unproductive cough, the following suggestions/introductions can help to reduce their cough (Chamberlain et al., 2013; Hough, 2020). Some advice to pass on to the patient includes:

1. Tell yourself that you don't need to cough
2. Swallow
3. Take sips of very cold water; if ice is available, have ice in the drink
4. If safe to do so try to suck on a lozenge
5. Try breathing in the following way:
   - breathe slowly and with very shallow breaths
   - breathe in gently through your nose
   - breathe out through pursed lips.

Mechanical aids such as the Cough Assist machine can be beneficial when the patient has a weak cough related to degenerative neuromuscular disease.

Summary

Cough is a frequent, debilitating symptom which can cause psychological distress in the context of cancer and non-cancer diagnoses. The focus of management should be on determining the underlying cause and treating appropriately. Early honest discussion with the patient regarding the goals of treatment is important to manage expectations.

Respiratory Secretions

Experience and impact

Retained respiratory tract secretions develop towards the end of life and are one of the most common symptoms observed in the final stages alongside pain, breathlessness, nausea and agitation. They have been noted in 23–92% of dying patients in palliative care units (Wildiers et al., 2002; Ellershaw et al., 1995), and onset has generally been found to occur around 60–70 hours prior to death (Wildiers et al., 2002; Ellershaw et al., 1995; Bennett, 1996; Wildiers et al., 2008; Morita et al., 2000). Relatives have described secretions as 'gurgling' and 'bubbly' (Wee et al., 2006b), and they are often referred to as 'death rattle'. The literature suggests that the sound is produced when pooled secretions in the oropharynx and trachea, which the patient can no longer clear by expectorating or swallowing, vibrate with inspiration and expiration (Twycross et al., 1999). However, the exact pathophysiology is not fully understood, and research is limited by the emotional and logistical difficulties associated with conducting studies in a palliative care population (Clark et al., 2009).

Several attempts have been made to classify retained respiratory tract secretions. Bennett proposed type 1 and type 2 secretions, the former being largely salivary and the latter being largely bronchial in origin (Bennett, 1996), and Wildiers et al., believed 'real' death rattle to be due to non-expectorated, non-pathological secretions and 'pseudo' death rattle to be due to bronchial or other secretions in the context of pulmonary disease (Wildiers et al., 2002). More recently, Clark et al., described a three-step mechanism whereby secretions accumulate due to an inability to cough or swallow, which causes partial airway obstruction evidenced by gurgling respirations, and this in turn causes further secretions to be produced (Clark et al., 2009).

> While retained secretions at the end of life are often referred to as 'death rattle' in the literature, it is best to avoid this phrase when speaking to relatives. Instead, consider explaining secretions in terms of 'moistness in the chest' or phlegm that the patient is no longer able to clear because of their reduced responsiveness. Reassure relatives that secretions rarely appear to be a source of distress to patients, and enable them to express concerns or ask questions. It should be explained that little evidence exists for the management of secretions, but treatment options are available if necessary.

Risk factors

A number of factors have been studied in an attempt to establish whether or not they are associated with an increased risk of developing retained respiratory tract secretions.

Artificial hydration

There is considerable anecdotal evidence that artificial hydration leads to a higher susceptibility to death rattle, and one study found that symptom scores for bronchial secretions significantly increased when patients were given parenteral fluids amounting to 1,000 ml or more per day (Nakajima et al., 2013). However, the majority of studies have demonstrated no such relationship (Ellershaw et al., 1995; Morita et al., 2005).

Cerebral pathology

Patients with cerebral malignancies have been identified to be at greater risk of developing death rattle (Bennett, 1996; Morita et al., 2000), perhaps due to the loss of cough and swallow reflexes and the subsequent dysphagia (Bennett, 1996; Morita et al., 2004; Wildiers et al., 2002).

Pulmonary pathology

An association between pulmonary pathology and death rattle has also been demonstrated (Ellershaw et al., 1995; Morita et al., 2004; Morita et al., 2000). Patients with chest infections or inflammatory conditions of the lung may have excessive bronchial secretions due to reactive changes in the epithelium, and severe bronchorrhoea may occur in some primary lung cancers or cancers metastatic to the lung (Clark et al., 2009). Mucus is often viscous and difficult to clear, and cilia are lost in the presence of infection and inflammation, and together this results in airway narrowing and obstruction (Clark et al., 2009).

Neuromuscular disorders

Hypersalivation and impaired swallowing lead to excess secretions gathering in the upper airways, again resulting in narrowing and obstruction (Clark et al., 2009). Patients with respiratory weakness due to neuromuscular disorders already have impaired compensatory mechanisms, and they are therefore at increased risk of developing death rattle (Clark et al., 2009).

Final midazolam dose

A recent study found that midazolam at a dose of 20 mg or more in 24 hours was associated with an increased likelihood of death rattle occurring (Kolb et al., 2018). When given at the end of life, it is possible that midazolam results in relaxation of the muscles involved in coughing and swallowing and thereby decreases the ability to clear secretions (Back et al., 2001). However, the statistical model used in the study cannot attribute causality (Kolb et al., 2018).

Anticholinergic load

Many drugs used in palliative care have anticholinergic properties. The cumulative effect of one or more medications with anticholinergic properties is called the anticholinergic load or burden (Fox et al., 2011), and Agar et al. found that the anticholinergic load of palliative patients increased over time, especially at the end of life (Agar et al., 2009). While anticholinergic (antimuscarinic) medication is used as the primary treatment for death rattle, one study demonstrated that higher anticholinergic load might increase the risk of death rattle developing (Sheehan et al., 2011), and another study found that the anticholinergic properties of medications were not protective against death rattle (Kolb et al., 2018).

Assessment

It is important to differentiate clinical scenarios in which respiratory tract secretions are a sign of impending death from those in which a more active approach may be appropriate (Clark et al., 2009). This involves assessing for other indications that the individual may be imminently nearing end of life, such as reduced consciousness, reduced mobility and reduced oral intake in the context of a known life-limiting illness. In terminally ill patients who do not appear to be imminently nearing end of life, likely prognosis should be considered alongside the potential benefits and burdens of any investigations and interventions.

There is no standardised tool to assess death rattle or to measure the intensity of secretions (Clark et al., 2009). In some research studies, noise scores – simple numeric or verbal scores of intensity – have been used (Wildiers et al., 2008; Back et al., 2001), although the majority have relied on single observer scores with the inherent issue of inter-observer bias (Clark et al., 2009); in day-to-day practice, interventions are largely initiated as subjective responses to the clinical situation (Clark et al., 2009).

Management

Non-pharmacological

Non-pharmacological management is generally recommended in the first instance. If patients are well enough, respiratory exercises with a physiotherapist may help to clear secretions from the airways (Regnard et al., 1998); in more poorly patients, passive repositioning to a lateral or upright position may aid postural drainage (Bennett et al., 2002), or the Scottish Palliative Care Guidelines recommend a head down position (Scottish Palliative Care Guidelines, 2020c). Oropharyngeal suctioning can also be considered, although this may exacerbate secretions in some cases (Scottish Palliative Care Guidelines, 2020c). No studies have documented the efficacy of non-pharmacological interventions at the end of life (Wee et al., 2008). While the reduction or cessation of parenteral fluids is a contentious issue, close monitoring of patients who are receiving parenteral fluids is certainly advisable.

Mucus clearance techniques would require referral to a physiotherapist. Physiotherapy services are usually available in the community as well as the hospital setting, dependent on local resources.

Positioning the patient comfortably and appropriately for aiding secretion clearance can be beneficial. Alternative side lying can be the most effective, if tolerated by the patient.

Active cycle of breathing (ACBT) and autogenic drainage (Agostini et al., 2007) are the most common techniques utilised to aid mucus clearance. In these situations, the techniques will often have to be modified, as frequently the patient will not have full concentration or stable airways. However, for patients who are fully alert and distressed by their secretions, these techniques can bring significant relief.

Pharmacological

Pharmacological interventions are available if conservative measures are ineffective. If patients remain able to cough, but sputum is tenacious, regular nebulised saline (5 ml of 0.9% sodium chloride four times daily) and a mucolytic agent (for example carbocisteine 750 mg orally three times daily) may help to aid expectoration (Regnard et al., 1998). In the case of secretions caused by respiratory infection, antibiotics may be appropriate if there are distressing symptoms – such as profuse, purulent sputum – and if the patient is willing and able to take oral medications (Regnard et al., 1998); antibiotic choice should be guided by local policy. In very ill patients, antibiotics do not greatly alter the course of events, and symptoms can be palliated in other ways (Regnard et al., 1998).

As previously mentioned, death rattle can be managed with antimuscarinic medication which antagonises acetylcholine and thereby blocks parasympathetic activity, leading to decreased production of airway secretions (Prommer, 2013). It has been suggested that antimuscarinic antisecretory drugs should be given promptly because they have little effect on secretions that have already developed (Twycross et al., 2017), and type 2 and 'pseudo' death rattle are said to be less likely to respond to antimuscarinic medications compared to type 1 and 'real' death rattle (Bennett, 1996; Wildiers et al., 2002).

The Scottish Palliative Care Guidelines (Scottish Palliative Care Guidelines, 2020c) recommend the following for the treatment of death rattle:

- First line: hyoscine butylbromide subcutaneously 20 mg, hourly as required (up to 120 mg/24 hours)
- Second line: glycopyrronium bromide subcutaneously 200 micrograms, 6 to 8 hourly as required
- Third line: hyoscine hydrobromide subcutaneously 400 micrograms, 2 hourly as required

All of these medications can be given as bolus injections or as a continuous subcutaneous infusion.

The efficacy of hyoscine butylbromide, glycopyrronium and hyoscine hydrobromide appears to be similar (Hughes et al., 2000), and indeed a Cochrane Review found no conclusive evidence of one drug being superior to another (Wee et al., 2008). The Review also found that no intervention was superior to placebo in the treatment of death rattle, and yet anticholinergic drugs may cause a dry mouth, urinary retention, visual disturbance and, occasionally, confusion (Wee et al., 2008).

While the majority of patients are semi-conscious or unconscious when they develop retained respiratory tract secretions and do not generally appear to be troubled by them, treatment is often initiated due to the perceived distress of relatives or carers. It is important to establish if distress is a real issue because most patients are not able to consent to intervention or report adverse effects, such as discomfort from suctioning or an excessively dry mouth from antimuscarinic drugs (Wee et al., 2006a).

It is widely presumed that relatives and carers are distressed by the sound of retained respiratory tract secretions. However, two studies by Wee et al. have demonstrated that this is not always the case. One study found that five of twelve relatives expressed explicit negative feelings about hearing 'death rattle' (Wee et al., 2006a) while the other found that ten of seventeen relatives were distressed by it (Wee et al., 2006b). Distress was often associated with concerns about the patient suffering (Wee et al., 2006a) or, more specifically, drowning or choking, a fear that was reinforced by witnessing fluid dribble from their loved ones' mouths (Wee et al., 2006b). On the other hand, some relatives stated that they had not been 'bothered' by the sound, and others regarded it as a helpful or even comforting indicator of impending death (Wee et al., 2006a). Careful exploration regarding the effect on relatives and carers of hearing retained respiratory tract secretions should therefore take place, and any decision to commence active management should be made thoughtfully (Wee et al., 2006a).

The Cochrane Review concluded that it is difficult to take a passive approach to death rattle in the face of heightened emotions at the end of life, and some treatments may be worth trying. However, patients need to be closely monitored for lack of benefit and adverse effects in order that futile or burdensome treatments can be discontinued (Wee et al., 2008).

Care of relatives

A better understanding of relatives' and carers' perceptions of retained respiratory tract secretions should allow healthcare professionals to direct their explanations and interventions more effectively (Wee et al., 2006a) and to dispel any unwarranted fears (Wee et al., 2006b); clear explanations may obviate the need for treatments that, at present, are without proven efficacy and may have adverse effects (Wee et al., 2006b). One possible means of reassuring relatives and carers is by accompanying them to the bedside and observing and identifying with them signs that indicate whether or not the patient is comfortable, placing particular emphasis on addressing concerns about drowning and choking (Wee et al., 2006b).

Respiratory Obstruction

Experience and impact

In patients with advanced malignancy affecting either lower or upper airways, the concept of airway obstruction can be a frightening prospect and one that needs to be treated as effectively as possible to alleviate distressing symptoms. In patients where obstruction is a possibility consideration should be given to having an established management plan involving the patient and significant others. When airway obstruction occurs as an end-of-life emergency and interventional treatments are not appropriate, it is important to treat acute respiratory distress swiftly to minimise the impact on both the patient and carers.

Mechanisms

Airway obstruction can affect upper or lower airways and in complete obstruction is a clinical emergency. Careful assessment of the patient is required to ascertain the cause of the obstruction to best guide appropriate management.

In upper airway obstruction it is important to identify if obstruction is from a foreign body, tumour causing extrinsic/intrinsic compression, secretions or another cause.

In lower airway obstruction the mechanism can be due to tumour, lymphadenopathy or underlying conditions such as chronic obstructive pulmonary disease, asthma or mucous plugging.

Assessment

It is important to properly assess the patient to achieve the best management plan moving forward. This will require review of the patient's diagnosis, co-morbidities, current medications, recent investigations, presenting history and examination. The important factors to consider are:

- Is this upper or lower airway obstruction? Look for clinical signs such as stridor in upper airway obstruction.
- Is the patient likely to have endobronchial obstruction/superior vena cava obstruction? Is further investigation of this appropriate?
- What is the patients' disease trajectory, expected prognosis and current performance status?
- Are there any previously discussed wishes/management plans around airway obstruction?
- Should the patient be in the last days of life and obstruction appears to be the terminal event, are there previously made anticipatory care or management plans.

Management

The treatment of airway obstruction will depend on the underlying cause, the patient's fitness and the patient's wishes.

Patients newly presenting with a mediastinal mass causing airway compromise should be investigated and treated as per local guidance with early discussion involving a respiratory physician, oncologist/haematologist, and anaesthetist as appropriate. This group of patients are not specifically covered in this chapter as they usually have a more active course of treatment.

Non-pharmacological

NICE and SIGN recommend early discussion with oncology/respiratory specialists to consider, in line with patient performance status, disease and wishes, palliative interventions such as:

For endobronchial obstruction –

- Consideration of external beam radiotherapy or endobronchial debulking or stent if endobronchial obstruction is impending (NICE, 2019).

For superior vena cava obstruction (SVCO) –

- In small cell lung cancer, systemic anticancer treatment (SACT) or radiotherapy with consideration of stenting for ongoing SVCO (SIGN, 2014).
- In non-small cell lung cancer, SACT/radiotherapy also for consideration but could consider primary treatment with stenting (SIGN, 2014).

In patients with head and neck cancers there may be some occasions in which radiotherapy, chemotherapy or surgery may be considered to improve quality of life in discussion with an ear, nose and throat consultant (Cocks et al., 2016). The multidisciplinary team will discuss the patient's performance status, and benefit versus burden of treatment should be considered. Careful consideration and previous discussion, along with palliative care involvement, can help achieve the best management plan for these patients (NICE, 2016b). If tracheostomy is indicated or an anticipated future care need, then local protocols are needed to help support this. However, surgical intervention such as tracheostomy for life-threatening airway compromise may not be appropriate and focus may be on treating distressing symptoms as discussed in pharmacological management (Cocks et al., 2016).

Non-pharmacological aspects for managing a patient with airways obstruction may depend on the cause of the obstruction: for example if it is secretions causing the issue, the information found in the respiratory secretion section may help.

Positive expiratory pressure (PEP) therapy can assist patients to stabilise airways by preventing their collapse (Müllauer, 2013). Although this therapy can help, it is not readily available in every clinical setting. In its absence, the best way to encourage stabilisation is by teaching your patient to breathe with pursed lips. This can ease the breathing in the occurrence of acute airway obstruction but is not as effective as using a PEP system.

Psychosocial and spiritual support

Consideration should be taken of an individual's needs, with a holistic approach to management, providing support as appropriate in the care environment the patient wishes to be cared for. A change in care package may be required; consideration of equipment such as a hospital bed may improve comfort. Discussions around the current situation, management plan, acknowledging the anxieties around the patient's symptoms and supporting their significant others remains paramount in trying to achieve the patient's priorities for care (See Chapter 7 – Psychosocial and Spiritual Aspects of Palliative and End-of-Life Care for more information).

Pharmacological

If there is evidence of superior vena cava obstruction in patients with established cancer diagnosis, steroids may be used to temporarily palliate symptoms before other more definitive treatment options are considered (if appropriate). However, the evidence around use of steroids is lacking (Scottish Palliative Care Guidelines, 2020c).

Palliation of breathlessness should also include consideration of an appropriate opioid on an as-required basis for intermittent breathlessness or regularly for persistent dyspnoea in accordance with the Scottish Palliative Care Guidelines. In the case of airway obstruction, parenteral route of administration would be required.

Oxygen may offer some symptomatic benefit in hypoxic patients (NICE, 2016b).

If airway obstruction is likely to be a terminal event then it is important to also consider anticipatory prescribing (see Chapter 5 – Drugs and Medication, 'Anticipatory Medicines' (p. 247)) and holistic assessment of the patient to prioritise comfort in the last hours and days of life (also Chapter 13 – Caring for People in the Last Days and Hours of Life).

Benzodiazepines such as midzolam 5–10 mg IM or IV should be considered in acute severe respiratory distress, in last days of life, to help alleviate symptoms more quickly (Care in last days of life, Scottish Palliative Care Guidelines, acute respiratory distress) (Scottish Palliative Care Guidelines, 2020c).

Scenario Recap

Acute breathlessness is a terrifying symptom – ABCD provides a solid therapeutic foundation from which both breathlessness and associated distress can be managed with non-drug and drug measures. Recognising dying is important but so is recognising that uncertainty is a part of life and illness. The best decisions are based on good communication, gathering the available information about the situation, and the patient's wishes. It is useful to ask yourself whether 'someone is sick enough to die' and whether you should be discussing the normal dying process with them and their family, if this has not already been done. Be positive in your approach to the escalation of end-of-life care. Do not use negative language of 'withdrawal of care' or 'not for'. Be clear that, in line with the principles of end-of-life care, the goal is to provide care that aims to support the person and their family:

1. Ensure optimal positioning for breathing; if the patient has a fan ensure airflow is provided; give medication for dyspnoea (opioid) and medication for fear (either lorazepam or midazolam). Allow time for medicines to provide relief and repeat if necessary.

2. If immediate acute breathlessness symptoms respond to first actions then discuss options with the patient and/or partner. Check the partner's expectations and understanding of the current situation, including the DNACPR form and previous anticipatory care planning discussions.

3. Discuss the patient's preferred place of care. If there is a wish to remain at home then ensure that an appropriate care package and medication is in place. Consider continuous subcutaneous infusion for symptom control. Ensure contact numbers are available and clear for the patient and his family. If admission is wished then seek this via the palliative care unit or hospital.

4. If there are no reversible acute issues, then recognise that the patient is likely to be at end of life. Take this opportunity to talk about other normal changes that can occur in the dying process, such as altered breathing patterns and pauses in breathing. Ensure the family feels supported, has the right contacts, and that clear information is available on electronic systems, and renew medicine supplies. Ensure this is underpinned by an ABCD approach to care.

References

Agar M et al. (2009) Changes in anticholinergic load from regular prescribed medications in palliative care as death approaches. *Palliative Medicine*, 23(3): 257–265.

Agostini P and Knowles N (2007) Autogenic drainage: the technique, physiological basis and evidence. *Physiotherapy*, 93(2): 157–163.

Ahmedzai SH (2004) Cough in cancer patients. *Pulmonary Pharmacology and Therapeutics*, 17(6): 415–423.

Back IN et al. (2001) A study comparing hyoscine hydrobromide and glycopyrrolate in the treatment of death rattle. *Palliative Medicine*, 15(4): 329–336.

Barnes H et al. (2016) Opioids for the palliation of refractory breathlessness in adults with advanced diseases and terminal illness. *Cochrane Database of Systematic Reviews*, 3: 1465–1858

Bausewein C et al. (2010) Individual breathlessness trajectories do not match summary trajectories in advanced cancer and chronic obstructive pulmonary disease: results from a longitudinal study. *Palliative Medicine*, 24(8): 777–786.

Bausewein C and Simon ST (2013) Shortness of breath and cough in patients in palliative care. *Deutsches Arzeblatt International*, 110(33–34): 563–572.

Bennett MI (1996) Death rattle: an audit of hyoscine (scopolamine) use and review of management. *Journal of Pain and Symptom Management*, 12(4): 229–233.

Bennett M et al. (2002) Using anti-muscarinic drugs in the management of death rattle: evidence-based guidelines for palliative care. *Palliative Medicine*, 16(5): 369–374.

Birring SS et al. (2003) Development of a symptom specific health status measure for patients with chronic cough: Leicester Cough Questionnaire (LCQ). *Thorax*, 58(4)**:** 339–343.

Booth S, Moosavi SH and Higginson IJ (2008)The etiology and management of intractable breathlessness in patients with advanced cancer: a systematic review of pharmacological therapy. *Nature Clinical Practice Oncology*, 5(2): 90–100.

Chamberlain S, Garrod R and Birring SS (2013) Cough suppression therapy: does it work? *Pulmonary Pharmacology and Therapeutics*, 26(5): 524–527.

Clark K and Butler M (2009) Noisy respiratory secretions at the end of life. *Current Opinion in Supportive and Palliative Care*, 3(2): 120–124.

Cocks H et al. (2016) Palliative and supportive care in head and neck cancer: UK national multidisciplinary guidelines. *The Journal of Laryngologoy and Otology*, 130(S2): S198–S207.

Ellershaw JE, Sutcliffe JM and Saunders CM (1995) Dehydration and the dying patient. *Journal of Pain and Symptom Management*, 10(3): 192–197.

Fisher J and O'Donnell D (2009) The clinical physiology and integrative neurobiology of dyspnea. *Respiratory Physiology and Neurobiology*, 167(1): 1.

Fox C et al. (2011) Anticholinergic medication use and cognitive impairment in the older population: the medical research council cognitive function and ageing study. *Journal of the American Geriatrics Society*, 59(8): 1477–1483.

French CT et al. (2002) Evaluation of a cough-specific quality-of-life questionnaire. *Chest*, 121(4): 1123–1131.

Galbraith S et al. (2010) Does the use of a handheld fan improve chronic dyspnea? A randomized, controlled, crossover trial. *Journal of Pain and Symptom Management*, 39(5): 831–838.

Gysels MH and Higginson IJ (2011) The lived experience of breathlessness and its implication for care: a qualitative comparison in cancer, COPD, heart failure and MND. *BMC Palliative Care*, 10(15): 1–10.

Hardinge M et al. (2015) Symptoms at presentation for treatment in patients with lung cancer: implications for the evaluation of palliative treatment. The Medical Research Council (MRC) Lung Cancer Working Party. *British Journal of Cancer.* 71(3): 633–36.

Hough A (2020) Respiratory Physiotherapy: Patient Leaflets. Available at: www.alexhough.com/patient-leaflets

Hughes et al. (2000) Audit of three antimuscarinic drugs for managing retained secretions. *Palliative medicine*, 14(3): 221–222.

Johnson MJ et al. (2017) Towards an expert consensus to delineate a clinical syndrome of chronic breathlessness. *European Respiratory Journal*, 49(5): 1–8.

Kamal AH et al. (2012) Dyspnea review for the palliative care professional: treatment goals and therapeutic options. *Journal of Palliative Medicine*, 15(1): 106–114.

Kolb H et al. (2018) A retrospective medical records review of risk factors for the development of respiratory tract secretions (death rattle) in the dying patient. *Journal of Advanced Nursing*, 74(7): 1639–1648.

LeGrand SB et al. (2017) Opioids, respiratory function, and dyspnea. *The American Journal of Hospice and Palliative Care*, 20(1): 57–61.

Macnaughton J and Carel H (2016) Breathing and breathlessness in clinic and culture: using critical medical humanities to bridge epistemic gap. In Whitehead A et al. (eds) *The Edinburgh Companion to the Critical Medical Humanities.* Edinburgh: Edinburgh University Press, pp. 294–309.

Mahler DA and Baird JC (2008) Are you fluent in the language of dyspnea? *CHEST*, 134(3): 476–477.

Moens K et al. (2014) Are there differences in the prevalence of palliative care-related problems in people living with advanced cancer and eight non-cancer conditions? A systematic review. *Journal of Pain and Symptom Management*, 48(4): 660–677.

Molassiotis A et al. (2010) A qualitative exploration of a respiratory distress symptom cluster in lung cancer: cough, breathlessness and fatigue. *Lung Cancer*, 71(1): 94–102.

Molassiotis A et al. (2011) The experience of cough in patients diagnosed with lung cancer. *Support Care Cancer* 19(12): 1997–2004.

Molassiotis A et al. (2015) Interventions for cough in cancer. *Cochrane Database of Systematic Reviews*, 5: CD007881.

Morice AH, McGarvey L and Pavord I (2006) Recommendations for the management of cough in adults, *Thorax*, 61: i1–i24.

Morita T et al. (2000) Risk factors for death rattle in terminally ill cancer patients: a prospective exploratory study. *Palliative Medicine*, 14(1): 19–23.

Morita T et al. (2004) Measuring the quality of structure and process in end-of-life care from the bereaved family perspective. *Journal of Pain and Symptom Management*, 27(6): 492–501.

Morita T et al. (2005) Association between hydration volume and symptoms in terminally ill cancer patients with abdominal malignancies. *Annals of Oncology*, 16(4): 640–647.

Mularksi RA et al. (2013) An official American Thoracic Society Workshop report: assessment and palliative management of dyspnea crisis. *Annals of the American Thoracic Society*, 10(5): 98–106.

Müllauer E (2013) Respiratory symptoms: dyspnoea/breathlessness from airway obstruction and impaired oxygen capacity in *Potential and Possibility: Rehabilitation at end of life*. Munich: Elsevier Urban & Fischer: 62–69.

Nakajima N, Hata Y and Kusumuto K (2013) A clinical study on the influence of hydration volume on the signs of terminally ill cancer patients with abdominal malignancies. *Journal of Palliative Medicine*, 16(2): 185–189.

NICE (2016a) Palliative care – dyspnoea. Available at: https://cks.nice.org.uk/palliative-care-dyspnoea

NICE (2016b) Cancer of the upper aerodigestive tract: assessment and management in people aged 16 and over. Available at: https://www.nice.org.uk/guidance/ng36

NICE (2019) Lung cancer: diagnosis and management. Available at: https://www.nice.org.uk/guidance/ng122

NICE CKS (2015) Palliative care – cough. Available at: https://cks.nice.org.uk/palliative-care-cough

Parshall MB et al. (2012) An official American Thoracic Society statement: update on the mechanisms, assessment, and management of dyspnea. *American Journal of Respiratory and Critical Care Medicine*, 185(4): 435–452.

Portenoy RK et al. (1994) Symptom prevalence, characteristics and distress in a cancer population. *Quality of Life Research*, 3(3): 183–189.

Prommer E (2013) Anticholinergics in palliative medicine: an update. *The American Journal of Hospice and Palliative Care*, 30(5): 490–498.

Regnard CFB and Tempest S (1998) *A Guide to Symptom Relief in Advanced Disease*, 4th edition. Cheshire: Hochland and Hochland Ltd.

Schwartzstein RM et al. (1987) Cold facial stimulation reduces breathlessness induced in normal subjects. *The American Review of Respiratory Disease*, 136(1): 58–61.

Scottish Palliative Care Guidelines (2020a) Breathlessness. Available at: https://www.palliativecareguidelines.scot.nhs.uk/guidelines/symptom-control/breathlessness.aspx

Scottish Palliative Care Guidelines (2020b) Cough. Available at: https://www.palliativecareguidelines.scot.nhs.uk/guidelines/symptom-control/Cough.aspx

Scottish Palliative Care Guidelines (2020c) Care in the Last Days of Life. Available at: https://www.palliativecareguidelines.scot.nhs.uk/guidelines/end-of-life-care/Care-in-the-Last-Days-of-Life

Scottish Palliative Care Guidelines (2021a) Renal Disease in the Last Days of Life. Available at: https://www.palliativecareguidelines.scot.nhs.uk/guidelines/end-of-life-care/renal-disease-in-the-last-days-of-life.aspx

Scottish Palliative Care Guidelines (2021b) Choosing and Changing Opioids. Available at: https://www.palliativecareguidelines.scot.nhs.uk/guidelines/pain/choosing-and-changing-opioids.aspx

Sheehan C et al. (2011) A retrospective analysis of primary diagnosis, comorbidities, anticholinergic load, and other factors on treatment for noisy respiratory secretions at the end of life. *Journal of Palliative Medicine*, 14(11): 1211–1216.

SIGN (2014) Management of lung cancer. Available at: https://www.sign.ac.uk/media/1075/sign137.pdf

Spathis A et al. (2017) The Breathing, Thinking, Functioning clinical model: a proposal to facilitate evidence-based breathlessness management in chronic respiratory disease. NPJ *Prim Care Resp Med* 27: 27.

Swan F et al. (2019) Airflow relieves chronic breathlessness in people with advanced disease: an exploratory systematic review and meta-analyses. *Palliative Medicine*, 33(6): 618–633.

Taylor DH et al. (2013)The effect of palliative care on patient functioning. *Journal of Palliative Medicine*, 16(10): 1227–1231.

Twycross RG and Lichter I (1999)The terminal phase. In Doyle D, Hanke G and MacDonald N (eds) *Oxford Textbook of Palliative Medicine*, 2nd edition. Oxford: Oxford University Press.

Twycross R, Wilcock A and Howard P (2017) *Palliative Care Formulary* (PCF6), 6th edition (UK). Nottingham: Palliativedrugs.com Ltd.

Wee BL et al. (2006a) The sound of death rattle I: are relatives distressed by hearing this sound? *Palliative Medicine*, 20(3): 171–175.

Wee BL et al. (2006b) The sound of death rattle II: how do relatives interpret the sound? *Palliative Medicine*, 20(3): 177–181.

Wee B and Hillier R (2008) Interventions for noisy breathing in patients near to death (review). *Cochrane Database of Systematic Reviews*, 2008(1): CD005177.

Wildiers H and Menten J (2002) Death rattle: prevalence, prevention and treatment. *Journal of Pain and Symptom Management*, 23(4): 310–317.

Wildiers H et al. (2008) Treatment of death rattle in dying patients. *Belgian Journal of Medical Oncology*, 2(5): 275–279.

Young RP et al. (2009) COPD prevalence is increased in lung cancer, independent of age, sex and smoking history. *European Respiratory Journal*, 34(2): 380–386.

4.4 MENTAL HEALTH

Paul Brown with Joanna Franz, Holly McGuigan and Nicola Watt

Learning Objectives

This section will help you to:

- Understand the main clinical features of common psychiatric conditions in palliative patients
- Understand how to assess and diagnose these conditions
- Develop knowledge of the pharmacological and non-pharmacological management options
- Develop awareness of special clinical considerations in this patient group
- Develop knowledge of the common criteria for referral to specialist services.

Scenario

Background

You are a GP trainee working in the care of the elderly ward of a district general hospital. Jacqui is a 77-year-old female who has been transferred from the cardiology ward. She has suffered from cardiac failure for six years, and regularly attended her local cardiology outpatient clinic. She has complied well with treatment and investigations, but despite this her cardiac symptoms have steadily deteriorated, especially over the last two years. She now has marked exertional breathlessness and she can only walk very short distances. The cardiologists have optimised her treatment as far as possible during this admission and she has now been transferred to geriatric care. She has always been fiercely independent and was usually the person helping other people in the family when in trouble. The nurses do not know her well and after 48 hours of transferring to the ward, they ask you to see her because she appears withdrawn with low mood, poor nutritional intake and a lack of any spontaneous interaction with patients or clinical staff.

Key points

- It is crucial to obtain a corroborative history for a patient like this. People who know the patient well (close family, GP, carers) can be invaluable in describing how the symptoms evolved, how they affect the patient, time course, associated features and previous psychiatric history.

- Never assume that the patient's mental state is somehow explainable by the difficult predicament that they are in. Always search for diagnosable psychiatric illness and treat this fully as it can make a real difference to the patient's palliative care journey. Always retain a broad differential diagnosis and remember that psychiatric co-morbidity is common, for example depression and hypoactive delirium at the same point in time. Always document a basic psychiatric risk assessment (especially around suicide) and if any doubts, discuss with liaison psychiatry. Ask about psychotic symptoms which are often found in severe depression. If present, the patient will require additional medication.

- Keep an open mind. Psychiatric symptoms can be caused by medical disorder and from side-effects of certain medications, and medical disorder can be exacerbated by mental disorder. In this particular case, there are some features which could also suggest hypocalcaemia. Whilst somatic symptoms may be caused by depressive illness, this should never be assumed. Only a comprehensive assessment, physical exam, and investigations will clarify the situation. The treatment of mental illness in palliative care has an expanding evidence base and professionals should endeavour to offer patients the range of options available including pharmacotherapy, psychotherapy and, if needed, specialist liaison psychiatric referral.

Timeline

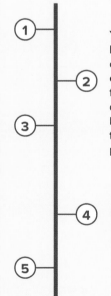

When you meet Jacqui, she appears lethargic, her sleep is poor and she constantly feels tense. She frequently murmurs that 'there's no point' and 'my time is up' throughout the day.

1

You take a comprehensive, precise, history of psychiatric symptoms coupled with a mental state examination. You speak to her heart failure nurse who advises that around a month before admission Jacqui no longer asked about her condition or treatment. She required increasing persuasion to take her medication.

2

Over the next day she becomes increasingly agitated, lies in her bed for most of the day and shows no interest in working with the nurses and allied health professionals.

3

Following assessment by the liaison psychiatric nurse she was started on antidepressants. On discharge home she benefited from a community psychiatric nurse who continued her cognitive behavioural treatment. Her psychosocial and spiritual needs were addressed in hospital and at home – this work was done alongside palliative care services who continued to review the patient at home.

4

You are really worried about her declining mental health and promptly make an urgent referral to liaison psychiatry services.

5

Key considerations

- What other clinical information would you need to know about this case?
- What is the differential diagnosis?
- What would make you suspect depression rather than a different cause for her presentation?
- If she is diagnosed with depression after your assessment, what are the management options?
- If you decide to prescribe medication, what would influence your choice of anti-depressant (bearing in mind the significant cardiac morbidity in this patient and the symptom profile of her mental disorder)?

Introduction

It is widely accepted that mental disorders are common in the palliative care population, yet they remain under-detected and under-treated. This chapter discusses the key details of psychiatric and neuropsychiatric disorders commonly encountered in palliative care patients. A major goal throughout the chapter is to provide clinical information in a way that is very accessible to the non-specialist which can be readily implemented in clinical settings to improve patient care.

Depression

Depression is a mood disorder with characteristic clinical features including (Rayner et al., 2010):

- Low mood, loss of enjoyment/interest and fatigue
- Additional features that may occur include loss of libido, poor (or increased) appetite, disturbed sleep, low self-esteem, feelings of guilt and worthlessness, agitation, slowing of thought and/or movement, poor concentration and suicidality.

Depression can be classified as follows:

- Mild depressive episode
- Moderate depressive episode
- Severe depressive episode (with or without psychotic features).

Estimates vary, but it is thought that around 20% of patients receiving end-of-life care experience major depressive disorder, with more experiencing depressive symptoms to various degrees (Rayner et al., 2011a). This can have a detrimental effect on quality of life. Depression deserves prompt identification and treatment.

Screening and assessment: finding cases

Patients may not volunteer their symptoms. Older patients in particular may not complain directly of low mood, presenting instead with agitation, loss of appetite and psychosomatic symptoms. You should have a low threshold for considering depression, particularly when other factors do not wholly account for the clinical picture easily. National guidelines suggest assessing for depression in this patient group. You should consider asking the following two questions (NICE, 2009):

- During the last month have you often been bothered by feeling down, depressed or hopeless?
- During the last month have you often been bothered by having little interest or pleasure in doing things?

Enquire further if the answer is 'yes' to either question.

The PHQ-9 screening tool is validated for use in primary care (though not specifically in this population) and could identify patients who require further assessment for mood disorder (Gilbody et al., 2007). Screening tools that emphasise physical symptoms may be less useful in depression with co-morbid physical disease.

Diagnosing depression

It is recognised that diagnosing depression in the palliative care population has its challenges (Rayner et al., 2011b). Some of the features of depression are shared with symptoms of end stage physical disease. These include sleep disturbance, loss of appetite and fatigue. Working out whether the degree of psychological distress is 'appropriate' to the life event of having a terminal diagnosis or whether it meets criteria for depressive disorder is not easy. Features such as low mood and feeling hopeless, feeling worthless or guilty, and suicidality may point to depression as the diagnosis, while physical symptoms of depression may be less useful. See Box 4.4.1 for some common examples of differential diagnoses in the palliative care setting.

Box 4.4.1 Differential diagnosis

Consider:
- Hypoactive delirium
- Adjustment disorder
- Anxiety disorders
- Hypercalcaemia
- Hypothyroidism
- Drugs that can cause depressive symptoms, for example L-dopa, beta blockers, interferon alpha, corticosteroids.

In the palliative population where pharmacological/medical complexity is the norm there may be difficulty in applying psychiatric criteria stringently; what matters most is the rapid identification of suspected depression/depressive symptoms and consideration of whether an evidence-based intervention can improve quality of life. Any identified contributing/causative factors should be corrected as far as possible.

Management

Depression in palliative care patients is treated similarly to the general population but there are special considerations, particularly in relation to physical co-morbidities and drug interactions.

- Mild depression – antidepressants are not recommended by NICE as first-line treatment; consider non-pharmacological management (NICE, 2018).
- Moderate/severe depression – consider antidepressant medication in addition to non-pharmacological measures.

Non-pharmacological management

- Optimise physical symptom control (for example pain, dyspnoea) as suboptimal symptom control can impact upon mood
- Consider guided self-help (NICE, 2018)
- Psychological therapies: consider cognitive behavioural therapy (CBT) or IPT (Inter-personal therapy) (NICE, 2018)
- Social support
- If the patient has a cancer diagnosis, resources such as Maggie's Centres offer practical, emotional and social support
- Spiritual care if appropriate to the individual.

Pharmacological management

No antidepressant has been shown to be more effective than another in this patient group (Scottish Palliative Care Guidelines, 2019).

Selective serotonin receptor inhibitors (SSRI)

An SSRI such as **sertraline, fluoxetine** or **citalopram** is usually first line (consult local formulary) in the treatment of depression. Sertraline is considered safe to use in cardiac disease.

Keep in mind that SSRIs are associated with:

- Increased risk of bleeding – especially if given to patients who are particularly at risk of this (for example GI ulcers or use of NSAIDS/anticoagulation). Consider gastro-protection in relevant patients.
- Increased risk of hyponatraemia.
- Serotonin syndrome (described in the management of agitation section). Patients who are on other medications with serotonergic properties (for example triptans, tramadol, other antidepressants) will be at higher risk of serotonin syndrome and need to be closely monitored. Where in doubt specialist advice should be sought.

In this patient group, drug interactions need to be considered.

Fluoxetine has many interactions (see the British National Formulary (BNF)) so may be less suitable in this population. Some relevant interactions are listed in Box 4.4.2. Dose adjustments may be required.

Box 4.4.2   Fluoxetine interactions

- Fluoxetine increases levels of amitriptyline and haloperidol
- Fluoxetine decreases efficacy of codeine, tramadol and tamoxifen
- Fluoxetine increases bleeding risk when used with NSAIDS or anticoagulants.

The MHRA advises against using **citalopram** in combination with other medications that have the potential to prolong the corrected QT interval (QTc) (UK Government, 2014) (see Box 4.4.3 for some examples; check the BNF for a full list). QTc prolongation increases the risk of serious cardiac arrythmias.

Box 4.4.3   Some medications that can prolong the QTc (avoid concomitant use with citalopram/escitalopram)

- Some antipsychotics, for example haloperidol, levomepromazine
- Some antibiotics, for example erythromycin, clarithromycin, moxifloxacin
- Some anti-arrhythmics, for example amiodarone
- Some anti-emetics, for example domperidone, ondansetron
- Some antihistamines
- Tricyclic antidepressants.

Escitalopram can also prolong the QTc. Electrolyte imbalances increase the risk of QTc prolongation when citalopram or escitalopram is given in that context.

Other medications

Mirtazapine

- May have a faster onset of action than some other antidepressants (Watanabe et al., 2011)
- Is known to have sedative effects and to increase appetite – this may be useful in this patient group
- There is also some evidence of an anti-emetic effect (Sung-Wan Kim et al., 2008).

Tricyclic antidepressants

- Amitriptyline – used for pain management and sedative effects, may be helpful in some patients
- Note that effective antidepressant dose is higher than that generally used in pain management.

Antipsychotics can be helpful in cases of depression with psychotic features (Wijkstra et al., 2015). These medications can also be used to augment the treatment of depression where there is treatment resistance.

When to refer

Consider referral to specialist care, for example Community Mental Health Team (CMHT) or liaison psychiatry in the following circumstances:

- Severe depression with or without psychosis
- Complex pharmacological approaches required (many other antidepressants are available that are generally prescribed with specialist direction)
- Treatment resistance
- Suicidality or other significant risks related to the mental state
- Diagnostic uncertainty.

Anxiety

Anxiety is a clinically important issue in palliative care. Spencer et al. (2010) using rigorous DSM-IV (a classification system of mental disorder widely used in the United States of America) criteria for anxiety disorders found that 7.6% of patients had a diagnosable disorder in the context of advanced cancer. Interestingly, they also demonstrated that anxiety disorder has a detrimental effect on the doctor–patient relationship which could hinder patient outcomes. Moreover, significant anxious symptoms falling short of formal psychiatric illness are also very common in palliative care, at rates of up to 48% (Stark et al., 2002).

Anxiety can of course be part of normal human experience, particularly before and during stressful or dangerous events and indeed fear is an ancient emotion that offers survival advantages.

In the palliative population, a certain degree of anxiety will be non-pathological and can be considered a natural response to life-limiting, serious illness. Having said that, it should never be 'assumed' that anxiety when present is simply a natural response especially when the level of anxiety is disproportionate to the situation, causes considerable distress or impairs functioning.

There are special challenges when assessing anxiety in palliative patients (for example, applying a judgement as to when anxiety is 'disproportionate' in the face of pervasive, incurable disease). More severe presentations are generally easier to differentiate.

Nonetheless, such challenges should not preclude high-quality assessment and treatment of anxiety in palliative patients. It should never be simply assumed that it is 'understandable' that the patient has anxious problems because of the palliative context; they may benefit from evidence-based intervention that could improve their quality of life.

Anxiety disorders have a set of clinical features which can be divided into three groups:

1. Physical symptoms – dyspnoea, palpitations, chest tightness, headache, dizziness, sweating, nausea, tremor, polyuria, insomnia and increased tension subjectively.

2. Mental state – dominated by worry, restlessness, hyper-vigilance, rumination, depersonalisation, derealisation, impaired concentration and various emotional changes (described below). Obsessions and compulsions will be prominent if the main diagnosis is obsessive-compulsive disorder (OCD).

3. Emotional (affective) component – fear, anger, irritability, apprehension, tearfulness, secondary dysphoria.

It is useful for the non-specialist to be aware of the common patterns and distribution of the above features because this guides diagnosis, and specific treatment can vary depending on the anxiety disorder diagnosed. Where in doubt, specialist advice should always be sought.

That said, in the palliative care population it can be difficult to rigorously apply stringent criteria in the diagnosis of psychiatric illness and what is more important is the prompt identification, investigation and treatment of suspected anxiety disorder or anxious symptoms per se, rather than getting too narrowly focused on which syndrome is present.

An example of some common syndromes that have anxiety as the prominent feature are detailed below to give the non-specialist an idea of how the nature and features of anxiety vary between recognised disorders.

Generalised anxiety disorder

Here the anxiety is characteristically free-floating fears, and worries about many different matters predominate (for example family, money, health, work). The anxiety is persistent, interferes with daily life is and not restricted to a particular situation.

Phobic anxiety disorders

The anxiety occurs in very specific circumstances. In specific phobia, common precipitants include blood, animals, needles and other medical associations. Anticipatory anxiety is common and this classically leads to the patient avoiding the stimulus. Social phobias indicate anxiety in social situations (for example eating in restaurants or public speaking) when the person feels observed by others and could be criticised by them. Patients with agoraphobia are anxious when outside home, in crowds or in situations where they cannot leave easily.

Panic disorder

The predominant feature of this disorder is panic attacks. Patients often worry about having another panic attack but in between episodes they do not have the free-floating anxiety seen in generalised anxiety disorder. Patients often complain of panic attacks but it is important to enquire exactly as to what they mean. A classical panic attack is a rapid onset of severe anxiety that is usually spontaneous without a specific trigger (although they can also occur in situations), lasting for 30–60 minutes with gradual resolution. Physical symptoms of anxiety predominate and include breathlessness, chest pain, palpitations, nausea, sweating, dizziness and flushes/chills. Cognitive accompaniments include a fear of dying, 'going crazy' or losing control. Patients experiencing recurrent panic attacks should be assessed for a diagnosis of panic disorder (or another mental illness).

Adjustment disorders

Although classified as stress-related disorders rather than anxiety disorders, adjustment disorder commonly presents with prominent anxiety (as well as low mood). The key feature is the direct link between the symptoms and a major stressor (a new life-limiting diagnosis or coping with a terminal illness) easily meet the criteria here. Patients can have anxiety, depression or a mixture of both falling short of the level required to diagnose either condition. Identifying this disorder facilitates a structured approach and offers a framework to work collaboratively with the patient to employ evidence-based interventions.

It is important to note that prominent anxiety of various kinds also occurs frequently in clinical depression. This condition should always be sought and treated. It is also common to find that the patient has a mixture of anxiety and depressive symptoms not neatly meeting the criteria of either syndromes; in such a scenario the diagnosis can be classified as mixed anxiety and depressive disorder. Patients may also have anxiety as part of another mental illness (for example psychosis or cognitive impairment) and so these features should also be considered.

Assessment

In common with psychiatry, palliative care embraces a holistic approach to assessment and treatment covering multiple dimensions.

For an anxiety disorder to be diagnosed, strictly speaking the anxiety must not be caused directly by any untreated medical disorders, organic brain disease or medications. Of course, challenges exist in applying psychiatric classifications to the palliative population and in palliative care, anxiety is often very multifactorial and frequently includes the above-mentioned factors as relevant aetiologies. In the palliative setting, a broad, pragmatic approach should be taken to the diagnosis and management of anxiety. In other words, if anxiety of any kind is present there should be, at a minimum, consideration of reversal of any causative factors and whether the patient would benefit from psychiatric treatment.

Box 4.4.4   Medical factors to be considered

- Untreated palliative symptoms – pain, breathlessness, nausea, sleep issues
- Cardiovascular disease – mitral valve disease, untreated arrhythmia, unstable cardiac failure, angina, hypotension
- Neurological disease – vestibular problems, temporal lobe epilepsy, cerebral tumour or metastasis, head injury, migraine, CNS infection, demyelination
- Endocrine/metabolic disease – hypoglycaemia, hypoparathyroidism, hypo/hypercalcaemia, phaeochromocytoma, hypo/hyperthyroidism, carcinoid tumour, hypo/hyperkalaemia
- Respiratory disease – Pulmonary embolism, uncontrolled COPD, uncontrolled asthma, pneumonia.

Patients may have a chronic pre-existing anxiety disorder which has been exacerbated by the palliative situation and treatment should be optimised as far as possible.

Initially, medical factors must be considered and excluded as correction of these may reduce or even ameliorate the anxiety. Examples are shown in Box 4.4.4 as well as a list of common medications implicated in anxiety in Box 4.4.5.

Box 4.4.5   Common medications implicated in anxiety

- Cardiovascular – anti-hypertensives and anti-arrythmics
- CNS drugs – anticonvulsants, antidepressants, antipsychotics, dopaminergic medication (for example Parkinson's disease medications), anticholinergics
- Respiratory – sympathomimetic drugs, for example alpha/beta agonists including salbutamol
- Miscellaneous – antibiotics, levothyroxine, caffeine excess, illicit substance misuse, NSAIDS, steroids
- Withdrawal states – alcohol, opioids, benzodiazepines, antidepressants.

Once medical factors have been addressed, assessment can proceed to attempting to identify the anxiety disorder present and how best to treat this.

A number of psychosocial dimensions are very important to consider in the assessment of anxiety. Clinical issues identified that may be at least in part driving the anxiety could allow these to be targeted via holistic interventions provided via psychological therapy and social/spiritual interventions. Box 4.4.6 lists some relevant psychosocial factors in anxiety.

<hr>

Box 4.4.6 Psychosocial factors relevant in anxiety

- Loss of social roles
- Loss of occupational roles
- Family and relationship dynamics
- Financial factors
- Existential issues
- Faith/religion/spirituality issues
- Uncertainty inherent in life-limiting serious illness
- Denial, guilt and anger
- Pre-existing personality traits – neuroticism, rigidity
- Unresolved issues from earlier trauma
- Alcohol and substance misuse.

A range of screening tools have been developed to help identify patients with significant anxiety who need more thorough assessment and treatment.

The Hospital and Anxiety Depression Scale ((HADS) Zigmond et al., 1983) is widely used and has demonstrated adequate psychometric properties in the palliative population (Vodermaier et al., 2009).

This scale can serve as a useful reminder for the non-specialist about some important features of anxiety (and depression). Screening tools can act as a primer for more detailed assessment and possible specialist referral.

The HADS can objectively score depressive and anxiety symptoms with 0–7 representing a normal score.

Management

The management of anxiety can be divided into pharmacological and non-pharmacological approaches.

Drug treatments would be more likely to be tried if the anxiety was severe, disabling and not responding to the range of non-pharmacological measures or if there is a strong patient preference for this approach. Drug treatments can be combined with psychological approaches and at least in some patients this may offer the best chance of achieving good outcomes, as is the case with depression.

In a significant number of patients (especially in those with milder anxiety problems) psychological therapy is strongly preferred as the initial approach for anxiety disorder. In the palliative population, considering patient fitness and access to therapies, treatment should be pragmatic and focused on improving quality of life when considering the range of pharmacological and psychological options.

Pharmacological

A recent Cochrane Review (Candy et al., 2012) concluded that there is insufficient evidence to make formal recommendations regarding pharmacological treatments for anxiety in palliative patients.

There is, however, a good evidence base for drug treatments in anxiety disorders in the non-palliative population and although there may be difficulties translating this to the palliative population, paucity of evidence should not stop a pharmacological trial if it can help improve quality of life.

Patients with a prognosis of days to weeks

In this scenario it would be practical to select a benzodiazepine, usually lorazepam, diazepam or midazolam.

The common problems with benzodiazepines are widely known (for example falls, ataxia, confusion, dependence) although these factors may be less of a concern for patients with a very short prognosis. It is worth mentioning that dependence is markedly more likely in patients with pre-existing personality disorders or addiction problems.

Patients with a prognosis of months or more

The usual initial treatment would be a trial of antidepressant therapy, with the SSRIs (selective serotonin reuptake inhibitors) being the first-line choice. Antidepressants have demonstrated efficacy in anxiety disorders even when there is no depression.

A typical selection would be sertraline, fluoxetine or citalopram. There are many SSRIs and each has their own set of advantages and disadvantages; prescribers should consult the BNF or obtain psychiatric advice if there are any doubts.

The SSRI may have to be combined with a benzodiazepine, at least initially as efficacy for treating anxiety can take several weeks with an SSRI and efficacy may only be seen at higher doses. If a benzodiazepine is also prescribed, use should be limited to a maximum of four weeks in the vast majority of patients. There is a small subgroup of patients with severe, intractable anxiety who may need longer term treatment with a benzodiazepine; psychiatric advice can be sought in this scenario.

It is important to encourage the patient to persevere with SSRI treatment and patients need to understand that the anti-anxiety effect will take several weeks to achieve on SSRIs. Patients should also be warned not to stop these medications abruptly and any reduction needs to be under medical supervision (as is also the case with benzodiazepines).

Box 4.4.7 lists some examples of other pharmacological options that would usually be prescribed after taking psychiatric advice. This is to illustrate that a wide range of treatment options (pharmacological and non-pharmacological) exist for patients and awareness of this should lower the risk of under-treatment. Patients with treatment resistance may require medication combinations under specialist supervision.

Box 4.4.7   Other pharmacological options

- Trazodone
- Venlafaxine
- Duloxetine
- Pregabalin
- Atypical antipsychotics, especially quetiapine
- Clomipramine
- Imipramine
- Mirtazapine.

Non-pharmacological

There are a number of non-pharmacological strategies available to manage anxiety. Anxiety often responds well to psychological treatment (if the patient is fit enough to undergo treatment and is psychologically minded) and in mild to moderate cases this would normally be the treatment of choice unless the patient has a strong preference for a pharmacological approach.

That said, effective implementation often requires access to a clinical psychologist or psychiatrist with provision varying across service locations which can pose a challenge.

Cognitive behavioural therapy (CBT) has a solid evidence base for many mental disorders and there is randomised controlled trial (RCT) level evidence suggesting that anxiety in the palliative population can improve with CBT (Moorey et al., 2009).

Other treatment approaches that can be helpful include:

- Counselling and group support
- Supportive psychotherapy
- Applied relaxation
- Complementary/alternative therapies
- Managing any co-morbid addiction problems
- Addressing psychosocial and spiritual issues including chaplaincy, befriending, financial assistance, charities, support groups.

You should consider referring in instances of:

- Severe anxiety states
- Co-morbid disorders complicating management

- Anxiety of lower severity not responding to typical first-line approaches
- Suicidality or other significant risks related to the mental state
- Diagnostic uncertainty
- Complex pharmacological approaches
- Consideration of formal psychological therapy.

Delirium

What is delirium?

Delirium is an acute neuropsychiatric syndrome characterised by disturbances in cognitive function, perception, consciousness and attention. Delirium is usually precipitated by a trigger and it is characterised by an acute onset and fluctuating course (NICE, 2019a). In older patients especially, multiple aetiological factors are responsible for the delirious episode and so comprehensive assessment is crucial.

Delirium varies in duration, mostly resolving within days, but in some people it can last weeks or months (SIGN, 2019). Up to 50% of delirium in advanced cancer is thought to be reversible, particularly if the underlying cause is related to medication or metabolic disturbance (Spiller et al., 2006).

Delirium is common with a prevalence of almost one-third of specialist palliative care inpatients. Hypoactive delirium is more common than hyperactive delirium in this population (Spiller et al., 2006). Most people who recover from delirium recall it as having been very distressing (Breitbart et al., 2002).

Delirium assessment

Delirium should be suspected in patients who exhibit an acute change in mental state over hours to days. Assessment should focus on reaching a diagnosis of delirium and identification of any reversible causes. Collateral history from someone who knows the patient is vital.

There are three different types of delirium:

1. Hyperactive delirium – the person is restless, agitated and hyper-alert.
2. Hypoactive delirium – the person is withdrawn, quiet, drowsy and hypo-alert.
3. Mixed delirium – the person has a mixture of hyperactive and hypoactive symptoms.

Psychotic features (delusions and hallucinations) are common in delirium and patients should be actively screened for psychosis. In hyperactive delirium, it is easier to identify these features but they can occur in any form of delirium. A patient with hypoactive delirium may quietly harbour very distressing psychotic beliefs or be experiencing hallucinations that could benefit from treatment.

4AT screening tool

Name:

Date of birth:

CHI number:

Date: / /

Zero time: :

Practitioner name:

Practitioner signature:

Designation:

Alertness	
This includes patients who may be markedly drowsy (eg. difficult to rouse and/or obviously sleepy during assessment) or agitated/ hyperactive. Observe the patient. If asleep, attempt to wake with speech or gentle touch on shoulder. **Ask the patient to state their name and address to assist rating.**	
Normal (fully alert, but not agitated, throughout assessment)	0
Mild sleepiness for <10 seconds after waking, then normal	0
Clearly abnormal	4

AMT4	
Age, date of birth, place (name of the hospital or building), current year.	
No mistakes	0
1 mistake	1
2 or more mistakes/untestable	2

Attention	
Ask the patient: **"Please tell me the months of the year in backwards order, starting at December."** To assist initial understanding one prompt of **"What is the month before December?"** is permitted.	
Achieves 7 months or more correctly	0
Starts but scores < 7 months / refuses to start	1
Untestable (cannot start because unwell, drowsy, inattentive)	2

Acute change or fluctuating course	
Evidence of significant change or fluctuation in: alertness, cognition, other mental function (eg. paranoia, hallucinations) arising over the last 2 weeks and still evident in the last 24 hours.	
No	0
Yes	4

4AT Score
4 or above: possible delirium +/- cognitive impairment
1-3: possible cognitive impairment
0: delirium or severe cognitive impairment unlikely
(but delirium still possible if [4] information incomplete)

Figure 4.4.1 The 4AT.

Source: Reproduced with the kind permission of Healthcare Improvement Scotland.

Consider using a screening tool, for example the 4AT Test (Figure 4.4.1). This test was developed and validated in Scotland in non-ICU settings and has now been widely adopted. A score of 4 or more suggests delirium. The 4AT does not require specific training; it is brief and easy to use and has wide applicability in various clinical settings (SIGN, 2019). A positive 4AT should trigger a comprehensive assessment and management pathway for suspected delirium which should be based on local and national guidelines.

Box 4.4.8 lists some common causes of delirium in palliative care.

Box 4.4.8 Common causes of delirium in palliative care

- Medications including opioids and steroids
- Withdrawal from drugs, including alcohol, nicotine, sedatives and antidepressants
- Infections
- Dehydration
- Hypoxia
- Constipation
- Urinary retention
- Uncontrolled pain
- Electrolyte abnormalities including hypercalcaemia and hyponatraemia
- Hypoglycaemia
- Organ failure.

The TIME bundle (Healthcare Improvement Scotland, 2014) sets out a series of clinical processes to be activated when a potential delirium diagnosis has been made. The TIME bundle is included in Figure 4.4.2 and serves as a very useful tool in the comprehensive assessment of patients with suspected delirium.

As a matter of good practice, even patients who are not delirious should be rigorously monitored and treated for known delirium risk factors and triggers, and the TIME bundle serves as a common reminder of common causes.

Time bundle

Name:
Date of birth:
CHI number:

Date: / /
Zero time: :

Practitioner name:

Practitioner signature:

Designation:

Initiate TIME within 2 hours (initial and write time of completion)	Assessed/ sent	Results seen	Abnormality found
Think exclude and treat possible triggers			
NEWS (think sepsis six)			
Blood glucose			
T Medication history (identify new medications/change of dose/medication recently stopped)			
Pain review (Abbey Pain Scale)			
Assess for urinary retention			
Assess for constipation			
Investigate and intervene to correct underlying causes			
Assess Hydration and start fluid balance chart			
Bloods (FBC, U&E, Ca, LFTs, CRP, Mg, Glucose)			
I Look for symptoms/signs of infection (skin, chest, urine, CNS) and perform appropriate cultures/imaging depending on clinical assessment (see sepsis six)			
ECG (ACS)			
M **Management Plan**			*Completed*
Initiate treatment of ALL underlying causes found above			
Engage and Explore (complete within 2 hours or if family/carer not present within 24 hours)			
E Engage with patient/family/carer – explore if this is usual behaviour. Ask: How would you like to be involved?			
Explain diagnosis of delirium to patient and family/carers (use delirium leaflet)			
Document diagnosis of delirium			

© Healthcare Improvement Scotland 2014

v3.0 Testing May 2014

Figure 4.4.2 TIME bundle.

Source: Reproduced with the kind permission of Healthcare Improvement Scotland.

General approach to the delirious patient

- Review of medications paying particular attention to recent changes to analgesia, steroids and sedatives.
- History and examination looking for evidence of the causes outlined above.
- Consider if blood tests are appropriate (remember to check calcium as hypercalcaemia is common in some cancers and is treatable).
- Consider using a tool such as the Abbey Pain Scale to assess pain in a patient who is unable to communicate due to delirium.
- Involve the family of the patient, for example by asking them to complete a 'Getting to Know Me' form to give the clinical team an insight into the patient and what matters to them.
- CT brain scan should not be used routinely but should be considered in patients presenting to hospital with delirium in the presence of: new focal neurological signs, a history of recent falls, a head injury (patients of any age) and anticoagulation therapy (SIGN, 2019).
- CT may also be appropriate in patients with non-resolving delirium where no clear cause is identified. It is likely that CT brain will be considered earlier in patients with advanced cancer due to the risk of brain metastases.

Non-pharmalogical management of delirium

- Avoid restraint including the use of indirect restraint, for example placing a table in front of a patient's chair to prevent them from getting up.
- Identify and address potential causes of delirium (remembering that multiple causes are common).
- Optimise sleep hygiene.
- Orientate regularly and minimise sensory deficits (for example ensure hearing aids working, ensure good lighting).
- Consider environmental factors: reduce noise and consider moving the patient to a single room if possible. Regular reassurance and consistency of staff members and their approach to the patient can be helpful.
- Optimise management of concurrent medical conditions.
- Specifically detect, assess causes of, and treat agitation and/or distress using non-pharmacological means only if possible, for example reassurance from staff or family members. Verbal and non-verbal de-escalation has an important role for every patient.
- Communicate the diagnosis to patients and carers, encourage involvement of carers and provide ongoing engagement and support.
- Aim to prevent complications of delirium such as immobility, falls, pressure sores, dehydration, malnourishment and isolation.

Pharmacological management of delirium

The pharmacological management of delirium is a controversial topic. A recent Cochrane Review concluded that antipsychotics did not reduce delirium severity, resolve symptoms or alter mortality in the acute care setting. The Cochrane Review also identified a large RCT of patients receiving palliative cancer care, which found that patients treated with either risperidone or haloperidol had worse delirium symptom scores than those receiving placebo (SIGN, 2019).

The recently published delirium SIGN guidelines (SIGN, 2019) found that there was insufficient evidence to support formally recommending the use of medication (anti-psychotics, benzodiazepines, dexmedetomidine and acetylcholinesterase inhibitors). However, it is important to present a balanced review of the evidence and SIGN did advocate on an expert opinion basis the use of medication in those that demonstrate intractable, severe distress and risk to themselves or others. The NICE guidelines on delirium published in 2010 previously recommended the use of the antipsychotics haloperidol or olanzapine in similar circumstances described above and when verbal/non-verbal de-escalation measures had failed. The newly updated NICE delirium guidance in March 2019 has removed olanzapine because haloperidol now has a licensed indication for acute delirium (NICE, 2019a). It is important to note that the above guidance is based on studies largely done on non-palliative populations.

The key point to convey, despite the controversies, is that distressed patients fitting the descriptions above (especially when distressing psychosis is present) should not be denied a pharmacological trial if indicated as this may have a significant impact on quality of life in the right patients. Treatment should be commenced at the lowest possible dose and titrated gradually if needed. This is especially important in frail and/or older adults. Typical initial doses in this population:

- Haloperidol 0.5 mg twice daily
- Olanzapine 2.5 mg at night
- Risperidone 0.25 mg twice daily.

There is a wide range of antipsychotic medication available (with marked side-effect profile variation) and various levels of evidence exist supporting the use of a number of different antipsychotics in delirium. Knowledge of the different properties of antipsychotics can be useful in choosing the optimal treatment for the patient. For example, olanzapine has more sedative properties than haloperidol and so may be a better choice if the patient is really distressed nocturnally. Specialist advice should be sought from palliative medicine, psychiatry or geriatric medicine if needed.

It must be borne in mind that antipsychotics have potent side-effects and risks; the balance of risk/benefit needs to be considered in every patient and there should be good communication with the family/power of attorney/guardians throughout the assessment and treatment process. An excellent approach to delirium assessment, medical treatment and non-pharmacological management should minimise the use of psychiatric medication, restricting it to patients who really need it.

Benzodiazepines in general should not be used in most cases of delirium. Notable exceptions would be end-of-life care and delirium related directly to alcohol/substance use disorders.

Advice around the use of other medication classes in delirium not detailed above should be in line with specialist psychiatric advice.

If commenced, antipsychotics prescribed for delirium should be reviewed on a daily basis and stopped as soon as the clinical situation allows, ideally within 1–2 days and up to one week. In situations where it is deemed safer to continue antipsychotic therapy for delirium beyond discharge or transfer from hospital, a clear plan for early medication review and follow-up in the community should be agreed.

Ethical and legal considerations

If a patient lacks capacity due to a delirium then an *Adults with Incapacity Act* (AWI) Section 47 Certificate of Incapacity should be completed (Mental Welfare Commission for Scotland, 2021) including an appropriate treatment plan. Make sure to check if your patient has named a power of attorney or has had a guardian appointed and involve them in decision making.

Medication can be given covertly under *Adults with Incapacity Act* legislation; this can represent a valuable route of treatment for a very distressed patient who will not take oral medication. For example, olanzapine can be given as an oro-dispersible preparation dissolved in water. Always follow local guidelines and seek specialist psychiatry/pharmacy advice when following covert treatment. It is important to involve power of attorney/ guardians in the decision-making process around covert medication.

Under most circumstances an AWI treatment certificate should be sufficient. If you are in any doubt about whether a patient needs to be detained under the *Mental Health Act*, seek advice from a psychiatrist.

Delirium at the end of life

Delirium is common at the end of life. This may either be delirium with a 'reversible cause' in a patient with a very limited prognosis who does not have the time needed to recover, or delirium secondary to the disease for which the patient is receiving palliative care.

In these patients the priority is managing the patient's distress. Specialist palliative care advice should be sought.

Delirium at the end of life is particularly challenging for the patient's family as they experience the loss of their loved one prior to bereavement. Delirium at the end of life is a significant risk factor for complex bereavement, and bereavement support should be offered if available.

Agitation

What is agitation?

Agitation has many definitions: it can be described as a state of excessive verbal and/or motor behaviour accompanied by distress. Agitation is a clinical sign and a search must be made to reach an underlying diagnosis. Agitation can be characterised by pacing, hostility, fidgeting, anxiety and restlessness (Chand, 2013). It can occur at any stage of illness and treatment. It is important for clinicians to avoid too readily prescribing psychotropic medication and to look instead for the underlying causes (Marie Curie, 2018).

Some diagnoses are more likely to present with agitation including (Pitman et al., 2018):

- Testicular tumours
- Parathyroid, adrenal and pituitary tumours
- COPD
- Heart failure.

Similarly, certain medications can be associated with agitation including (Pitman et al., 2018):

- Corticosteroids
- Benzodiazepines – this is known as paradoxical reaction
- Seratonergic agents
- Azacitidine.

Causes and aetiology

As in delirium, the causes of agitation can be multiple and are not always easily identifiable. A comprehensive approach should be taken in the assessment of agitation to identify underlying diagnoses. Initially medical factors are sought and corrected/reversed.

Every patient with agitation should be considered for an underlying psychiatric diagnosis including agitated depression, anxiety disorder, delirium, dementia or other mental illness (eg. psychosis). Specialist advice should be obtained if necessary. The reader can refer to the specific sections in this manual including depression, anxiety and delirium and if the agitation is associated with any of these conditions, then treatment should follow the principles in the relevant section.

Box 4.4.9 details examples of common causes of agitation in the palliative setting.

Box 4.4.9 Common causes of agitation in the palliative setting

Biological

- Delirium (see 'Delirium' section for more information)
- Substance withdrawal – nicotine, alcohol and medications both prescribed and illicit
- Pain or opioid toxicity
- Urinary retention
- Constipation
- Dehydration
- Hypoxaemia

- Metabolic – hypercalcaemia is the most common life-threatening metabolic disorder in cancer patients
- Raised intracranial pressure: metastasis or bleeds.

Social
- Loss of role, relationship changes
- Financial worries
- Work concerns.

Psychological and spiritual
- Grief
- Anger
- Adjustment
- Existential concerns
- Religious and spiritual issues.

(NHS, 2017; Chand, 2013; Puchalski, 2006)

Serotonin syndrome

Serotonin syndrome is a common cause of agitation and palliative care patients are at higher risk. The syndrome results from serotonin (5HT) toxicity often due to polypharmacy of medicines with serotonergic effects. It causes autonomic, motor and neurological features including:

- Diarrhoea and increased bowel sounds
- Agitation
- Tachycardia
- Autonomic instability – temperature and blood pressure
- Tremor
- Clonus
- Hyperreflexia
- Shivering
- Mydriasis.

Box 4.4.10 details common drugs with serotonergic effects.

Box 4.4.10   Common serotonergic agents

- Antidepressants
- Antipsychotics
- Tramadol
- Gabapentin and pregabalin
- Oxycodone
- Carbamazepine and valproate
- Ondansatron and other anti-emetics
- Drugs of abuse.

Serotonin syndrome can be treated with withdrawal of causative medications if mild. If severe, patients can require cooling, dantrolene, benzodiazepines and would require specialist medical care (Buckley et al., 2014).

The link to changes in established patterns of living

Significant changes in physical circumstances, such as a change of accommodation or an inability to continue usual routines, can unmask otherwise unrecognised alcohol or nicotine use leading to agitation. Signs of withdrawal from nicotine can include: irritability, psychomotor restlessness, concentration problems and anger. Signs of alcohol withdrawal include tremor, anxiety, sweating, tachycardia, mild hyperthermia, and more severely hallucinations and disorientation. These are easy to treat if identified promptly with nicotine replacement (NICE, 2019b) or benzodiazepines for alcohol withdrawal (NICE, 2019c).

The link to spiritual or psychological distress

There may be spiritual and psychological reasons for the patient's experience of agitation and distress. This can be harder to uncover if there is impaired consciousness. Older adults are more likely to develop agitation and it is hypothesised this is due to pre-morbid organ dysfunction, increased polypharmacy and pre-existing cognitive impairment (Hosker et al., 2016).

Terminal phase agitation

Agitation is commonly experienced at the end of life, both in the pre-active and active dying phases. Described variously as 'terminal agitation', 'terminal restlessness' and 'terminal anguish', estimates have suggested that between 25% and 85% of patients experience it in some degree in the weeks before death. It manifests both physically and psychologically and can lead to ambivalent feelings in carers and professionals. Studies have found terminal agitation can increase the distress experienced by families and carers, while conversely the use of medications to ameliorate it can be perceived negatively by family members as reducing the ability of the patient to communicate and indeed to shorten their life (Brajtman, 2003). Studies have shown appropriate use of midazolam and haloperidol did not alter survival rates over those who received neither (Radha Krishna, 2012).

Risk factors for the development of terminal agitation include extremes of age, male gender, rapid disease progression and previous trauma. If risk factors are present with early signs of agitation consider early referral to specialist palliative care team.

A diagnosis of terminal agitation should be considered whenever there is a change in presentation in a patient. It can present with myoclonic jerks, irritability and impaired consciousness (Brajtman, 2003). Other symptoms can include hallucinations, paranoia, confusion and disorientation. It can be seen in the context of delirium or as a separate clinical entity. It is postulated that biochemical abnormalities linked to organ failure can cause the biological agitation. Most research conducted related to agitation is in the context of delirium resulting in a poor evidence base for treatment choice (NHS, 2017).

Assessment

A careful history should be taken drawing on carer, nurse and family observations. Features such as onset, changes to treatment plan or the environment can be helpful in identifying possible causes. A full systematic enquiry should be undertaken to look for signs of treatable illness or disease progression. Physical examination and investigations should be considered and the level of invasiveness of the intervention is based upon the clinical picture and the patient's wishes.

If possible the clinician should engage with the patient to elicit any concerns, screen for delirium (Scottish Delirium Association, 2019) or for changes to symptoms. It has been found that carers, families and health professionals can all avoid discussion of these issues leaving an unmet need. Openness in listening to worries, fears and spiritual experiences without providing false reassurances or certainties is key (Puchalski, 2006; Mitchell, 2008). Open questions should be used to facilitate a dialogue about psychological or spiritual concerns and needs (See Chapter 7 – Psychosocial and Spiritual Aspects of Palliative and End-of-Life Care – for more information on spiritual assessment tools (p. 298)).

Other frameworks such as 'What matters to you' (What Matters to You, 2019) and 'Goal setting in palliative care' (Hospice UK, 2019) can help start a dialogue about what is important to the patient and help find alternative ways to approach symptoms and target the symptoms most important to the patient.

Important legal Issues

It is important to ensure that any anticipatory care plans, advance directives or written wishes about location, treatment or interventions are taken into consideration when making a management plan. Consider if use of the *Adults with Incapacity Act* is appropriate and whether the medication is being used for a licensed indication. If the patient lacks capacity and is non-concordant with medication which is causing distress and harm, covert medication could be considered (Mental Welfare Commission, 2017).

Treatment

A key principle of treatment is to control the symptoms without producing unwanted side effects. As always non-pharmacological treatments should be trialled first if there is not an immediate risk to patients or others (NHS, 2017). Review all medications carefully and discontinue any non-essential drugs that may be contributing to the presentation.

Non-pharmacological

It is important not to ignore the non-pharmacological management of distress. This can be something as straightforward as repositioning the patient or making simple changes to the environment. For example, having companionship, ensuring personal photographs or memorable objects are visible or reorientation can improve the situation (Marie Curie, 2018). Lucid intervals can be used to discuss any psychological or spiritual issues the patient identifies as well as confirming their wishes for treatment at the end of life. Consider using resources such as healthcare chaplaincy or any religious figures in the patient's life if this is welcomed by the patient. Healthcare chaplaincy services are an integral part of the healthcare system. Patients do not need to be explicitly religious or of a particular faith for a referral (Scottish Government, 2009; Marie Curie, 2018). For other sources of support, including financial, peer and social, consider signposting to third-sector organisations such as Maggie's Centres for malignant diagnoses and disease specific organisations for non-cancer diagnoses.

Table 4.4.1   Pharmacological treatments and dosages for agitation.

Symptom	Treatment
Intermittent agitation	Midazolam subcutaneous 2–5 mg, hourly, as required Maximum 6 doses per 24 hours Consider advice if further doses required
Persistent agitation	Midazolam subcutaneous 10–20 mg over 24 hours by syringe pump Further 5 mg an hour as required
If not controlling distressing symptoms	Consider specialist advice Titrate midazolam Consider adding levomepromazine subcutaneous 10–25 mg 6–12 hourly as required

Treat any reversible causes with an intervention level which is appropriate to the person's wishes. Ensure good oral care, hydration, urinary and bowel care as this can reduce or prevent agitation.

Pharmacological

Clinicians can consider medications to help relieve distress and symptoms (Table 4.4.1). Palliative sedation may be helpful for those with advanced disease at the end of life. The aim is to control distress while dying, not to hasten it. Consideration of such sedation should prompt referral for specialist palliative medicine expertise (Hosker et al., 2016).

Consider the most appropriate routes of medication:

- Poor swallowing ability can be a sign of the active dying phase.
- Choice of oral, sublingual or injectable medication should be made in discussion with the patient and in line with any advance directive.

Consider haloperidol or another antipsychotic if delirium is a major diagnosis in the overall clinical picture – start with lower doses if the patient is medication naive or frail/older adult (Scottish Palliative Care Guidelines, 2020). Please see the 'Delirium' section for more information (p. 205).

Scenario Recap

In the scenario at the beginning of this chapter, Jacqui developed increasingly severe depressive illness. Prompt psychiatric assessment ensured that this was detected and she was offered evidence-based pharmacological and psychological interventions. Broad differential diagnoses were kept in mind, with medical and other psychiatric illnesses which could cause depressive symptoms excluded. Obviously, there is some symptom overlap with cardiac failure and somatic features of depression, but even allowing for the heart failure and the stress the patient was under, it was obvious that she had developed superadded mental illness that deserved an attempt at treatment. Palliative care services worked with psychiatry to explore all of her psychosocial, psychiatric and spiritual needs. This facilitated a discharge from hospital and an improved quality of life in the community. The GP trainee's awareness that a psychiatric problem was highly likely and their prompt referral to specialist services made a positive difference in the outcome of this case.

References

Brajtman S (2003) The impact on the family of terminal restlessness and its management. *Palliative Medicine*, 17(5): 454–460.

Breitbart W, Gibson C and Tremblay A (2002) The delirium experience: delirium recall and delirium-related distress in hospitalized patients with cancer, their spouses/caregivers, and their nurses. *Psychosomatics*, 43(3): 183–194.

Buckley NA, Dawson AH and Ibister GK (2014) Serotonin syndrome. *BMJ*, 348: g1626.

Candy B et al. (2012) Drug therapy for symptoms associated with anxiety in adult palliative care patients. *The Cochrane Database of Systematic Reviews*, 10: CD004596

Chand S (2013) Dealing with the dying patient – treatment of terminal restlessness. *The Pharmaceutical Journal*. DOI:10.1211/PJ.2021.1.73912

Gilbody S, Richards D and Barkham M (2007) Diagnosing depression in primary care using self-completed instruments: UK validation of PHQ–9 and CORE–OM. *British Journal of General Practice*, 57(541): 650–652.

Healthcare Improvement Scotland (2014). Think delirium. Available at: http://www.widgetlibrary.knowledge.scot.nhs.uk/media/WidgetFiles/1010435/Delirium%20toolkit%20v3.1%20testing%20sep%20(web).pdf

Hosker CM and Bennett MI (2016) Delirium and agitation at the end of life. *BMJ*, 353: i3085.

Hospice UK (2019) Resources for rehabilitative palliative care. Available at: https://www.hospiceuk.org/what-we-offer/clinical-and-care-support/rehabilitative-palliative-care/resources-for-rehabilitative-palliative-care

Marie Curie (2018) Agitation. Available at: https://www.mariecurie.org.uk/professionals/palliative-care-knowledge-zone/symptom-control/agitation

Mental Welfare Commission for Scotland (2017) Good practice guide: covert medication. Available at: https://www.mwcscot.org.uk/sites/default/files/2019-06/covert_medication.pdf

Mental Welfare Commission for Scotland (2021). Adults with incapacity Act. Available at: https://www.mwcscot.org.uk/law-and-rights/adults-incapacity-act

Mitchell D (2008) Spiritual and cultural issues at the end of life. *Medicine*, 36(2): 109–110.

Moorey S et al. (2009) A cluster randomized controlled trial of cognitive behaviour therapy for common mental disorders in patients with advanced cancer. *Psychological Medicine*, 39(5): 713–723.

NHS (2017) Guidelines for the management of agitation in the last weeks of life. Available at: https://www.nwcscnsenate.nhs.uk/files/1515/0583/4923/Agitation_Revised_Presentation_14th_Sept_2017.pdf

NICE (2009) Depression in adults with a chronic physical health problem: recognition and management. Available at: https://www.nice.org.uk/guidance/CG91/chapter/1-Guidance#step-1-recognition-assessment-and-initial-management-in-primary-care-and-general-hospital

NICE (2018) Depression in adults: recognition and management. Available at: https://www.nice.org.uk/guidance/cg90

NICE (2019a) Delirium: prevention, diagnosis and management. NICE guideline (CG103). Available at: https://www.nice.org.uk/guidance/cg103

NICE (2019b) Smoking cessation. Available at: https://bnf.nice.org.uk/treatment-summary/smoking-cessation.html

NICE (2019c) Alcohol dependence. Available at: https://bnf.nice.org.uk/treatment-summary/alcohol-dependence.html

Pitman A et al. (2018) Depression and anxiety in patients with cancer. *BMJ*, 361: k1415.

Puchalski CM (2006) *A Time for Listening and Caring: Spirituality and the Care of the Chronically Ill and Dying*. Oxford: Oxford University Press, pp. 5–7.

Radha Krishna LK, Poulouse VJ and Goh C (2012) The use of midazolam and haloperidol in cancer patients at the end of life. *Singapore Medical Journal*, 53(1): 62–66.

Rayner L et al. (2010) *The Management of Depression in Palliative Care: European Clinical Guidelines*. London: Department of Palliative Care, Policy and Rehabilitation.

Rayner L et al. (2011a) The clinical epidemiology in palliative care and the predictive value of somatic symptoms: cross-sectional survey with four-week follow-up. *Palliative Medicine*, 25(3): 229–241.

Rayner L et al. (2011b) Expert opinion on detecting and treating depression in palliative care: a Delphi study. *BMC Palliative Care*, 10(10): 1–9.

Scottish Delirium Association (2019) SIGN delirium guideline. Available at: http://www.scottishdeliriumassociation.com/

Scottish Government (2009) Spiritual care and chaplaincy. Guidance on spiritual care in the NHS in Scotland. Available at: https://www.gov.scot/publications/spiritual-care-chaplaincy/pages/2/

Scottish Palliative Care Guidelines (2019) Depression. Available at: https://www.palliativecareguidelines.scot.nhs.uk/guidelines/symptom-control/depression.aspx

Scottish Palliative Care Guidelines (2020). Delirium. Available at: https://www.palliativecareguidelines.scot.nhs.uk/guidelines/symptom-control/delirium.aspx

SIGN (2019) Risk reduction and management of delirium. Available at: https://www.sign.ac.uk/media/1423/sign157.pdf

Spencer R et al. (2010) Anxiety disorders in advanced cancer patients: correlates and predictors of end-of-life outcomes. *Cancer*, 116(7): 1810–1819.

Spiller J and Keen J (2006) Hypoactive delirium: assessing the extent of the problem for inpatient specialist palliative care. *Palliative Medicine*, 20(1): 17–23.

Stark D et al. (2002) Anxiety disorders in cancer patients: their nature, associations, and relation to quality of life. *Journal of Clinical Oncology*, 20(14): 3137–3148.

Sung-Wan Kim et al. (2008) Effectiveness of mirtazapine for nausea and insomnia in cancer patients with depression. *Psychiatry and Clinical Neuroscience*, 62(1): 75–83.

UK Government (2014) Citalopram and escitalopram: QT interval prolongation. Available at: https://www.gov.uk/drug-safety-update/citalopram-and-escitalopram-qt-interval-prolongation

Vodermaier A, Linden W and Siu C (2009) Screening for emotional distress in cancer patients: a systematic review of assessment instruments. *Journal of the National Cancer Institute*, 10(21): 1464–1488.

Watanabe N et al. (2011) Mirtazapine versus other antidepressive agents for depression. *Cochrane Databases of Systematic Reviews*, 7(12).

What Matters to You (2019) Available at: https://www.whatmatterstoyou.scot/#services

Wijkstra J et al. (2015) Pharmacological treatment for psychotic depression. *Cochrane Database of Systematic Reviews*, 30(7): CD004044.

Zigmond AS and Snaith RP (1983) The hospital anxiety and depression scale. *Acta Psychiatrica Scandinavica*, 67(6): 361–370.

4.5   MANAGING OTHER SYMPTOMS COMMON TO PALLIATIVE PATIENTS

Maire O'Riordan with Mairi Armstrong, Alana Brown-Kerr, Margaret Rose Key, Margaret Rice, Michelle Salmon, Marie Todd and Ruth Yates

Learning Objectives

Within palliative care, there are many other symptoms that can be very problematic for patients with progressive illness. In this section we will discuss lymphoedema, sweating, pruritus and fatigue but recognise that this list cannot be exhaustive and that there are many other less common but distressing symptoms that patients can experience.

This section will enable you to:

- Define what is meant by lymphoedema, sweating, pruritus and fatigue in palliative patients
- Identify and define the common causes of lymphoedema and these named symptoms in palliative care
- Understand the impact of lymphoedema and these named symptoms on the palliative care patient
- Enable the reader to be confident in providing a comprehensive assessment of the patient
- Suggest potential management options
- Discuss palliative pharmacological and non-pharmacological treatment options.

Lymphoedema

Scenario

Background

Seema is a 35-year-old woman who has brain metastases from a primary breast cancer. She has been on long-term steroid therapy and as a result has gained a significant amount of weight, is spending most of her time in a chair, and doesn't go to bed. She presents with grossly swollen legs with superficial ulceration and chronic exudate. Seema lives alone with daily visits from siblings. Community nurses are visiting three times a day to apply a dressing to mop up the exudate but the dressing is soaked through at each visit, causing wet clothing, footwear and carpets.

Key points

- Advanced disease with complications secondary to treatment – brain metastases, weight gain, immobility and swollen legs, possible cognitive impairment
- Detailed assessment of symptoms and impact (both physical and psychological) on patient and family/carers
- Guidance for patient and family/carers on management of swollen legs and ways of avoiding further complications and patient distress

Timeline

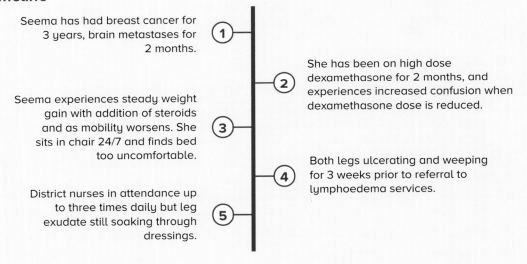

Seema has had breast cancer for 3 years, brain metastases for 2 months.

(1)

(2) She has been on high dose dexamethasone for 2 months, and experiences increased confusion when dexamethasone dose is reduced.

Seema experiences steady weight gain with addition of steroids and as mobility worsens. She sits in chair 24/7 and finds bed too uncomfortable.

(3)

(4) Both legs ulcerating and weeping for 3 weeks prior to referral to lymphoedema services.

District nurses in attendance up to three times daily but leg exudate still soaking through dressings.

(5)

Key considerations

- Is it possible to safely manage this situation at home?
- What other services are available to help manage this patient's symptoms?
- What further complications should be anticipated?

Pathophysiology

Lymphoedema is swelling in any part of the body but mainly the limbs caused by obstruction or failure of the lymphatic system, and results in net capillary filtration in the relevant anatomical site exceeding lymphatic drainage.

In palliative patients the causes include:

- Surgical removal of lymph nodes
- Radiotherapy to nodal areas
- Obstruction by tumour
- Combination of above.

However, lymphoedema can also affect patients with advanced non-malignant disease (Box 4.5.1). Palliative patients often also have other co-existing problems that may or may not be related to the initial diagnosis. Many of the manifestations of these or their management can have an impact on the development or the management of the swelling (Box 4.5.2) (Keeley, 2000).

Box 4.5.1 Advanced non-malignant disease

- Chronic cardiac failure
- End stage renal disease
- Advanced neurological disease
- Advanced liver disease
- End stage chronic respiratory disease.

Box 4.5.2 Contributing factors of lymphoedema

- Venous obstruction will cause oedema. The obstruction can be the result of external pressure from tumour or internally from thrombo-embolism.
- Some drugs are known to have fluid retaining properties (steroids, NSAIDs, calcium channel blockers, gabapentin, etc.).
- Hypoproteinaemia – the reduction in plasma protein levels caused by liver disease or nutritional deficiency in advanced disease.
- Reduced mobility and function can be a result of many of the problems associated with advancing disease, for example fatigue, pain, the swollen limb, bone metastases, or neurological impairment. Other co-morbidities, for example arthritis, chronic respiratory problems, may compound the problem. Prolonged dependency and a reduction in muscular activity can cause or exacerbate lymphoedema.
- Fungating lesions can make management of lymphoedema more difficult if situated close to the swollen limb. Severe swelling and problems with mobility of the limb may also restrict access to the lesion especially if in the axilla or in the groin.
- Renal, hepatic or cardiac failure.

Patients may experience one or many of the factors shown in Boxes 4.5.1 and 4.5.2, making overall management of the palliative patient more challenging (Williams, 2004).

Impact on patients and their families

Lymphoedema can be an extremely distressing and uncomfortable condition for patients with advanced disease and is reported as being the fourth most common symptom in this patient group, ahead of nausea and vomiting (Kaye, 1994). The swollen limb(s) can become very heavy and uncomfortable, reducing mobility and function. The ability to wear usual clothing and footwear can also be restricted. If the swelling extends into the trunk, this can add to the discomfort by making positioning difficult and affecting the ability to sleep, bathe and use the toilet. The oedema is usually very soft and pitting, making the skin fragile, and if broken can cause lymph to leak onto the surface of the skin (lymphorrhoea). This lymphorrhoea can cause maceration of the skin, soaking clothing, slippers, furniture and bedding, and can be very cold and upsetting for the patient (Renshaw, 2007). Managing lymphorrhoea also adds to the need to move the patient. The impact on patients' carers is often overlooked. Caring for a relative who is dying can cause tremendous psychological and physical strain, and can make the carer feel overwhelmed or powerless (Neale, 1991; Munck et al., 2008). Many aspects of lymphoedema can add to the carer's workload, for example increased laundry from lymphorrhoea. Patients may then also worry about this impact on their loved ones.

Because of the impact of lymphoedema on the physical, psychological and social well-being in patients (Tobin et al., 1993), a holistic approach to assessment is required to ensure the correct cause of swelling is identified. It is also important to ascertain the impact of swelling on the patient and his/her family to ensure the appropriate needs-based treatment plan is developed.

Management

Managing lymphoedema in palliative patients can be very challenging for healthcare professionals. Practitioners often have to deal with swelling that is unresponsive to treatment, unrealistic patient expectations, and difficulty in planning workload because of uncertainty of duration of treatment.

In palliative patients a holistic approach is fundamental and practitioners use modified treatment regimes depending on need and ability to comply.

Skin care

In palliative patients the skin can become very fragile and the aim is to prevent any damage. Care should be taken to wash and dry thoroughly, especially between the digits and any skin folds. Apply an unscented moisturiser to prevent drying of the skin. If compression hosiery is being applied, care should be taken to prevent damage during application. Any breaks in the skin will cause lymphorrhoea. Mild lymphorrhoea can be treated with an absorbent dressing and continuing with compression hosiery. If this fails to control the leakage, then more specialized dressings, for example Aquacel, and light compression bandaging may be required. In some cases the management is purely palliative and bed rest advised as bandaging may not stop the lymphorrhoea, especially if there is prolonged dependency of the limb.

There is a high risk of infection, especially when there is a break in the skin, in lymphoedema patients. Details of the concensus document on the treatment of cellulitis in lymphoedema can be downloaded from the British Lymphology Society at www.thebls.com.

Exercise

Normal use of the limb can be sufficient to assist lymphatic flow but even normal use may be restricted in palliative patients. Pain, weight of the limb, fatigue, or neurological impairment will impact on limb mobility. Elevation of the limb will help reduce the gravitational component of the swelling, for example supporting the arm on a pillow or cushion to prevent pooling at the elbow. Care should be taken to ensure the arm is not allowed to hang by the side when sitting, in bed, or walking. The arm could be supported in a sling if necessary. This will also reduce the pulling weight on the shoulder and neck muscles.

Compression therapy

There is a wide range of compression products available but these must be prescribed by an appropriately trained healthcare professional to ensure any contraindications to compression are identified and the correct pressure, size and style of compression is selected. Poorly fitted garments can damage the skin and push fluid to areas that have no compression applied, for example fingers. There is a range of donning aids available to assist the application of hosiery, for example the Actiglide, which is available on drug tariff. There are some patients, however, who are too ill or uncomfortable for hosiery or bandaging. In these cases simple measures may be adopted, for example elevation or a cotton liner.

Massage

While massage may not be clinically effective in palliative patients, they may benefit from the soothing hands-on effect from gentle massage or simply the application of a mild unscented moisturiser to the swollen area and beyond.

Other therapies used in the management of palliative lymphoedema

Palliative radiotherapy and/or chemotherapy can often reduce the metastatic tumour volume and thus help control lymphoedema. Although fluid retention is a side-effect of steroid therapy, these drugs may also help reduce the peritumour oedema. Analgesia should always be considered for relief of pain associated with any swelling and the presence of infection (cellulitis) requires prompt antibiotic therapy (see British Lymphology Society consensus document at www.thebls.com). Diuretics are generally avoided in lymphoedema management but can be useful if there is co-existing low-protein oedema associated with progressive disease.

Summary

Palliative lymphoedema can be caused or exacerbated by many of the co-existing problems palliative patients face. It is a distressing visible symptom and standard treatment modalities often should be modified to meet patients' needs. Practitioners caring for palliative patients can deliver these basic cornerstones of lymphoedema management to help reduce the impact of this condition.

Scenario recap

The district nurses contacted the local lymphoedema service and, following assessment of Seema by lymphoedema nurses, compression bandaging was applied daily to reduce the swelling and stop the lymphorrhoea. As the lymphorrhoea reduced, the bandages were changed less frequently until finally compression hosiery could be applied when the lymphorrhoea subsided completely. Carers attended Seema twice daily to help her with application of compression hosiery.

Seema was also being seen at the day therapy unit in the local hospice where she was assessed and provided with walking aids by the physiotherapist. Seema and her family were advised and given written information on skin care and prevention of infection and in the letter from the lymphoedema service, the GP was signposted to the British Lymphology Society consensus document on the management of cellulitis in lymphoedema as the patient was still considered to be at risk of this. Seema could mobilise small distances at home for the next 7 weeks and then required admission to the hospice as confusion and mobility worsened. She died in the hospice 2 months later.

Sweating

Experience and impact

Sweating is a normal physiological function designed to regulate body temperature and prevent hyperthermia. Hyperhidrosis (excessive sweating) is defined as that which exceeds this usual thermoregulatory requirement. This may involve drenching night sweats. Within palliative care this is a potentially overlooked and under-reported symptom which can cause significant burden and distress to patients (Mercadante et al., 2013). It is estimated that 10–20% of patients with advanced cancer will suffer from excessive sweating (Scottish Palliative Care Guidelines, 2020a).

Hyperhidrosis can be classified as primary or secondary. Primary hyperhidrosis is defined as excessive sweating with no identified underlying cause. The causes of secondary hyperhidrosis are listed in Table 4.5.1. Secondary hyperhidrosis can be further separated into generalised or focal. In the majority of cases in palliative care we will be dealing with generalised hyperhidrosis. However, it is worth considering that focal hyperhidrosis may occur in peripheral neuropathy or complex regional pain syndromes (CRPS).

Secondary causes

It is common for palliative care patients to have a number of factors contributing to excessive sweating (for example, liver metastases, hormone therapy and opioids prescribed for pain relief). This can make finding an effective treatment challenging.

Assessment

Full assessment of the patient is key to diagnosing the cause of excessive sweating and establishing an appropriate management plan. This should include disease history, past medical history, current medications, recent investigations and a physical examination. Specific symptoms which should be discussed include pain, weight loss, anxiety, 'hot

Table 4.5.1   Secondary causes of excessive sweating.

Malignancy	Lymphoma and other haematological malignancies, disseminated malignancy, liver metastases
Endocrine disturbance	Thyrotoxicosis/hyperthyroidism, diabetes mellitus (hypoglycaemia), acromegaly, menopause
Infective	Sepsis (consider risk of neutropenia), any infective process, endocarditis
Medications	Selective serotonin reuptake inhibitors (SSRIs) Hormone therapies (for example tamoxifen, aromatase inhibitors, gonadorelin analogues) Opioids

flushes', sleep disturbance, fever and other symptoms or signs suggestive of infection. An understanding of the disease trajectory and expected prognosis will be helpful in order to guide decision making on the appropriateness of more invasive investigation.

Time should be taken to address the patient's ideas, concerns and expectations. How is the sweating affecting their daily life? Do they have to do extra loads of washing, and is this causing fatigue? Are they embarrassed and is this affecting their social interactions? Do they require social support to help with washing clothing and bed linen?

Treatments

Non-pharmacological

In the first instance non-pharmacological interventions should be trialled. These include increasing ventilation of the patient's room, use of a handheld fan, use of cold compresses or tepid sponging and wearing loose-fitting, cotton clothing. Encourage adequate oral intake to prevent dehydration.

Acupuncture for sweating and hot flushes in breast cancer has anecdotal evidence, but randomised controlled trials (RCTs) have failed to demonstrate statistical significance compared to sham acupuncture (Deng et al., 2007).

Pharmacological

Treatment of the underlying cause (if identified) should be a priority. Consider opioid rotation if the patient is taking regular opioids. Review and switch other medications as appropriate.

If non-pharmacological strategies are ineffective, pharmacological interventions are available. The evidence base for all pharmacological strategies in managing excessive sweating is small, relying on case reports/series. There is currently no Cochrane Review on the subject. The Scottish Palliative Care Guidelines (2020a) recommend the treatments shown in Table 4.5.2 for excessive sweating. The use of all of the medications in this context is outside current marketing authorisation/off licence.

Table 4.5.2 Suggested pharmacological treatments of sweating with/without pyrexia.

Sweating with pyrexia	Sweating without pyrexia (associated with tumour)
Paracetamol 500 mg–1 g, 6 hourly[1]	NSAID
NSAID[2]	Amitriptyline 10–50 mg at night
	Cimetidine 400–800 mg once daily
	Venlafaxine 37.5 mg (modified release, once daily), increasing to 75 mg once daily if tolerated[3]

[1] Dose depending on body weight (if <50 kg, give 500 mg paracetamol 6 hourly).
[2] No difference reported in effect when indomethacin, naproxen and diclofenac were compared (Tsavaris et al., 1990).
[3] Venlafaxine should only be started in this context under specialist palliative advice.
Based on Scottish Palliative Care Guidelines, 2020a.

In a febrile patient a decision on the appropriateness of investigation and treatment of fever should be made. Antibiotics (oral or intravenous) may help to control a fever, but this should be considered within the goals of care of the individual.

Sweating associated with hot flushes

A number of treatments for breast cancer and prostate cancer work by hormone blockade, mimicking the menopause. These include tamoxifen, letrozole, exemestane, anastrozole and gonadorelin analogues. Side-effects of these drugs include hot flushes and excessive sweating. These can be so severe that treatment is discontinued with implications for recurrence of disease and survival (Cella et al., 2008).

Clonidine (an α_1 and α_2 agonist) may improve sweating and hot flushes in patients with breast cancer who are on hormone therapy (Pandya et al., 2005). The recommended starting dose is 50 micrograms orally twice daily, which can be increased to 75 micrograms twice daily after two weeks. The side-effects of clonidine may be intolerable to some patients: dry mouth, sedation, dizziness, postural hypotension and pruritus are all common (>10% of patients) (Twycross et al., 2017).

RCT evidence has also shown benefit from the use of gabapentin to treat hot flushes in patients with breast cancer (Pandya et al., 2005). The drug was effective at a dose of 900 mg per day, but not at a lower dose of 300 mg per day, so therefore adequate dose titration is required to see full effect. A systematic review found that patients reported a preference in taking venlafaxine (a serotonin and noradrenaline re-uptake inhibitor (SNRI)) for hot flushes above gabapentin (Johns et al., 2016).

Summary

In conclusion, sweating in a palliative care patient with advanced illness can be multi-factorial, and a thorough history, examination and medication review is necessary to elucidate possible causes. The treatment approach should be focused on the underlying cause and supportive, non-pharmacological strategies. Where these are not effective, a number of pharmacological strategies can be tried, but with careful consideration of the benefit and burden of the medications and reflection on potential drug interactions.

Pruritus (Itch)

Introduction

Pruritus was defined in 1660 by a German physician, Samuel Hafenreffer, as 'an unpleasant sensation associated with the desire to scratch' (Han et al., 2014). It is not a disease but a symptom of both localised and systemic pathologies. Chronic pruritus can be associated with low mood, anxiety and social isolation (Schneider et al., 2006). The prevalence of pruritus in palliative care is dependent on the underlying cause: over 70% of dialysis patients report chronic itch, 3–30% of patients with haematologic malignancies are affected and 1% of people suffer pruritus as a side-effect of systemic opioid use (Siemens et al., 2016).

Pathophysiology

The pathophysiology of pruritus helps to guide management and can be classified as:

1. Prurioreceptive – originates in the skin and the sensation is carried to the brain by the spinothalamic tract where it is perceived as itch. This stimulates the motor reflex to scratch, which blocks the sensation of itch (Yosipovitch et al., 2003). Histamine is the most well-known chemical mediator in this process but opioids, serotonin and cytokines can also play a role (Seccareccia et al., 2011).

2. Neuropathic – occurs when there is damage to afferent pathways, for example post-herpetic itch.

3. Neurogenic – centrally mediated by serotonin and opioid receptors and therefore unresponsive to antihistamines. Both uraemic and cholestatic itch are examples of neurogenic pruritus (Seccareccia et al., 2011).

4. Psychogenic – related to psychiatric disorders and is the least common.

Causes

Cholestatic pruritus

Very common in cholestasis but pathogenesis remains unclear. There is no correlation between bile acid levels and severity of pruritus and therefore cholestyramine is often ineffective.

Chronic kidney disease

Uraemic pruritus presents regardless of whether patients are receiving dialysis and can be generalised, localised, intermittent or continuous. Most patients with uremia also have dry skin.

Table 4.5.3   Possible causes of pruritus in palliative care.

Primary skin disease	Infection	Medication	Systemic disease
Atopic dermatitis	Scabies	Opioids	Cholestatic jaundice
Contact dermatitis	Lice	SSRIs	Chronic kidney disease
Psoriasis	Candidiasis	Ace inhibitors	Iron deficiency anaemia
		Statins	Leukaemia
		Chemotherapy	Paraneoplastic
		Monoclonal antibodies (many other medications can also cause pruritus)	Primary biliary cirrhosis
			Thyroid disease
			Multiple myeloma
			Polycythaemia
			Diabetes mellitus

Opioid induced

More common with spinal opioids than systemic opioids. The mechanism is unclear but thought to be mediated by μ-opioid receptors.

Solid tumours

Solid tumours can be associated with pruritus caused by a paraneoplastic process (immunologic response to tumour-specific antigens which can sometimes precede diagnosis). The presenting itch can be generalised or localised (for example peri-anal itch in colorectal cancer). See Table 4.5.3 for more information on possible causes of pruritus in palliative care.

Assessment

- Medical history
- Medication history
- Thorough skin examination – looking for local and systemic causes
- Consider investigations such as full blood count, ferritin, urea and electrolytes, liver function tests, thyroid function tests and blood glucose, depending on the suspected cause of pruritus.

Management

Many patients will have more than one factor at play in the cause of their pruritus. It is a symptom involving the skin, immune system, peripheral and central nervous system and therefore will often need a multifaceted management approach. There is no 'magic bullet' treatment for pruritus and it may be necessary to advise the patient that although the condition may be difficult to fully resolve, their symptom will be taken seriously and treated as such. A break down of general advice in managing pruritus is outlined in Table 4.5.4.

Table 4.5.4   Management of pruritus in palliative care.

General management/advice	<ul><li>Review drug causes and stop if possible</li><li>Treat any skin infections present</li><li>Patient should be advised to avoid vasodilators, for example caffeine, alcohol and spices</li><li>Advise loose, non-irritating clothing and if itching is uncontrolled, at night especially, suggest trimming fingernails and wearing cotton gloves.</li></ul>
Skin care (dry skin is often present alongside all causes of pruritus in palliative patients, and therefore general skin care advice is essential)	<ul><li>Emollients should be applied regularly (ensure that patient has help with this if required, for example a carer to apply creams to back)</li><li>Advise bathing in tepid water</li><li>Use of an unscented soap or soap substitute is recommended</li><li>Avoid heavily scented cosmetics.</li></ul>

Non-pharmacological management

- UVB phototherapy can be useful in uraemic pruritus. In theory, it works by reducing the number of mast cells and free nerve endings in the skin (Twycross et al., 2003). However, it is often impractical for patients nearing the end of their lives. A referral to dermatology would be necessary for this.
- In pruritus secondary to cholestatic jaundice where biliary obstruction is present, stenting can ease symptoms and negate the need for medications.

Pharmacological management

Topical agents to help manage pruritus include the following:

- **Emollients** – refer to local pharmacy/guidelines. Ensure patients understand the importance of frequent and persistent application.
- **Other topical agents** – emollients containing 1% menthol can substitute itching for a cooling sensation. Similarly, capsaicin 0.025% cream can be helpful for smaller areas of itch. For very localised patches of pruritus, mild to moderate potency corticosteroids can be helpful (ensure area is not infected) but must be reviewed regularly (Twycross et al., 2003).

Table 4.5.5 contains medications that may be recommended by a specialist. Please seek advice before initiation (adapted from the Scottish Palliative Care Guidelines, 2019).

Table **4.5.5**   Recommended medicines for pruritus in palliative care.

Cause	Treatment 1st line	2nd line	3rd line
Cholestasis	Rifampicin 300–600 mg once daily Sertraline 50–100 mg once daily Cholestyramine 4 g up to four times daily	N/A	N/A
Uraemia	Gabapentin 100 mg to 300 mg daily slowly – caution as accumulates in renal impairment. Dose and/or frequency may need adjustment.	Naltrexone 50 mg daily (uraemic itch could involve endogenous opioid peptides and, therefore, antagonism of this system may help. More effective in severe pruritus. Extreme caution should be taken if patient is prescribed opioids)	Mirtazapine 15–45 mg daily – caution as accumulates in renal impairment and doses as low as 7.5 mg may be suitable
Lymphoma	Prednisolone 10–20 mg three times daily	Cimetidine 400 mg twice daily	Mirtazapine 15–30 mg at bedtime
Systemic opioid-induced pruritus	Chlorphenamine 4–12 mg (if benefit 4 mg three times daily)	If no benefit switch opioid	Ondansetron 8 mg twice daily
Paraneoplastic	Paroxetine 5–20 mg once daily	Mirtazapine 15–30 mg at bedtime	

Summary

- Histamine release is often not the cause of pruritus observed in the palliative care patient population and therefore antihistamines are often ineffective.
- Emollients should always be prescribed if there is dry skin present – this is often a contributing factor in pruritus in palliative patients.
- Pharmacological treatment is often necessary for patients with systemic causes of pruritus and therefore it is important to understand the cause(s) in order to ensure that the patient receives the appropriate management.

Fatigue

Introduction

Fatigue is a symptom described by many within the general population in addition to those who are living with identified physical or psychological illness such as cancer, neurological disorders, heart or lung diseases, anxiety or depression. In the palliative care population, it is likely the most common symptom experienced (Radbruch, 2008) and often described by patients as their worst symptom, impacting on all aspects of their life, physical, psychosocial and spiritual. It is under-recognised, under-assessed and under-treated (Radbruch, 2008), complicated by the fact that patients are often reluctant to disclose this symptom. It is important, therefore, that clinicians become familiar with enquiring about this symptom at the beginning of a palliative diagnosis and continue to do so throughout the illness trajectory. Research shows that fatigue is rarely an isolated symptom. It is often more commonly associated with other symptoms including depression, breathlessness, oedema and pain (Herr, 2014).

Clinicians working within a multinational society should also be aware that the word fatigue is only common to the French and English language, therefore any enquiry in relation to this symptom is best described in conjunction with terms such as 'weakness' or 'tiredness'. However, the term fatigue will be used throughout this text.

What is fatigue?

There is no one identified definition of fatigue but most definitions contain similarities. The majority of research around fatigue has taken place within the field of oncology, where fatigue has been identified as cancer-related fatigue (CRF). Cancer-related fatigue is defined as a distressing persistent, subjective sense of physical, emotional and/or cognitive tiredness or exhaustion related to cancer or cancer treatment that is not proportional to recent activity and interferes with usual functioning (NCCN, 2018). The research further states that CRF also results in a poor quality of life and a reduction in treatment efficacy (Wang et al., 2019; Pyszora, 2017). CRF is also considered to be more severe and disabling when related to insomnia or over-exertion.

In a recent systematic review into the experience of fatigue in heart failure (HF), the following aggregated description of fatigue was agreed: 'A pervasive and unignorable bodily experience.' It also suggests that people with HF describe three different types of fatigue: lacking in physical and mental energy, lacking physical strength and unforeseen drowsiness (Schjoedt et al., 2016). This following definition for HF demonstrates real similarities with that of CRF: a subjective, unpleasant symptom which incorporates total body feelings ranging from tiredness to exhaustion, creating an unrelenting overall condition which interferes with the individual's ability to function at a normal level (Ream et al., 1996). These experiences are also found within many other life-limiting conditions, including chronic obstructive pulmonary disease (COPD), motor neurone disease (MND), multiple sclerosis and human immunodeficiency virus (HIV).

The International Classification of Diseases 10th revision (ICD-10) (Table 4.5.6) criteria for the definition of fatigue may be a useful tool to refer to.

Table 4.5.6 Definition of fatigue in the International Classification of Diseases (ICD 10) (Cella, 2001).

The ICD-10 definition of Fatigue includes A1, and at least five out of A2–A11 have been present for most days in at least two consecutive weeks in the past month (Cella, 2001).

A	
A1	Significant fatigue, diminished energy or increased need to rest, disproportionate to any recent change in activity level
A2	Generalised weakness, limb heaviness
A3	Diminished concentration or attention
A4	Decreased motivation or interest to engage in usual activities
A5	Insomnia or hyper-insomnia
A6	Experience of sleep as unrefreshing or nonrestorative
A7	Perceived need to struggle to overcome inactivity
A8	Marked emotional reactivity (such as sadness, frustration, irritability) to feeling fatigued
A9	Difficulty completing daily tasks attributed to feeling fatigued
A10	Perceived problem with short term memory
A11	Post exertional malaise lasting several hours
B	The symptoms cause clinically significant distress or impairment in social, occupational or other important areas of functioning
C	Evidence from history, physical examination or laboratory findings, that symptoms are a consequence of cancer or cancer treatment
D	Symptoms are not primarily a consequence of comorbid psychiatric disorders such as major depression, somatisation disorder, somatoform disorder or delirium

Prevalence

Fatigue is identified as one of the most common symptoms/side-effects found in patients with advanced cancer (Ghoshal et al., 2017) and is suggested to affect approximately 60–90% of these patients. It has been described as a problem by 99% of patients who have received radiotherapy or chemotherapy (Lawrence et al., 2004; Servaes et al., 2002). Approximately 50% of patients living with multiple sclerosis (MS) report fatigue as a significant issue and an even higher percentages of patients living with COPD and HF (Radbruch et al., 2008).

Pathophysiology

Researchers acknowledge that they continue to struggle with identifying the aetiology and classification of fatigue within different illness groups. However, it is recognised that many of the elements described below relating specifically to CRF are similar for other palliative conditions but have been less researched. Being aware of the multidimensional physical and psychosocial mechanisms contributing to fatigue will enable the clinician both to understand and be able to describe to patients why the management of this condition is complicated.

Disease specific factors include (primary fatigue):

- Tumour by-products
- Pro-inflammatory cytokine-induced cachexia
- Muscle loss
- Deconditioning.

(NCCN, 2018)

Other, possibly more general factors include (secondary fatigue):

- Co-morbidities
- Medical complications such as anaemia
- Side-effects of other medicines and treatments including chemotherapy and radiotherapy
- Other physical and psychological factors.

(Radbruch et al., 2008)

Assessment

Subjective self-evaluation is agreed to be the best assessment of fatigue and there are multiple tools available to assist this process (NCCN, 2018), but the use of simple tools are suggested for patients who are palliative. Two simple tools have been provided:

1. The Edmonton Symptom Assessment Tool (Figure 4.5.1) (Multivariate)
   - Enabling assessment of other possible related symptoms
2. The Brief Fatigue Inventory (Univariate)
   - Providing more specific detail in relation to both the extent of the fatigue and its impact on quality of life
   - Patient's rate their level of fatigue on a scale of 0 (no fatigue) to 10 (as bad as you can imagine)
   - Patients score how fatigue has affected their general activity, mood, walking ability, work, relationships, and enjoyment of life on a scale of 0 (does not interfere) to 10 (completely interferes)
   - Fatigue scoring is described as following:
     - Mild 1–3
     - Moderate 4–6
     - Severe 7–10
   - Some patients may prefer to use the words mild, moderate and severe in preference to using numbers.

(NCCN, 2018; Radbruch et al., 2008)

Please circle the number that best describes how you feel NOW:

No Pain	0	1	2	3	4	5	6	7	8	9	10	Worst Possible Pain
No Tiredness (Tiredness = lack of energy)	0	1	2	3	4	5	6	7	8	9	10	Worst Possible Tiredness
No Drowsiness (Drowsiness = feeling sleepy)	0	1	2	3	4	5	6	7	8	9	10	Worst Possible Drowsiness
No Nausea	0	1	2	3	4	5	6	7	8	9	10	Worst Possible Nausea
No Lack of Appetite	0	1	2	3	4	5	6	7	8	9	10	Worst Possible Lack of Appetite
No Shortness of Breath	0	1	2	3	4	5	6	7	8	9	10	Worst Possible Shortness of Breath
No Depression (Depression = feeling sad)	0	1	2	3	4	5	6	7	8	9	10	Worst Possible Depression
No Anxiety (Anxiety = feeling nervous)	0	1	2	3	4	5	6	7	8	9	10	Worst Possible Anxiety
Best Wellbeing (Wellbeing = how you feel overall)	0	1	2	3	4	5	6	7	8	9	10	Worst Possible Wellbeing
No _____ Other Problem (for example constipation)	0	1	2	3	4	5	6	7	8	9	10	Worst Possible _____

Figure 4.5.1 Edmonton Symptom Assessment Tool (Revised Version) (ESAS-R).

Source: Reproduced with the kind permission of the University of Alberta. Originally published in Bruera E et al., (1991) The Edmonton Symptom Assessment System (ESAS): a simple method for the assessment of palliative care patients. *Journal of Palliative Care, 7:* 6–9.

As fatigue is recognised as having both physical and cognitive dimensions, it is important that the questions used in any assessment recognise both of these elements. Where patients are cognitively impaired, the views of carers or staff members should be taken into consideration, remembering that carers will often overestimate symptoms and staff often underestimate (Radbruch et al., 2008).

Fatigue in heart failure

Fatigue is often the first symptom experienced by patients with heart failure and along with dyspnoea, it is described as the most distressing. Its impact on daily living is complicated by its unpredictability, fluctuating intensity and direct impact on physical capacity (Herr et al., 2014). Fatigue due to its relation with other symptoms, including depression, dyspnoea, oedema and pain, is also identified in the literature as a syndrome (Radbruch et al., 2008).

Literature on HF emphasises the necessity for an echocardiogram to take place to confirm that the presenting symptoms truly do relate to HF as this will influence the subsequent management decisions (Hagglund et al., 2007).

Patients with HF may experience different types of fatigue, such as:

- Lack of physical and mental energy
- Lack of physical strength
- Unforeseen drowsiness.

Fatigue assessment therefore must include detail around:

- Frequency
- Variation
- Severity
- Relationship to activity
- Impact on everyday life
- What the patient may do to prevent or relieve this symptom.

Gaining this information will help the clinician to know how aware the patient is of this symptom and how they personally cope with it.

Whether utilising assessment tools or not, the priority for the clinician is to recognise that fatigue is likely to be present and the patient needs encouragement, support and permission to disclose this often overwhelming symptom.

Management

Following recognition and assessment of fatigue, the evidence would support a multidisciplinary approach to management of this multifactorial symptom. A person-centred approach is essential.

Clinical considerations in the management of fatigue

Remember to reverse the reversible:

- Use of antibiotics for the treatment of identified infection.
- Use of antidepressants taking into consideration prognosis and potential side-effect profiles.
- Blood transfusion for the treatment of symptomatic anaemia.
- There is limited evidence to support the use of erythropoietin in patients receiving palliative chemotherapy, and any potential benefit has to be measured alongside the side-effect profile and the individual patient's prognosis.
- Management of pain, nausea, sleep problems or other troubling symptoms (see local palliative care guidelines). It has been recognised that managing other symptoms co-existing with fatigue can improve the patient's quality of life even though it may not directly impact on the experience of fatigue.
- Ongoing review to ensure the management is effective and not causing more burden than benefit.

Non-pharmacological management of fatigue

This is where the best evidence is currently available.

- Multidisciplinary approach:
  - Qualitative evidence supports a multidisciplinary approach for palliative care patients. One study where improvement of fatigue was measured as significant showed that this was enabled by patients knowing that their carers were receiving support, and that having the input from social workers and dieticians improved psychosocial and other non-medical elements of pain, fatigue and anxiety (Koesel et al., 2019).
- Rehabilitation and exercise:
  - There is some evidence in cancer patients but also in HF, COPD and neurological conditions for the use of exercise programmes and rehabilitation interventions in improving fatigue, mood, functional independence, breathlessness and pain (Wittry et al., 2018). Aerobic exercise has greater evidence but other exercise is also described. The duration and the location of the exercise also vary depending on the needs of the patient.
  - Patients may benefit from using an activity/fatigue diary to help them identify when they are most fatigued and any particular elements which may be contributing (Scottish Palliative Care Guidelines, 2020b).
  - HF patients are advised to refrain from activities that have previously worsened fatigue and instead focus on identifying activities that are more realisable (Schjoedt et al., 2016).

- Psychosocial interventions:

  These have already been referred to briefly but the benefits achieved by these interventions cannot be underestimated. These interventions may include:
  - Stress/anxiety management
  - Relaxation/complementary therapies
  - Indulging in positive thinking
  - Involvement in moderate social activity
  - Counselling
- Sleep hygiene advice:
  - Stimulus control, that is going to bed when sleepy, regular timing of going to bed and rising
  - Comfortable, dark quiet sleeping environment
  - Avoid long or late afternoon naps
  - Avoid caffeine after noon
  - Avoid use of interactive technology for several hours prior to sleep.
- Written and audio materials.

Pharmacological management of fatigue

There is limited evidence to support any specific drug therapy for the management of fatigue.

- Consider medicines, including over the counter medications that the patient is currently taking which could be impacting on fatigue, for example beta blockers, narcotics, antidepressants, antihistamines. Polypharmacy can also be an issue and may benefit from overall review.

- Limited evidence supports short-term improvement of fatigue in patients commenced on corticosteroids (dexamethasone) but the side-effect profile of long-term use of steroids does not support their use specifically for fatigue. However, steroids are often commenced for other symptoms, for example pain or anorexia, and initially patients often experience a boost in energy and an improvement in their quality of life. Short duration of treatment will prevent patients developing issues such as myopathy and possibly steroid-induced diabetes.

- There have been trials using stimulant drugs such as methylphenidate and modafinil but the quality of evidence does not support their recommendation in this group of patients.

- The use of antidepressants to address concomitant depression in patients with fatigue showed evidence of improvement in depression but no evidence supporting any impact on fatigue.

- Hypnotic medication should be reserved for transient and short-term insomnia and its use reviewed regularly (Hugel et al., 2004)

(Radbruch et al., 2008; Scottish Palliative Care Guidelines, 2020b; NCCN, 2018)

Summary

Fatigue is a common and complex multidimensional symptom in both cancer and non-cancer end-of-life conditions. Its impact on a patient's quality of life is not always recognised by healthcare professionals and it has also been relatively neglected in end-of-life research. Management includes screening, assessment and a team approach using non-pharmacological and pharmacological modalities.

References

Bruera E et al. (1991) The Edmonton Symptom Assessment System (ESAS): a simple method for the assessment of palliative care patients. *Journal of Palliative Care*, 7(2): 6–9.

Cella D et al. (2001) Cancer-related fatigue: prevalence of proposed diagnostic criteria in a United States sample of cancer survivors. *Journal of Clinical Oncology*, 19(14): 3385–3391.

Cella D and Fallowfield LJ (2008) Recognition and management of treatment-related side effects for breast cancer patients receiving adjuvant endocrine therapy. *Breast Cancer Research and Treatment,* 107(2): 167–180.

Deng G et al. (2007) Randomized, controlled trial of acupuncture for the treatment of hot flashes in breast cancer patients. *Journal of Clinical Oncology,* 25(35): 5584–5590.

Ghoshal A et al. (2017) Impact of symptom control on fatigue in patients with advanced cancer: A prospective observational study. *Progress in Palliative Care*, 25(2): 63–74.

Hagglund L et al. (2007) Fatigue and health-related quality of life in elderly patients with and without heart failure in primary healthcare. *European Journal of Cardiovascular Nursing*, 6(3): 208–215.

Han L and Dong X (2014) Itch mechanisms and circuits. *Annual Review of Biophysics,* 43(1): 331–355.

Herr JK et al. (2014) Heart failure symptom relationships. A systematic review. *Journal of Cardiovascular Nursing*, 29(5): 416–422.

Hugel H et al. (2004) The prevalence, key causes and management of insomnia in palliative care patients. *Journal of Pain and Symptom Management*, 27(4): 316–320.

Johns C et al. (2016) Informing hot flash treatment decisions for breast cancer survivors: a systematic review of randomized trials comparing active interventions, *Breast Cancer Research and Treatment,* 156(3): 415–426.

Kaye P (1994) *A–Z Pocketbook of Symptom Control*. Northampton: EPL Publishers.

Keeley V (2000) Oedema in advanced cancer. In Twycross R, Jenns K and Todd J (eds) *Lymphoedema*. Oxford: Radcliffe Medical Press, pp. 338–358.

Koesel N et al. (2019) Symptom distress: implementation of palliative care guidelines to improve pain, fatigue, and anxiety in patients with advanced cancer. *Clinical Journal of Oncology*, 23(2): 149–155.

Lawrence DP et al. (2004) Evidence report on the occurrence, assessment, and treatment of fatigue in cancer patients. *Journal of the National Cancer Institute Monograph*, 2004(32): 40–50.

Mercadante S et al. (2013) Orphan symptoms in advanced cancer patients followed at home. *Supportive Care in Cancer*, 21(12): 3525.

Munck B, Fridlund B and Martensson J (2008) Next of kin caregivers in palliative home care from control to loss of control. *Journal of Advanced Nursing*, 64(6): 578–586.

NCCN (National Comprehensive Cancer Network) (2018) NCCN clinical practice guidelines in oncology (NCCN Guidelines) cancer-related fatigue, version 2. NCCN.org. Available at: https://oncolife.com.ua/doc/nccn/fatigue.pdf

Neale B (1991) Informal palliative care: a review of research on needs, standards and service evaluation. Occasional Paper 3. Sheffield: Trent Palliative Care Service.

Pandya KJ et al. (2005) Gabapentin for hot flashes in 420 women with breast cancer: a randomised double-blind placebo-controlled trial. *Lancet,* 366(9488): 818–824.

Pyszora A (2017) Physiotherapy programme reduces fatigue in patients with advanced cancer receiving palliative care: randomized control trial. *Supportive Care in Cancer*, 25(9): 2899–2908.

Radbruch L et al., and the Research Steering Committee of the European Association for Palliative Care (EAPC) (2008) Fatigue in palliative care patients – an EAPC approach. *Palliative Medicine*, 22(1): 13–32.

Ream E and Richardson A. (1996) Fatigue: a concept analysis. *International Journal of Nursing Studies*, 33(5): 519–529.

Renshaw M (2007) Lymphorrhoea: 'leaky legs' are not just the nurse's problem. *British Journal of Community Nurses*, 12(4): 18–21.

Schjoedt I, Sommer I and Bjerrum MB (2016) Experiences and management of fatigue in everyday life among adult patients living with heart failure: a systematic review of qualitative evidence. *Joanna Briggs Institute Database of Systematic Reviews and Implementation Reports*, 14(3): 68–115.

Schneider G et al. (2006) Psychosomatic cofactors and psychiatric comorbidity in patients with chronic itch. *Clinical and Experimental Dermatology,* 31(6): 762–767.

Scottish Palliative Care Guidelines (2019) Pruritus. Available at: https://www.palliativecareguidelines.scot.nhs.uk/guidelines/symptom-control/Pruritis.aspx

Scottish Palliative Care Guidelines (2020a) Sweating. Available at: https://www.palliativecareguidelines.scot.nhs.uk/guidelines/symptom-control/sweating.aspx

Scottish Palliative Care Guidelines (2020b) Weakness/Fatigue. Available at: https://www.palliativecareguidelines.scot.nhs.uk/guidelines/symptom-control/weakness-fatigue.aspx

Seccareccia D and Gebara N (2011) Pruritus in palliative care: getting up to scratch. *Canadian Family Physician Medecin De Famille Canadien* 57(9): 1010–1013, e316–319.

Servaes P, Verhagen C and Bleijenberg G (2002) Fatigue in cancer patients during and after treatment: prevalence, correlates and interventions. *European Journal of Cancer*, 38(1): 27–43.

Siemens W et al. (2016) Pharmacological interventions for pruritus in adult palliative care patients. Edited by the Cochrane Pain, Palliative and Supportive Care Group. *Cochrane Database of Systematic Reviews*, November 16.

Tobin MB et al. (1993) The psychological morbidity of breast cancer related arm swelling. *Cancer*, 72(11): 3248–3252.

Tsavaris N et al. (1990) A randomized trial of the effect of three non-steroid antiinflammatory agents in ameliorating cancer-induced fever. *Journal of Internal Medicine*, 228(5): 451–455.

Twycross R et al. (2003) Itch: scratching more than the surface. *QJM: Monthly Journal of the Association of Physicians*, 96(1): 7–26.

Twycross R, Wilcock A and Howard P (2017) *Palliative Care Formulary* (PCF6), 6th edition (UK). Nottingham: Palliativedrugs.com Ltd.

Wang CH et al. (2019) Karnofsky performance status as a predictive factor for cancer-related fatigue treatment with astragalus polysaccharides (pg2) injection – a double blind, multi-centre, randomized phase iv study. *Cancers*, 11(2): 128.

Williams AF (2004) Understanding and managing lymphoedema in people with advanced cancer. *Journal of Community Nursing*, 18(11): 30–37.

Wittry SA, Lan NY and McNally T (2018) The value of rehabilitation medicine for patients receiving palliative care. *American Journal of Hospice and Palliative Medicine*, 35(6):889–896.

Yosipovitch G, Greaves MW and Schmelz M (2003) Itch. *Lancet*, 361(9358): 690–694.

Chapter 5

Drugs and Medication

Paul Wilson with Leza Z Quate

Learning Objectives

This chapter will enable you to:

- Identify what is meant by polypharmacy and the triggers for a medication review
- Identify tools and priorities for carrying out a medication review
- Understand the rationale for anticipatory medicines and what and when to prescribe them
- Understand the rationale, advantages and disadvantages for using alternative routes of administrations
- Take account of challenging patient groups and some of the specific issues which they can present with.

Scenario

Background

Kamal, a 73-year-old male, has been diagnosed with bowel cancer with several areas of local and distant metastases. He has recently been told that he is for no further curative treatment and is for best supportive care. He is currently taking:

- Alendronic acid 70 mg once weekly
- Adcal D3 chewable 1 (twice daily)
- Aspirin 75 mg (once daily)
- Carvedilol 12.5 mg (twice daily)

- Losartan 50 mg (once daily)
- Furosemide 20 mg (once daily)
- Eplerenone 25 mg (once daily)
- Rosuvastatin 10 mg (at night)
- Omeprazole 20 mg (once daily)
- Paracetamol 1 g (four times a day)
- Mirtazapine 15 mg (at night).

Kamal is currently reporting symptoms of occasional pain mostly on movement and some dizziness on standing, but is otherwise near his baseline. His pain is usually in the abdomen and groin area but he is mostly pain free at the moment.

Key points

- Patients that have advanced disease and a limited prognosis should have their medication reviewed.
- Patients that currently have a number of symptoms that are ongoing and not controlled should have their medicines reviewed.
- If a patient is already taking a significant number of medicines, which are likely to be added to, they should have their medicines reviewed.

Timeline

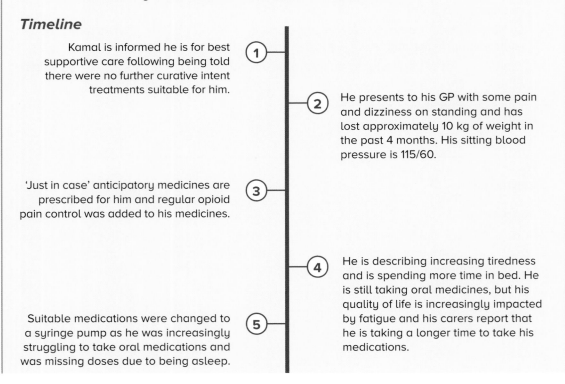

1 Kamal is informed he is for best supportive care following being told there were no further curative intent treatments suitable for him.

2 He presents to his GP with some pain and dizziness on standing and has lost approximately 10 kg of weight in the past 4 months. His sitting blood pressure is 115/60.

3 'Just in case' anticipatory medicines are prescribed for him and regular opioid pain control was added to his medicines.

4 He is describing increasing tiredness and is spending more time in bed. He is still taking oral medicines, but his quality of life is increasingly impacted by fatigue and his carers report that he is taking a longer time to take his medications.

5 Suitable medications were changed to a syringe pump as he was increasingly struggling to take oral medications and was missing doses due to being asleep.

Key considerations

- Does Kamal have any indications of potential complicating factors relating to medication?

- Polypharmacy is an ongoing process and when patients are being treated with palliative intent the risk versus benefit consideration is always changing. Do you think that Kamal is benefiting from the therapy he is receiving and is he able to safely manage it?

- When considering Kamal's care, how would you plan ahead?

- Therapies can rapidly become complex and multi-morbidities add to that complexity as well as the volume of medicines which can overwhelm patients and carers. What would you do to manage the complexity of polypharmacy in a palliative patient?

Polypharmacy and Realistic Medicines

Polypharmacy means, in a literal sense, many medicines but in a practical sense we should be considering appropriate polypharmacy. It will mean assessing if there is still a purpose for the, often multiple, medications that are being prescribed. Medication is the most common form of medical intervention and palliative care is no different in this respect. Individual symptoms or therapies can often require multiple medicines. Polypharmacy is not inherently wrong, but as treatments are added it should trigger a response in you to look at what is now no longer required, as well as what is. When anyone is nearing a double-digit list of medications, do they really know what they are all for and if they are actually working?

Appropriate polypharmacy means:

- The patient agrees to the therapeutic aims and is motivated and able to take the medication as intended.

- The therapeutic aims are being achieved or are achievable.

- The dosing is optimised to maximise effectiveness while minimising the adverse effects of the therapy.

Medication review

Medication review is a core part of ensuring appropriate polypharmacy, but how do you identify the patients most at risk, and achieve the greatest benefit when managing a significant medication burden? The Scottish Government document *Polypharmacy Guidance: Realistic Prescribing* (Scottish Government Polypharmacy Model of Care Group, 2018) identifies factors which should trigger a review.

These are:

A. Those aged 50 years and older and resident in a care home, regardless of the number of medicines prescribed.

B. Those approaching the end of their life. Adults of any age, approaching the end of their life due to any cause, are likely to have different medication needs. The risk versus benefit discussions will often differ from healthy adults with longer expected life spans.

C. Those who are prescribed ten or more medicines.

D. Those on high-risk medication, regardless of the number of medicines taken. High-risk medicines have a proven benefit but have also been identified as having adverse drug reactions, potentially causing/contributing to hospital admissions (they are listed in Table 5.1).

Palliative care patients meet criteria B, but commonly will also be on high-risk medication (opioids, benzodiazapines or Z-drugs (zopiclone and zolpidem)) and will often also require ten or more prescribed medications. Pain control treatment can create five medications alone: regular and as required (PRN) opioid, paracetamol, adjuvant (for example gabapentin), laxative and, as required, anti-emetic. Patients who are receiving palliative care, not just end-of-life care, need regular medication review. The balance of risk versus benefit of prescribed medication alters throughout the progression of a disease. Therefore, medications that may be of value early on in the disease may be less beneficial and more burdensome later on in the disease journey.

Table 5.1   Examples of high-risk drugs.

British National Formulary section	Examples
2.1 Positive inotropic medicines	Digoxin
2.2 Diuretics	Bendroflumethiazide, spironolactone, furosemide
2.5 Hypertension/heart failure	Ramipril, enalapril, losartan
2.8 Anticoagulants and protamine	Warfarin, rivaroxaban, edoxaban, apixaban, dabigatran
2.9 Anti-platelets	Clopidogrel, dipyridamole
4.1 Hypnotics and anxiolytics	Benzodiazepines, Z-drugs
4.2 Antipsychotic/antimanic drugs	Amisulpride, risperidone
4.3 Antidepressants	Amitriptyline, fluoxetine, paroxetine
4.7.2 Opioid analgesics	Tramadol, co-codamol, morphine, fentanyl
10.1 Rheumatic diseases and gout	NSAIDs, corticosteroids, methotrexate

Source: Scottish Government Polypharmacy Model of Care Group, 2018.

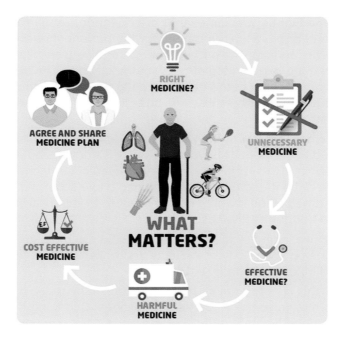

Figure 5.1 7 steps to appropriate polypharmacy: what matters?

Source: Scottish Government Polypharmacy Model of Care Group (2018) *Polypharmacy Guidance, Realistic Prescribing*, 3rd edition. Edinburgh: Scottish Government.

How do you carry out a medication review

The *Polypharmacy Guidance: Realistic Prescribing* guidelines provide a seven-step process to follow that guides healthcare professionals (HCPs) through a review of a patient's medicines. The process starts with, and must retain throughout, what matters to the patient. If medication reviews are to be successful and maximise effectiveness then the patient has to be involved and in agreement with the process. The seven steps to appropriate polypharmacy have the patient and their priorities at its centre and give a starting point to reviewing each of the medicines that are prescribed. It can also be used to determine if it is appropriate to start new medicines (Figure 5.1).

The steps

Always start a review by asking the patient what their priorities for their medication therapies are and what problems they are having, if any, with their current medication regimen. Then work along the steps (Scottish Government Polypharmacy Model of Care Group, 2018):

- **Essential medicines**: either essential replacement medicines (i.e. levothyroxine) or medicines that prevent rapid symptomatic decline (heart failure or epilepsy medications).

- **Unnecessary medicines**: medicines that are no longer required, have limited benefit in general or have limited benefit for the patient under review (i.e. long-term prophylactic medicines in patients with a relatively short prognosis, statins in patients with a life expectancy of a few months). They can also be medicines that are no longer needed at the dose currently prescribed and can be reduced to lower doses (i.e. blood pressure medicines if the patient has lost weight due to other disease states).

- **Effective medicines**: are therapeutic targets being met and do increases in medication need to be made? Medication review is not just about reducing medicine burden – it is about maximising effectiveness of medicines. If cholesterol control is important to the patient and the patient is taking a low dose of a statin but is not meeting local targets, then it would be appropriate to increase the dose of statin to try and achieve better effectiveness.

- **Harmful medicines**: high-risk medicines in Table 5.1 are a reasonable starting point, but any medicine can have adverse effects and frailer patients are at greater risk of being impacted by adverse drug reactions.

- **Cost effective**: this is not about stopping a medicine because it is expensive but about trying to maximise the value from medicines. Changing medicines for cost should only be done if safety, effectiveness and compliance are not compromised. The least cost-effective medicines are the ones that are sitting unused in a patient's home because the patient cannot or does not want to take the medicine. Cost effectiveness can be improved by ensuring there are not any unnecessary costly formulations of a product prescribed (i.e. particular branded products or costly formulations that are not actually needed). Patients may have needed a liquid or dispersible formulation at one point due to an acute episode that has now resolved and may be able to take normal formulations now that the episode has passed.

- **Agree and share the plan**: patient agreement to the plan is essential to achieving the desired outcomes and benefits. If a patient does not wish to stop or start a medicine then there is likely to be a failure in the intended outcomes.

Polypharmacy-led medicine reviews and considerations taken during any prescribing are NOT about saving money. They are about efficient, outcome-driven and patient-focused prescribing to improve the patient's quality of life, with the occasional outcome that money is saved. They are a collaborative process. When carrying out a review if there are multiple opportunities agreed for improving a patient's medicines it is sensible to carry out one or two things at a time. This may mean that the plan is not fully enacted after a single consultation or at that time, but it does mean that if there are any adverse impacts of the changes to medicines then it is easier to identify which change has triggered the negative outcome.

The polypharmacy review could also be an opportunity to check concordance of the patient with their medicines. This may involve investigating if there are any difficulties inhibiting the patient from taking the prescribed medicines and looking at appropriate tactics for easing the concordance with medicines taking. These could include tablet splitters (for large or difficult to swallow tablets), setting alarms on phones to remind the patient to take their medicines or self filled pill bibles. Monitored Dosage Systems (MDS), also known as blister packs or NOMADs, can be useful where oversight is needed or in relatively fixed drug regimens where the patient can't, or chooses not to, take part in their medicines. They are not always ideal for patients given the additional workload involved in getting them to the patient. Local community pharmacies can help with services offered to aid a patient with taking their medicines.

Anticipatory Medicines

Anticipatory medicines, often also called 'just in case' medicines, are medicines which are prescribed in advance and in anticipation of a patient requiring them later. This advanced prescribing minimises unnecessary delays in supply and administration of the medicines to manage the symptoms. This reduces stress and distress on both the patient and the carers, both professional and unpaid.

These medicines are intended to improve the most common symptoms experienced at end of life. These are pain, breathlessness, anxiety, nausea and respiratory secretions. The most commonly used drugs are morphine, midazolam, hyoscine butylbromide and levomepromazine, but local practice may vary. There is an ongoing dialogue around when is the best time to put these medicines into a patient's home. It can be a difficult decision and is a risk versus benefit issue. A practical approach is that the correct time is at the point where you think a patient may need these medicines in the next few weeks to months. This may seem very early for some, but the biggest advantage of having these medicines in a patient's home is that it can give everybody involved a sense of comfort in the knowledge that those medicines are available if they are needed. This can help to avoid patients suffering distressing symptoms while HCPs organise a prescription, obtain the medicines and finally administer them. HCPs can often find managing a palliative care patient stressful enough, without the added stress of knowing what they should do, but are unable to do because the medicines are not available to them when they visit. Reasons for not putting these medicines in place early could be because there is a risk of misuse by the patient, a risk of diversion of the drugs by a friend or carer, or a risk to other members of the household, such as young children.

The Scottish Palliative Care Guidelines (Scottish Palliative Care Guidelines, 2014a) has a guideline on anticipatory prescribing which highlights the five main symptoms that the four medicines (morphine, midazolam, hyoscine butylbromide and levomepromazine) can treat. These core medicines, among other medicines, will often be stocked by community pharmacies contributing to local community pharmacy palliative care networks which will be able to offer enhanced stockholding, advice and support to their local communities.

Prescribing opioids

Table 5.2 outlines the doses and advice for opioid-naive patients. The dose, and the opioid, will change if the patient is already on regular opioids. 'The as-required' dose will be the approximate equivalent dose to 1/10th to 1/6th of the usual regular dose. This may require some calculation if the patient is on regular oral opioids or not on subcutaneous administration already (Scottish Palliative Care Guidelines, 2020).

Table 5.2   Anticipatory prescribing symptoms and medications.

Anticipatory prescription	The prescription should include the four medications that might be required for end-of-life symptom control, plus diluent Note: It is important that prescription wording for controlled drugs meets the legal requirements to reduce delays in dispensing
Opioid for pain and/or breathlessness (for opioid naive patient)	Morphine sulfate injection (10 mg/ml ampoules) Dose: 2 mg subcutaneous, repeated at hourly intervals as needed for pain or breathlessness If three or more doses have been given within 4 hours with little or no benefit seek urgent advice or review If more than six doses are required in 24 hours seek advice or review Supply ten 1 ml ampoules* Note: Some NHS boards may use diamorphine
Anxiolytic sedative for anxiety or agitation or breathlessness	Midazolam injection (10 mg in 2 ml ampoules) Dose: 2 mg SC, repeated at hourly intervals as needed for anxiety/distress If three or more doses have been given within 4 hours with little or no benefit seek urgent advice or review If more than six doses are required in 24 hours seek advice or review Supply ten ampoules of 2 ml* Midazolam can be used in massive terminal haemorrhage Note: if the patient is already on large background doses of benzodiazepines, a larger dose may be needed (if they are frail, a smaller dose may be sufficient) Levomepromazine can be used in terminal agitation or agitated delirium under specialist advice at a different dose
Anti-secretory for respiratory secretions	Hyoscine butylbromide injection (Buscopan®) (20 mg/ml ampoules) Dose: 20 mg SC, repeated at hourly intervals as needed for respiratory secretions Maximum of 120 mg in 24 hours. Supply ten ampoules*
Anti-emetic for nausea and vomiting	Levomepromazine injection (25 mg/ml ampoules) Dose: 2.5 to 5 mg SC, 12 hourly as needed for nausea. May need to be given more frequently initially, for example hourly, to control symptoms. If three or more doses have been given within 4 hours with little or no benefit seek urgent advice or review. If more than six doses are required in 24 hours seek advice or review. Supply ten ampoules* Levomepromazine can be used in terminal agitation or agitated delirium under specialist advice at a different dose

*Some Health Boards may recommend smaller quantities as appropriate.

Source: Scottish Palliative Care Guidelines, 2014a.

Kamal, discussed above, is on 40 mg twice daily of oxycodone modified release (MR) orally with 13 mg orally as required, using the liquid. The likely anticipatory dose for this patient is therefore oxycodone 6 mg subcutaneously hourly as required for pain or breathlessness. The things to note about this are:

Where possible use the same opioid for as-required dosing as for regular dosing (this is not practical for fentanyl patches, so consider the last used opioid or morphine).

The dose should be rounded to a practically administrable dose (1/6th to 1/10th is advised). In the above example the dose can be calculated either by dividing the total daily oral dose by 6 then converted to subcutaneous equivalent by dividing by 2 (e.g. 80/6 then divide by 2 = 6.666667 mg). Alternatively you could use the current oral as required dose, of 13 mg, and convert that to an equivalent subcutaneous dose, in this case divide by 2 (for example, 13 divided by 2 = 6.5 mg). Both methods would give a decimal place. It is good practice to avoid this where possible, and not give a volume that is difficult to measure. Oxycodone is available in 10 mg/ml, so simply rounding down to 6 mg eliminates the decimal place in the dose and eases administration without having any likely impact on patient care (any whole number between 4 and 7 mg in this case would be sensible, depending on clinical assessment).

Alternative Routes of Administration Including Syringe Pumps

The primary method of administering medications in palliative care is orally. It is the simplest and most widely available method of drug delivery and barring any confounding factors it is the route of choice. However, in palliative care there are often factors which can mean that the oral route is either not available or is not in the best interest of the patient (see Box 5.1).

Box 5.1 Examples of reasons to use alternative routes in palliative care

1. Persistent nausea and/or vomiting
2. Dysphagia
3. Bowel obstruction and malabsorption or drug kinetics
4. Significant tablet burden and patient preference/care
5. Reduced level of consciousness, such as in the last days of life.

The most widely used alternative route of medication administration is a syringe pump (currently the most common device is a T34™ or Bodyguard™ T syringe pump – see Figure 5.2) which allows medication to be administered over 24 hours via subcutaneous injection. The use of a subcutaneous pump does not deliver better symptom control than oral therapies unless there is an issue with either absorption or administration of the medicine.

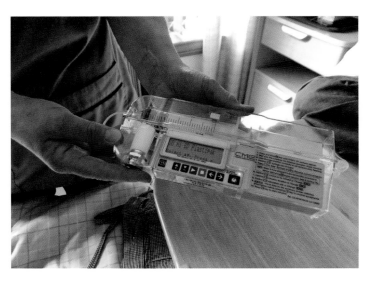

Figure 5.2 T34™ Syringe pump.

The use of the pump is not necessarily because the patient is nearing end of life. It is worth discussing and reinforcing this with patients and their carers, as people often associate the use of the pump with 'end of life' and a 'one way' procedure rather than managing symptoms and poor or unpredictable oral intake, which may or may not be related to end-of-life care.

The pump delivers small volumes (approximately 30 ml maximum) over a period of 24 hours and can contain single or multiple medications diluted with either water for injection or sodium chloride 0.9% (local practices may vary). The administration of medicines via this route is almost always 'off-label' and when multiple medicines are used it is always off-label use. There are a number of sources of advice around which combinations of medicines can and cannot be mixed in a single syringe. One of the most widely available is the Scottish Palliative Care Guidelines (Scottish Palliative Care Guidelines, 2014b), 'Syringe Pumps' section, which contains tables covering dozens of combinations of medicines with maximum quantities known to be compatible.

The use of 'off-label' medicines, which occurs commonly in palliative care, should always be carried out mindful of the risks and benefits to the patient. It also changes the legal liability related to these medicines. Higher liability lies with the prescriber, rather than the manufacturer, and prescribers should be aware of this.

Alternative routes of administration can also be used when a patient is transitioning away from oral routes for any reason. These can be as simple and straightforward as using transdermal patches (i.e. fentanyl or hyoscine hydrobromide). Bolus subcutaneous injections can be particularly suited to medicines which can be given once daily (i.e. levomepromazine or dexamethasone). Less commonly used options are buccal or sublingual administration. These routes are more limited and only some medications and some formulations will work. Advice may be required by the generalist from their local palliative care team. A combination of some or all the available options may be required for an individual. This can add to the complexity of the patient's medications and can be taken as an opportunity, as discussed above, to rationalise them.

For patients with enteral feeding tubes, administering medicines through the tube is a complicated process involving prescribers, pharmacists, nursing staff, patients and carers (if they are involved in administering any of the medicines). This route can impact the licensed status of a medicine, often making it off label. It runs the risk of blocking feeding tubes and medicines can also be absorbed by the tube, so each medicine that is to be administered via an enteral tube should be assessed individually to ensure it is safe and effective. Information can be found in consultation with pharmacy colleagues and also in textbooks like *Handbook of Drug Administration via Enteral Feeding Tubes* (White and Bradnam, 2007).

A recent trend in marketed medications has been the use of 'melt' tablet formulations. These can be very useful as a means of getting patients to take medicines they are having difficulty swallowing but they are limited in that the formulations still need to be swallowed and are not buccally or sublingually absorbed. These tablets can be relatively delicate and require an amount of manual dexterity to manage and remove from their packaging: it is often a peel off type rather than a simpler push through type of packaging. Their advantage is that the tablet 'melts' into sufficiently small granules that the patient doesn't notice swallowing the medication along with their saliva. An example of this would be lansoprazole 'melt' tablets which consist of tiny enteric coated granules and have to actually be swallowed and get through the stomach and into the duodenum before they are absorbed.

Challenging Patient Groups

Renal impairment

The patients most significantly impacted by renal impairment will be those with stage 4 or 5 (Estimated Glomerular Filtration Rate (eGFR) <30 ml/min) acute or chronic kidney disease (Renal Association, 2020). For renal impairment we have a good measure, the eGFR, of how we can expect the kidneys to handle the elimination of medicines. This can be very useful in guiding how we approach the therapy of a patient. It is quick and convenient, usually part of standard biochemistry results. However, in patients with advanced disease the eGFR can be inaccurate and show 'false' renal function (Glassock and Winearls, 2008). A patient who is severely cachectic may have very little muscle mass so is producing very little creatinine and therefore renal function (eGFR) may be calculated as artificially healthy. The best way of adjusting is by calculating the creatinine clearance using the Cockcroft–Gault equation and using this figure as the basis dose adjustments rather than the eGFR.

The general principles of drug therapy in renal impairment are to give small and cautious doses with a reduced frequency. This is broad advice, and specific advice is usually found in the British National Formulary (BNF) (NICE, 2021). Look to treat any reversible causes of the renal impairment (i.e. dehydration or infection). The use of anticipatory medicines, beyond opioids, is not significantly altered by renal impairment and standard dosing is advised (Scottish Palliative Care Guidelines, 2013). With opioids, usual first choices are morphine, diamorphine and oxycodone which are all excreted by the kidneys, and all have renally excreted active metabolites.

Alfentanil and fentanyl are both not excreted via the kidney and are good options for use in renal failure, but both also have limitations in practical use. Alfentanil comes as an injection and has a very short half-life of approximately 90 minutes (EMC, 2020). This can be limiting both in that a syringe pump would be required, and that sometimes the use of alfentanil 'as required' does not last very long. This is useful for short-lasting incident pain but sometimes is not long enough for normal breakthrough or uncontrolled pain. Alfentanil does have a high strength formulation which can allow for very high opioid equivalent doses (5 mg alfentanil injection = 150 mg oral morphine) to be administered in a syringe pump (Scottish Palliative Care Guidelines, 2020). Fentanyl is available in transdermal patches for regular background analgesia, but with their inherent limitations: slow titration, relatively high 'lowest dosing' and occasional patch displacement. Injections, which are limited by concentration but can be used in a syringe pump (specialist use only), and the various formulations of rapid acting buccal, sublingual and nasal fentanyl, which again are short acting (2–3 hours), are also very potent, with the lowest strength of these products equivalent to around an oral morphine dose of 10–15 mg (Scottish Palliative Care Guidelines, 2020).

For opioid-naive, renally impaired patients the best advice is to use low doses of the most convenient opioid, with longer than normal dosage intervals and the avoidance of long-acting preparations, until pain control is stable. This could mean, for a patient able to take oral medications, oxycodone (probably slightly better than morphine) 1 or 2 mg, two or three times daily and 1 mg as required, with small and cautious dose increases as needed. You would only consider changing to MR tablets if the patient was tolerating sufficiently large doses (over 10 mg/24 hours) and is stable on the dose. Alfentanil, a better drug in renal impairment, could be chosen if a syringe pump is thought to be appropriate and longer-term administration is not a factor, but still starting at low doses of 200–500 micrograms/24 hours with 100 micrograms as required.

For patients already on opioids who have an acute kidney injury or slowly deteriorating renal function, the usual advice would be to change the opioid if there are signs of opioid toxicity and not solely because they have renal impairement. With this group of patients, one of the first signs to look out for is, odd though it may sound, an improvement in pain control as indicated by a reduction in the number of 'as-required' doses they are taking. This can indicate that the drug is accumulating in the body before the patient shows symptoms of toxicity. In this scenario consider reducing the dose by 25–50% but not changing the drug. If the patient had started showing signs of toxicity, both reduce the equivalent dose and switch the opioid administered.

With renal impairment the simple advice is titrate up slowly and cautiously, but titrate down and switch opioids quickly and aggressively, always trying to get to a better tolerated opioid that is suitable for that individual patient's circumstances. Don't switch opioids if the patient is already on and tolerating an opioid but do monitor them for toxicity.

Drugs, the liver and the variability of metabolism

About 75% of medicines are partly or completely metabolised by Cytochrome P450 (CYP450) which is significantly concentrated in the liver (Guengerich, 2008). There are multiple factors which influence and affect a response to medications, including genetics and environmental influences. Medications will interact with the CYP450 enzymes in three ways:

1. They can be a *substrate* and are metabolised by the enzymes.
2. They can *inhibit* the enzyme meaning they prevent or reduce metabolism by that enzyme.
3. They can *induce* the enzyme meaning they can increase the metabolism by that enzyme.

We have no simple and direct way of determining what a person's baseline CYP450 function is and how it is changed by the administration of a medicine. There are, however, broad guidelines and there is a growing understanding of which medicines cause which effects.

Substrates are metabolised by a specific or multiple CYP450 enzymes.

Inhibitors tend to bond to a specific or multiple CYP450 enzymes and then block the ability of the enzyme to carry out its activity. This can be either temporary and occurs while the drug is present, or permanent and only stops when the enzyme is itself replaced. This will show an impact within a few days of the inhibiting drug being administered and will usually lose effect a few days after the inhibiting drug is stopped.

Inducers will tend to increase the production of the CYP450 enzyme involved and not make the enzyme more efficient. This increased production of an enzyme increases the body's ability to metabolise medicines. This effect will show an impact in 1–2 weeks and will tend to lose effect over 1–2 weeks after the inducer is removed from the system (Wilcock et al. 2020)

Medicines can have several interactions with the CYP450 system. For example, carbamazepine is both a substrate and an inducer of several CYP450 enzymes and omeprazole is a substrate and an inhibitor of CYP450 enzymes. How this impacts the person being treated is the main question that we need to answer. Unfortunately, there is no simple answer: being aware of these potential interactions, minimising the impact by discontinuing unnecessary medicines and responding to the effects of the medicines that are being administered are the best we can do. As stated earlier we do not have a good simple measure of the enzymatic activity that is going on in the body. Good sources of information on which drugs interact with the CYP450 enzyme system can be found in the BNF and the Palliative Care Formulary (PCF) (Wilcock et al., 2020). This information can be used to help predict what may happen to a medicine that a patient is taking but, as with many things in palliative care, the best thing you can actually do is try to minimise the risks and respond to the person in front of you.

The following is an example of what can happen:

Patient X is taking omeprazole (substrate and inhibitor), midazolam (substrate), oxycodone (substrate) and dexamethasone (substrate and inducer).

There is a lot potentially going on with the enzymes of Patient X but it may only become noticeable when a part of the puzzle changes. If omeprazole was changed to lansoprazole (not an inhibitor) this change could lead to the patient experiencing more pain, having a seizure, or increasing anxiety over a few days as relative enzymatic activity increases. This is due to increasing metabolism of the oxycodone or midazolam, but could also be progression of the disease. The opposite could happen over the next few weeks if the dexamethasone is stopped, leading to increased sedation or opioid toxic effects as enzymatic activity decreases. Again, this could be similar to disease progression. We cannot really tell so we can only respond and alter what we can, and deal with the symptoms that are in front of us.

Drug misuse and palliative care

Drug misuse is found across society, but those who are likely to be excluded from society and those living in deprived areas are most affected. This is compounded by the fact that those living in deprived areas are also more likely to suffer from serious health sequelae as a consequence of their drug misuse (Audit Scotland, 2009).

In 2010, Beynon et al. found that 77% of deaths in drug users over 40 are not drug related (Beynon et al., 2010). More recently Public Health Scotland reported that just over half of people assessed for specialist drug treatment were from older age groups. In 2019/20 the percentage of people who were aged 35 years or over was 54%, a large increase from 29% in 2006/07 (Public Health Scotland, 2021). This shows that there is a growing population of ageing patients with ongoing or past addiction issues, who have an increased risk of developing a life limiting illness (drug and non-drug related).

Providing assessment and care for this group can be challenging, not only because of the pharmacological issues, but because they often present with late-stage disease and engage poorly with HCPs. This is complicated further by high levels of deprivation, chaotic lifestyles, being socially isolated and often estranged from families and other forms of support (British Pain Society, 2007). Pain and symptom management of patients who are also receiving treatment for addiction, or have addictive personalities, usually requires specialist input.

The basic principles of symptom management – taking a complete history and communicating openly with the patient – are not changed because a patient is receiving opioid replacement therapy. There needs to be a focus on communication both with the patient and with the various specialties involved in their care (palliative care, addiction services and primary care). Early involvement of both the Addictions team, and Specialist Palliative Care team, should be a priority for the generalist. Currently there is no clear guidance (*Pain and Substance Misuse: Improving the Patient Experience*, British Pain Society 2007, is currently under review) on what is the best way to manage patients receiving opioid maintenance therapy who require analgesia.

Currently there is little evidence or guidance available to guide prescribing practice. However, it is widely accepted that the current approaches, detailed below, can be helpful.

Methadone maintenance therapy (MMT)

The generalist would be strongly advised to seek advice form a specialist experienced in the management of patients who are taking methadone. There are two ways of approaching methadone therapy patients (Neerkin et al., 2009):

1. For a patient who is on a methadone maintenance programme, the dose of methadone should continue and not be altered. Treat the methadone as a separate prescription that is not involved in their pain management. The methadone dose should not be titrated for pain. Treat the patient's pain as if they are relatively opioid naive and titrate, probably with morphine, as you would any other patient. This is particularly useful for short term acute or post-surgical pain as titration to the pain requirements is more 'normal'. The MMT, as a single daily dose, is a therapy to reduce opioid craving and is not to be considered part of the pain control regimen. If the oral route is not available, the oral methadone maintenance treatment can be converted to a syringe pump preparation and, as before, should be kept separate from other opioids. This must be done under the guidance of a Specialist Palliative Care service.

2. The analgesic effects after a single dose of methadone are usually much shorter than would be expected, given its half-life. The methadone dose can be divided into two daily doses and titrated for pain control. While methadone is a very effective analgesic it has challenges in titration and signs and symptoms of toxicity. Therefore this method would only be advisable where a specialist prescriber has experience in managing pain using methadone.

Buprenorphine

Buprenorphine (sublingual tablet) is sometimes used in the management of opioid addiction. Buprenorphine has both partial opioid agonist and partial antagonist properties. It is an antagonist of the kappa opioid receptor which means that it provides a less euphoric and less sedating effect when compared to methadone. Because of its higher affinity for opioid receptors, it reduces the effect of additional use of opioids, and at higher doses has a prolonged duration of action, allowing for alternate day dosing. If patients require opioids for the management of pain, it is advisable that the buprenorphine is converted to methadone. This should be done by liaising with the local Addictions team (Neerkin et al., 2009).

Management of pain

It is advised that the generalist involves the Specialist Palliative Medicine team early.

In general, it is advised to still use the WHO Analgesic Ladder (See Chapter 4.1 – Pain), even if the person is actively misusing opioids or on a methadone programme. If there is no contraindication, start with low dose, long-acting morphine (Neerkin et al., 2009). These are less likely to be abused compared to normal or immediate release preparations.

Some patients taking MMT may be reluctant to take opioids. Clear communication and information needs to be given regarding the purpose of opioids for analgesia rather than recreational use.

Titrate the dose as normal but try to titrate the doses with controlled release preparations rather than normal or immediate release preparations, again to avoid abuse if possible (Neerkin et al.).

Some practitioners will limit the dose of as-required opioids per 24 hour period. Only do this if there will be frequent clinical review.

Breakthrough analgesia

As before it is encouraged that the generalist involves the Specialist Palliative Medicine team. The appropriate breakthrough dose of an opioid is best calculated according to the current analgesic regime only, and it is important that the current methadone dose is not incorporated into the background dose for use in any calculations. There is no current evidence to suggest that incorporating methadone doses into calculations for breakthrough analgesia confers a benefit, whilst doing so will incur a significant risk for a calculation error. Be aware of excessive breakthrough use (Human et al., 2015). Ask yourself, why? Is this misuse, or is it that pain is under treated? Consider the possibility that if their pain is undertreated, there may be a risk of the patient seeking illicit drugs to help the pain. Seeking advice and working collaboratively with the local Addictions and Palliative Medicine team is again strongly advised.

Co-adjuvants

Non-opioid analgesics should be used as adjuvants when appropriate, but not as substitutes for strong opioids (Neerkin et al., 2009).

Be aware that there is still potential for abuse of co-adjuvants (e.g. gabapentin or pregabalin), and there is great street value to these drugs. Consider amitriptyline as first line use if you are very concerned about misuse and a co-adjuvant is appropriate.

Non-pharmacological interventions such as radiotherapy, surgery and anaesthetic techniques should be considered where appropriate (Neerkin et al., 2009).

Other considerations

Ensure good and timely communication between all HCPs involved. Have a single point of prescribing and prescribe analgesic medication weekly. A relative can be nominated as the person to collect methadone and analgesics when the patient is too frail.

Consider installing a Locked Box. Even if there are no concerns about the patient/family misusing medications, they may become vulnerable because of the community they live in.

Ensure the out-of-hours provider is aware of substance misuse issues to prevent additional prescriptions being issued.

Ask about naloxone. Often the patient may have this at home from the Addictions Service. If they do, re-assess if it is still appropriate.

As you can see there is no clearly correct pharmacological method of managing this challenging group of patients. The most effective method is clear communication and decision making between the various health professionals involved in their care. Individual circumstances will dictate a variation in approach, incorporating expected progression of the pain and disease, and also taking into account risks of drug misuse.

Scenario Recap

Oral morphine 2 ml (4 mg) was initiated for pain to see if it was helpful. A discussion with Kamal was carried out around the implementation of a 'just in case' (JIC) box. The emphasis was very much that it was not required at the moment, and might never be needed, but that it might be useful if a further deterioration occurred. He agreed to getting a JIC box. The medications in the JIC box were only needed at the end of life as fatigue became a more significant issue.

Kamal benefited from a reduction in their carvedilol dose, preventing further postural hypotensive events. A discussion took place with Kamal's cardiology team to discuss what the next step might be if hypotensive events continued. The cardiac medicines were discontinued gradually as per the advice from cardiology.

The rosuvastatin was stopped to reduce his tablet burden and the adcal D3 and alendronic acid were continued at that time as they may have been playing a role in preventing bone pain. Kamal died peacefully 3 months after initial assessment.

References

Audit Scotland (2009) Drug and Alcohol Services in Scotland. Available at: https://www.audit-scotland.gov.uk/docs/health/2009/nr_090326_drugs_alcohol.pdf

Beynon C et al. (2010) Older and sicker: changing mortality of drug users in treatment in the North West of England. *International Journal of Drug Policy*, 21(5): 429–431.

The British Pain Society (2007) *Pain and Substance Misuse: Improving the Patient Experience*, A consensus statement prepared by The British Pain Society in collaboration with The Royal College of Psychiatrists, The Royal College of General Practitioners and The Advisory Council on the Misuse of Drugs, August 2007. London: The British Pain Society.

EMC (2020) Alfentanil 5mg/ml solution for injection. https://www.medicines.org.uk/emc/product/6430#

Glassock RJ and Winearls C (2008) Screening for CKD with eGFR: doubts and dangers. *Clinical Journal of the American Society of Nephrology*, 3(5): 1563–1568.

Guengerich FP (2008) Cytochrome P450 and Chemical Toxicology. *Chemical Research in Toxicology*, 21(1): 70–83.

Human S, Walker G and Sykes J (2015) Palliative Care Prescribing for Patients Who Are Substance Misusers. *Rowcroft Hospice*. Available at: https://rowcrofthospice.org.uk/wp-content/uploads/Rowcroft-Hospice-Palliative-Care-Prescribing-For-Substance-Misusers.pdf

Neerkin J, Cheung C and Stirling S (2009) Guidelines for Cancer Pain Management in Substance Misusers. Available at: https://www.palliativedrugs.com/download/100615_Substance_misuse_pain_guidlines_final.pdf

NICE (2021) Prescribing in renal impairment. *British National Formulary (BNF)*. Available at: https://bnf.nice.org.uk/guidance/prescribing-in-renal-impairment.html

Public Health Scotland (2021) Scottish Drug Misuse Database: A National Statistics publication for Scotland. Available at: https://beta.isdscotland.org/find-publications-and-data/lifestyle-and-behaviours/substance-use/scottish-drug-misuse-database/

Renal Association (2020) CKD Stages. Available at: https://renal.org/health-professionals/information-resources/uk-eckd-guide/ckd-stages

Scottish Government Polypharmacy Model of Care Group (2018) *Polypharmacy Guidance: Realistic Prescribing*, 3rd edition. Edinburgh: Scottish Government.

Scottish Palliative Care Guidelines (2013) Renal Disease in the Last Days of Life. Available at: https://www.palliativecareguidelines.scot.nhs.uk/guidelines/end-of-life-care/renal-disease-in-the-last-days-of-life.aspx

Scottish Palliative Care Guidelines (2014a) Anticipatory Prescribing. Available at: https://www.palliativecareguidelines.scot.nhs.uk/guidelines/pain/anticipatory-prescribing.aspx

Scottish Palliative Care Guidelines (2014b) Syringe Pumps. Available at: https://www.palliativecareguidelines.scot.nhs.uk/guidelines/end-of-life-care/syringe-pumps

Scottish Palliative Care Guidelines (2020) Choosing and Changing Opioids. Available at: https://www.palliativecareguidelines.scot.nhs.uk/guidelines/pain/choosing-and-changing-opioids.aspx

White R and Bradnam V (2007) *Handbook of Drug Administration via Enteral Feeding Tubes*. London: Pharmaceutical Press.

Wilcock A, Howard P and Charlesworth S (2020) *Palliative Care Formulary,* 7th edn. London: Pharmaceutical Press.

Chapter 6

Specific Conditions

Alexandra Little with Shalini Bhola,
Andrew Collier, Claire A Douglas, Alice Radley,
Michael K Sullivan, Fiona Finlay, Gillian Foster,
Karen J Hogg, Alistair McKeown,
Yvonne Millerick and Ian Morrison

Learning Objectives

By reading this chapter you will understand how to recognise and manage the following conditions:

- End stage heart failure
- End stage respiratory disease
- Motor neurone disease
- Diabetes
- End stage liver disease
- Kidney failure.

End Stage Heart Failure

What is heart failure?

Heart failure is a clinical syndrome characterised by symptoms of breathlessness and fatigue which is commonly associated with physical signs of peripheral oedema, pulmonary crackles and raised jugular venous pressure. These signs and symptoms usually originate from a structural and/or functional cardiac abnormality resulting from a reduced cardiac output and/or elevated intracardiac pressures at rest or during stress (Antman et al., 2016). Heart failure very seldom comes in isolation and is often accompanied with multiple co-morbid disorders, particularly in the older age group. Although there are a wide range of effective evidence-based heart failure treatments which improve clinical outcomes, the prognosis is poor and the symptom burden remains high with many symptoms often left unmanaged. The quality of life for many patients is poor, exacerbated by frequent and prolonged hospital admissions often resulting with death in hospital regardless of the patient's preferences of care. The social burden and carer strain are also high often contributing to further hospital admissions.

Heart failure has an unpredictable disease trajectory which is characterised by patients experiencing many years of cardiac ill-health, which inevitably leads to uncertainty regarding a definitive diagnosis of 'end stage heart failure'. Although many people would prefer to be cared for at home, in the absence of early identification and coordination of supported care, the reality is that many will often experience multiple hospital admissions associated with deterioration, inevitable decline and death in hospital. The economic and personal cost of heart failure is significant, with costs being largely driven by frequent and prolonged hospital admissions.

Heart failure significantly impacts on patients, family and caregivers as the unpredictable trajectory is exhausting and often leads to many life and death experiences. Most people living with advanced heart failure do not get the opportunity for advance care planning which could help address their evolving needs and care preferences. A fundamental barrier to palliative care access is a poor understanding of heart failure as a life-threatening illness (Antman et al., 2016).

The 'uncertainty' surrounding heart failure makes healthcare professionals reluctant to initiate meaningful conversations about disease progression and prognostication, appropriate goals of care and evolving care plans that might prepare patients and their caregivers for inevitable decline and potential death. This reluctance stems from a professional fear of taking away hope when further deterioration is uncertain and from historical views on the meaning of a palliative approach to care.

Supportive and palliative care needs

Patients with heart failure have less understanding of their illness; many die in hospital while still receiving intensive and often invasive medical intervention, as no other options have been discussed or offered. This invariably leads to less access to supportive and palliative care throughout their illness trajectory (Exley et al., 2005; Macdonald et al., 2016; Murray et al., 2002).

Unlike cancer, a diagnosis of heart failure may not always be considered as a devastating diagnosis by the general public, patients, family members or even some healthcare professionals. People with heart failure may feel extremely ill but look reasonably well in contrast to patients living with cancer whose predictable decline is often clearly visible. Only 7% of those dying from heart failure were registered on the GP palliative care register with a third of this number being entered the week of their death. This is not timely enough for professionals to support and facilitate patients' care preferences (Gadoud et al., 2014).

Integrating core components of care into everyday heart failure care management may improve the current inequity of access to palliative care, with the focus on patients' unmet needs and much less on prognostication.

Integrating core components of care into everyday heart failure clinical practice can support professionals to provide optimal care management in response to evolving patient care needs despite an uncertain trajectory.

Core components

1. Early identification of patients who are New York Heart Association (NYHA) Classification III/IV, with an escalating symptom burden and unmet needs despite being on optimal evidence-based treatments.
2. Comprehensive assessment to determine cardiological, co-morbidity and holistic care outcomes.
3. Meaningful discussion, documentation, communication and facilitation of realistic goals and preferences of care across all care boundaries.
4. Multidisciplinary working to ensure that optimal and proactive care is provided in a timely and realistic manner regardless of the care environment.

Heart failure medications

Patients with heart failure will be on a combination of evidence-based, disease-modifying and symptom-relieving medication. These medications will often continue while they provide clinical benefit impacting on quality of life even if they no longer have an impact on the quantity of life. However, at times dosing may be altered or the drug stopped if the effects become disadvantageous to symptom control and quality of life. These medications may include angiotensin-converting-enzyme inhibitors (ACE), beta blockers (BB), mineralocorticoid receptor antagonists (MRA), angiotensin receptor blockers (ARB), ivabradine, sacubitril/valsartan (Entresto), hydralazine and/or digoxin.

Diuretics are routinely used and dose adjusted frequently to relieve patient symptoms associated with fluid retention. Low dose opioids may be used to minimise exertional breathlessness whilst benzodiazepines may help to minimise anxiety-induced symptoms which may precipitate increased breathlessness. Antidepressants may also be introduced to minimise the symptoms associated with depression and anxiety. Consideration should always be given to the benefit versus burden of any medications that are being introduced. Patients with heart failure often have other more generic symptoms such as fatigue, itch or pain. These symptoms which are often ignored must be assessed and managed appropriately.

Cardiac transplantation

Heart transplantation can be a life-sustaining intervention for a small number of heart failure patients. Nonetheless, the risk of deterioration whilst waiting for a donor organ is significant. Supportive and palliative care principles should run parallel to life-sustaining intervention and treatments.

Anticipatory care planning

Meaningful conversation with patients and their caregivers to elicit realistic expectations and facilitation of care preferences is essential. Professionals should consider this as an evolving conversation which reflects changing care needs throughout the illness trajectory.

Key areas for discussion with heart failure patients may include timely planning and deactivation of their cardiac device. In doing so, patients will not be at risk of experiencing inappropriate or distressing defibrillator shocks at end of life.

Cardiac devices

Device therapy has revolutionised heart failure management improving patients' symptoms, hospitalisations and prognosis. As such, many patients will have an implanted cardiac defibrillator (ICD) or cardiac resynchronisation therapy (CRT-pacing (CRT-P)/defibrillator) in situ. It is important that anticipatory care planning takes into account a number of clinical considerations such as the appropriateness of a patient's device remaining active and, if so, involving the patient in a device plan. A device plan allows the patient the opportunity to receive information, discuss concerns and to take an active role in their own anticipatory care planning and end-of-life care, even if that is not felt to be imminent. A greater emphasis over time will be placed on providing device deactivation discussions with patients at the time of consent rather than keeping these discussions only for a time associated with imminent death. The latter approach tends to mean that these discussions never take place, which risks unwanted shocks prior to death. Patients who do not have a defibrillator and have a CRT-P or pacemaker only do not require deactivation of either. In fact, an active CRT-P may help to alleviate heart failure symptoms including prior to death.

End-of-life care

Despite an uncertain illness trajectory, the principles of providing high-quality end-of-life care for patients with heart failure is synonymous with all other life-threatening conditions.

Identifying patients earlier, undertaking comprehensive assessment to minimise unmet care and symptom needs, engaging in meaningful conversation to empower and enable patients to share their care preferences, including place of care and place of death, and working cross-boundary with the multidisciplinary teams (MDTs) to facilitate care preferences can only contribute to an optimal end-of-life experience for patients and family.

End Stage Respiratory Disease

Background

Advanced and progressive non-malignant respiratory diseases can be one of the most challenging areas in which to provide good quality palliative care. There are a wide range of pathologies and diagnoses and these diseases often have a chronic and unpredictable course. Advanced chronic obstructive pulmonary disease (COPD) is the most frequently encountered in the UK, and is the fifth most common cause of death in Scotland (National

Records for Scotland, 2017), but other pathologies such as interstitial lung disease, pulmonary hypertension, pulmonary fibrosis, alpha-1-antitrypsin deficiency and cystic fibrosis, to name but a few, are all life-limiting and progressive conditions with evidence of significant physical symptoms and social/psychological burden.

A number of key documents (NICE, 2018a; NICE, 2017; Maddocks et al., 2017) now actively advocate for extension of palliative care provision into patients with non-malignant respiratory disease. It is increasingly recognised that this group have a symptom burden similar to those with cancer, as well as high levels of depression and distress, and often have poor access to palliative care services.

Joint working and identification

Due to the complex nature and variety of end stage respiratory illness, joint working is essential in all advanced lung conditions. Optimal medical and surgical management of the patient's underlying disease processes and working in partnership with respiratory specialists is key to both identifying patients for whom a more palliative care-centred approach is appropriate, and in managing their symptoms and formulating appropriately informed anticipatory care plans.

Identification of patients for palliative care input and approach is challenging – the Supportive and Palliative Care Indicators Tool (SPICT) (University of Edinburgh, 2019) and Gold Standards Framework Proactive Identification Guidance (Gold Standards Framework, 2016) provide some useful indicators but, again, close working with the relevant specialists may help with identification. There may be disease-specific documents and tools available, or local working practices that can be developed, for example specific lung function parameters, listing for lung transplantation or recurrent admissions to hospital.

Medications

Medication choices for management of symptoms such as pain, breathlessness and cough are not different in end stage respiratory illness from other disease processes and are outlined elsewhere in this book. However, close working with other members of the healthcare team and consideration of benefit/burden of medications should always be considered as with any patient. For example, opioids may increase the risk of bowel dysfunction in patients with cystic fibrosis who are already at risk of complications in this area, but can be highly beneficial for symptom control of dyspnoea. Benzodiazepines may be associated with increased morbidity in COPD patients (Ekstrom et al., 2014) but have an important role in anxiolysis in a symptomatic population. Finally, as prognostication can be challenging, the impact of higher-dose opioids being used in the potentially longer term should be carefully considered. Decisions should be made on a case-by-case basis.

Lung transplantation

Lung transplantation adds complexity to the overall situation and may be an option for a small number of patients. The possibility of significant improvement in patient prognosis, even very late in respiratory disease, means that clarity around levels of intervention in the event of deterioration are essential, as well as other anticipatory care planning (ACP) decisions. Some services have specific ACP documents (such as the Cystic Fibrosis Trust) that help with recording such discussions and sharing them with the healthcare teams involved in patient care (Cystic Fibrosis Trust, 2019).

Anticipatory care planning

Anticipatory care planning for patients with respiratory disease can be challenging, but appropriate documentation and communication of wishes is essential. This should ideally be facilitated by an individual who knows the patient well and understands the interventions available, and can communicate their positive and negative aspects. Use of non-invasive ventilation (NIV) is commonplace for a range of respiratory conditions and can support patients late in their disease trajectory – but some patients find it intolerable. Extracorporeal membrane oxygenation (ECMO) can provide a bridge to transplantation in a small number of patients, such as some with cystic fibrosis – but is highly invasive and only an option for a few patients. As with any other area, liaison with the respiratory team for guidance around these areas can be helpful.

End-of-life care

Providing good quality end-of-life care in patients with advanced respiratory disease is similar to general care for any patient with a life-limiting condition. The basic tenants of good quality holistic care, with attention paid to physical, psychological, social and spiritual domains, are key. Patients with poor lung function may have significant anxiety around what end of life will be like – concerns around 'gasping for breath' and 'drowning' are frequent, and reassurance around appropriate use of anxiolytics and other medications during the dying process can be important.

Motor Neurone Disease

What is motor neurone disease?

Motor neurone disease (MND) refers to a spectrum of neurodegenerative conditions that predominantly affect the motor neurones. The most common manifestation of MND is amyotrophic lateral sclerosis (ALS), which results in progressive involvement of the upper and lower motor neurones. However, other conditions that are classified as motor neurone diseases include:

- Primary lateral sclerosis (PLS) – predominantly upper motor neurone signs.
- Progressive muscular atrophy (PMA) – predominantly lower limb motor neurone signs.
- Progressive bulbar palsy – weakness of bulbar muscles.
- Pseudobulbar palsy – weakness and spasticity of bulbar muscles.
- Monomelic amyotrophy – muscular atrophy of a limb, usually upper limb.

Cognitive change can also occur in approximately 50% of patients with MND. Around 35% have mild cognitive changes, with deficits in executive function, language or social cognition.

Others either have fronto-temporal dementia (FTD), either at diagnosis or develop this in their illness, or have FTD first then develop MND after their diagnosis of dementia (Bak, 2010).

Recent evidence suggests that MND prevalence in Scotland is around 7.61/100,000 of the population, with a standardised incidence of 3.42/100,000. A recent study suggests the incidence has increased by 36% over a 25-year period, although the reasons for this are uncertain (Leighton et al., 2019). The exact pathophysiology is unclear but is likely to be multifactorial and includes genetic and environmental risk factors (Al-Chalabi and Hardiman, 2013; Al-Chalabi et al., 2014).

Patients can present with a variety of symptoms, depending on the muscles involved or cognitive profile:

- Functional effects of motor weakness, for example, loss of dexterity, falls or trips; or direct muscle symptoms including wasting, fasciculations and cramps
- Speech or swallowing problems, or tongue fasciculations
- Respiratory issues
- Behavioural change or memory issues.

Although the average life expectancy of MND is quoted as 36 months, the clinical heterogeneity of the illness means that life expectancy is more variable depending on the duration and severity of symptoms at diagnosis (Turner et al., 2003). Some patients can survive many years with the illness.

At the moment, there is no cure for MND with the only available medical treatment (riluzole) slowing the progression of the illness during the latter stages of the disease (Dharmadasa and Kiernan, 2018). From the outset, treatment of MND is therefore palliative, to maintain quality of life for the patient and their families. However, the heterogeneity of the illness and progressive nature mean the needs of a patient will vary during the illness. For example, once the diagnosis is given, time will be spent adjusting to the diagnosis, explaining the illness and adapting work/life balance to reflect the implications of the illness. During the terminal phase, care is predominantly directed to management of end-of-life care; and during 'crises', intervention is based on addressing sudden care needs.

It is therefore important to recognise that patients with MND are unique and their needs will vary depending on type of MND, presentation, clinical signs and symptoms, and stage of illness. Managing a patient's care, as summarised in the excellent article by David Oliver (Oliver, 2002), is based on addressing physical, psychological, social and spiritual needs.

Care team

A recent increase in funding in Scotland has doubled the number of MND nurse specialists, providing a model for the delivery of coordinated care that can address the lack of experience in MND care in community settings (MND Scotland, 2018). The use of a care team, ideally led by either a medical or nurse specialist in MND, is crucial to deliver the most effective care and coordinate the specialist services required to effectively palliate patients (Figure 6.1).

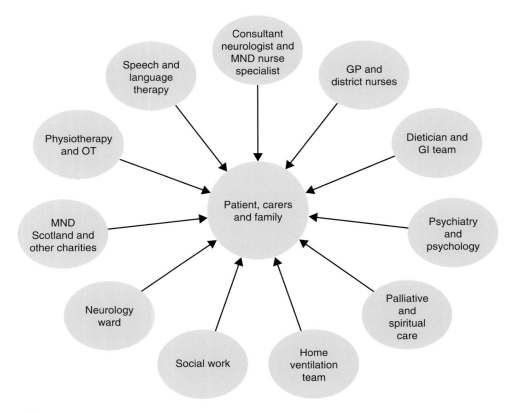

Figure 6.1   Aspects of a palliative care team.

Physical aspects of care

Breathlessness

MND can affect respiratory muscles, causing increased respiratory effort with associated breathlessness and respiratory failure. It is a common symptom in up to 85% of patients and worsens with disease progression (Oliver, 1996).

If respiratory failure is suspected, assessment using overnight oximetry is usually recommended initially. Simple interventions including postural change, particularly reclining the back of a wheelchair slightly, can be helpful alongside specialist input from physiotherapy and occupational therapy (Howard and Orrell, 2002).

Some patients may require non-invasive positive pressure ventilation (NIPPV), particularly overnight, and there is evidence this can reduce the symptoms of respiratory failure and improve quality of life. However, patients require the use of their hands for this intervention as displacement of the mask overnight can be uncomfortable and distressing if not re-sited easily. It may not be appropriate if patients have only limited use of their upper limbs.

The use of NIPPV can potentially increase to 24-hour respiratory support. It is therefore important to discuss management of further respiratory failure at the initiation of NIPPV, particularly deterioration in the terminal phase and the increased burden on the patients and their families that may result, and develop a strategy to withdraw the treatment if it becomes impractical or distressing.

It is also important to discuss the potential role of tracheostomy and its implications at an early stage, rather than during a sudden deterioration. Tracheostomy can be used to maintain respiratory support in patients requiring long-term ventilation but progressive weakness elsewhere in the body could lead to a patient becoming 'locked in' (Oliver, 2002), which should be discussed with the patient frankly at the onset of ventilation.

If non-invasive ventilation is not possible or poorly tolerated, low-dose opioids can be used to manage any symptoms of respiratory distress.

Dysphagia

Dysphagia is a common symptom, affecting up to 87% of patients with MND (Oliver, 1996). Early assessment and regular follow-up by speech and language therapy (SALT) throughout the illness is essential to alter the consistency of the diet to maintain safe eating (Kirker and Oliver, 2003).

In some instances, particularly patients with prominent bulbar symptoms, it may not be possible to maintain body weight through oral intake, at which point gastrostomy could be considered. Although gastrostomy has been shown to improve survival (Mazzini et al., 1995), care should be taken when selecting patients for this intervention as there is an increased risk of death post-gastrostomy in patients who are older or recently diagnosed (Gorrie et al., 2019). It is also recommended that patients have a forced vital capacity (FVC) greater than 50% before the procedure. As a result of these limitations, gastrostomy should be discussed at an early stage and, in certain instances, may need to be inserted before it is used for feeding (Miller et al., 1999).

Secretion management

Hypersalivation can be present in up to 23% of patients (Oliver, 1996), often due to difficulties with swallowing, and is a very distressing symptom for patients. It can be treated with atropine drops, hyoscine, either sublingually or via a transdermal patch, or tricyclic antidepressants. In more difficult cases, subcutaneous infusions of glycopyrronium or hyoscine may be necessary (Oliver, 2002) or even injection of botulinum toxin A into the salivary glands (Squires et al., 2014).

Patients may also experience a very dry mouth and excellent oral hygiene is required to prevent infections and discomfort through oral ulceration. Simple techniques like regular sips of water or the use of pastilles can stimulate salivation, or alternatively artificial salivary products can be used.

Muscle weakness

At the moment, there is no treatment that can significantly influence the onset and progression of muscle weakness in MND. Any input is therefore supportive, with regular physiotherapy and occupational therapy to minimise complications from muscle weakness and to maximise existing power to limit disability.

Mobility aids such as sticks, wheelchairs and transfer devices, in conjunction with aids to assist with self-care around the house, can be offered to maintain independence and reduce the impact of any muscle weakness.

Pain

Pain is a common symptom in MND and, while not directly related to nerve injury, is often associated with the complications of muscle weakness or spasticity. Patients can also experience joint pain or skin pressure pain due to muscle weakness and altered activity, and physiotherapy to manage the associated muscle weakness is most helpful. If the cause cannot be identified or easily treated, analgesia should be offered for symptom control, including the use of low-dose opioids where necessary.

Spasticity

Spasticity is a common symptom in ALS that can lead to distressing muscle cramps. Baclofen, tizanidine or dantrolene can be helpful in reducing the discomfort from spasticity (Ng et al., 2017). Early trial data also suggest that nabiximols (Sativex – a form of cannabis delivered by oral spray) may also help to reduce symptoms relating to spasticity (Riva et al., 2019).

Communication

Progressive bulbar dysfunction may result in deterioration in the quality of a patient's speech. Regular review by SALT and the use of communication aids is important to maintain effective communication (Elliott et al., 2019). These aids can be limited when upper limb function is impaired, although devices using eye movements are available.

Other physical symptoms

Cough

Cough may be a sign of significant disease progression and usually suggests a failure to clear respiratory secretions as a consequence of bulbar weakness or respiratory muscle weakness. It may also arise as a consequence of an underlying chest infection. Treatment of the cough should be directed to the underlying cause. If necessary, opioids may be required (Oliver, 2002).

Constipation

This is a common symptom that can arise through dietary changes, immobility or medication including opioids. Prevention of constipation is important and may require alteration in diet or laxatives.

Psychological

Emotional lability

This is often present in up to 23% of patients and may be due to frontal lobe dysfunction, although the exact pathogenesis is unclear (Oliver, 1996; Borasio et al., 1997). Equally, the strain of living with MND can cause significant mood disturbance, leading to psychiatric symptoms including emotional lability. Although it is a common symptom, there is no consensus on its management. If FTD or psychiatric co-morbidity is suspected, early referral to psychiatry is recommended, with additional involvement from neuropsychology to fully evaluate the symptoms. If a psychiatric diagnosis is confirmed, additional input from occupational therapy may be necessary to adapt to these symptoms at home, alongside the use of antidepressants or anxiolytics. Family members are likely to find these symptoms equally distressing and support should be offered to them either through neuropsychology or spiritual care.

Adjustment

Considerable psychological distress can occur following the diagnosis and the adjustment that is required thereafter. In particular, concerns about loss of independence, dying, disability and issues of sexuality can lead to significant fear and psychological upset. Recognition of these concerns and open discussions where any stigma, prejudice or misconception can be addressed are important from the outset. Where necessary, additional psychological or spiritual counselling can be offered.

Loss of employment and the additional financial demands following diagnosis can lead to fiscal concerns, and involvement of MND charities or social workers with expertise in accessing benefits may help to offset these issues to an extent.

Terminal phase

It is difficult to predict the onset of the terminal stage of MND, with some patients experiencing a gradual decline while others progress rapidly over hours or days. The cause of death can be variable, with Neudert suggesting the cause of death is respiratory failure (86%), heart failure (6%), pneumonia (4%), suicide (1%) and other causes (3%) (Neudert et al., 2001).

It is important to minimise distress at the end of life where possible, and effective palliative care, including management of secretions, respiratory issues and pain, is critical. The use of 'just in case' boxes is a useful adjunct for acute palliation in the event of rapid deterioration.

Assisted dying and anticipatory care planning

Both euthanasia and assisted dying are illegal in the United Kingdom. Although assisted dying is possible in other countries, helping a patient to access these facilities could result in criminal prosecution in the United Kingdom.

It is important to discuss the terminal phase of the illness and address any concerns about symptom management and the palliative process openly with patients and their families, particularly addressing any misconceptions about distress towards the end of life and symptom control. It is also useful to plan for future care by discussing and documenting the patient's wishes for escalation of care and end-of-life management, in addition to potentially creating a lasting power of attorney if appropriate.

Bereavement

The progressive nature of MND and relentless loss of abilities can lead to an almost continual bereavement reaction for patients and their families throughout the illness, as they mourn the loss of their previous life. Particular care should be given to this with counselling and spiritual support offered throughout the illness that is directed to managing these issues.

When a patient eventually dies, particularly following a long illness, family members often experience difficulty disengaging from the carer role and may require support to re-adjust to independent living. They may also have established close relationships with the MND care team and disengagement should be undertaken gradually and sympathetically, often in a staged manner, to avoid any worsening of bereavement symptoms.

Perhaps unsurprisingly, the strain of a prolonged illness can lead to a confusing and distressing sense of relief for family members when a patient eventually dies. Recognition and reassurance is important if this occurs, and in this instance, spiritual support can be helpful in managing these challenging emotions.

Diabetes

A person is defined as approaching the end of life if they are considered likely to die within 12 months. Diabetes management decisions at this stage change and should focus on individualised glycaemic targets with the aim of symptom control plus preventing medication side-effects. Hyperglycaemia and hypoglycaemia should be avoided. Additionally, it is important to prevent dehydration and complications such as pressure sores, particularly for bed-bound individuals.

Glycaemic targets

There is no established evidence for blood glucose levels or HbA_{1c} target levels. Expert discussion has led to the target range of blood glucose levels to be no less than 6 mmol/l and no greater than 15 mmol/l. A target HbA_{1c} level of 53–64 mmol/l is appropriate but a target of up to 70 mmol/l is acceptable. Achieving these levels involves adjustment of the individual's diabetes medication while considering their nutritional intake, change in weight, stage of illness, changes in communication, cognition, ability to swallow, functional decline, decreased mobility and presence of organ dysfunction.

Individuals should be monitored for hypoglycaemia, especially in those who are unable to communicate and may present with uncharacteristic behaviours.

Adjusting diabetes medication

- Sulphonylurea dosage should be reduced or the medication stopped due to the risk of hypoglycaemia.
- Metformin does not increase the risk of hypoglycaemia; dose reduction is required in renal impairment and cessation if the eGFR is <30 ml/min/1.73 m^2.
- Pioglitazone should be withdrawn in the presence of heart failure.
- SGLT-2 inhibitors should be stopped if there is evidence of reduced oral intake or dehydration.
- GLP-1 analogues should be withdrawn if there is weight loss or changes to patterns of eating.

Insulin

Insulin should not be stopped in individuals with type 1 diabetes. With a reduction in food intake, fast acting insulin may be withheld in both type 1 and type 2 diabetes. In type 2 diabetes, insulin could be combined with an oral antiglycaemic agent, but insulin alone is preferred in advanced disease with either a single daily or twice daily regime. The administration of insulin should be reviewed in those who develop problems with dexterity, vision, physical limitations or require carer assistance. To detect possible hypoglycaemia glucose measurements should be undertaken just prior to insulin administration. Further glucose measurements should be undertaken only when absolutely necessary, for example if the patient is symptomatic. For those on continuous subcutaneous insulin infusion, multiple daily injections or flash glucose monitoring (i.e. FreeStyle Libre) is often appropriate to simplify the regimen.

Most individuals with diabetes requiring enteral feeding require insulin, usually a long-acting insulin with bolus short-acting insulin for bolus feeds. Steroid use can lead to new onset diabetes in those not previously known to have diabetes and in established diabetes can lead to worsening control. These patients often require insulin therapy.

Last days of life

In the last days of life, blood glucose monitoring should be discontinued for all patients with type 2 diabetes not on insulin. All oral agents and GLP-1 analogues should be stopped. Insulin should be continued in type 1 diabetes. The dose of insulin should be reduced, and blood glucose levels aimed at 6–15 mmol/l with the aim of avoiding hypo- and hyper-glyaecemic symptoms. In type 2 diabetes insulin can often be discontinued. Monitoring urine glucose is simple and blood glucose monitoring should only be performed if urinalysis demonstrates more than 2+ glucose. If the blood glucose is above 20 mmol/l, a short-acting insulin could be administered and if required more often, a once or twice daily insulin should be considered.

It is vital to manage the expectations of the individual and their carers and to prevent feelings of futility and anxiety surrounding any changes. Patients should be supported and, where possible, maintain empowerment in their diabetes self-management (Diabetes UK, 2018).

End Stage Liver Disease

What is end stage liver disease?

Cirrhosis is the end result of long-term fibrosis of the liver, which occurs with ongoing exposure to a toxic insult. The three commonest causes of liver disease in the UK are alcohol, obesity and viral hepatitis. For this reason, liver disease is considered to be 90% preventable. Mortality rates have increased by over 400% since 1970, in contrast to deaths from most other illnesses, including cerebrovascular disease, respiratory disease and cancer, which have reduced (Williams et al., 2014). It is largely a disease of socioeconomic deprivation and is the third commonest cause of death in people of working age in the UK.

Illness trajectory – compensated to decompensated

Cirrhosis in its early stages is hard to diagnose. Due to the ability of the liver to function relatively well despite permanent damage, many people are asymptomatic of their liver disease. This is 'compensated cirrhosis'. Liver function tests may be normal despite cirrhosis.

The pathophysiological hallmark of cirrhosis is portal hypertension, which drives many of the complications of advanced liver disease: ascites, variceal haemorrhage, and hepatic encephalopathy. When these occur, this phase of the illness is termed 'decompensated cirrhosis' and is associated with a much poorer prognosis.

Diagnosis of cirrhosis is often made late, once decompensation occurs, and often this is during an unscheduled admission to hospital. Between 20 and 30% of patients presenting to hospital with their first decompensation will not survive to discharge, and the 1-year mortality rate after hospital admission with decompensated liver disease is 50%. This is poorer than the prognosis associated with many forms of cancer.

Once decompensated cirrhosis occurs, illness trajectory is often characterised by sudden, unpredictable deteriorations in health, resulting in frequent admissions to hospital, with intensive medical treatments focused on recovery, followed by discharge home as soon as possible if recovery occurs. This often hampers the ability to plan future care for a group of patients at high risk of deterioration and death in the coming months (Hudson et al., 2018).

A diagnosis of cirrhosis markedly increases your risk of hepatocellular cancer (HCC): one third of patients with cirrhosis go on to develop HCC. Patients with cirrhosis are therefore regularly screened for evidence of HCC, with regular blood testing for alpha fetoprotein (AFP) and abdominal ultrasound scanning. People with cirrhosis are much more likely to be referred for specialist palliative care input if they have cirrhosis and concurrent hepatocellular cancer (Poonja et al., 2014)

There is added complexity in managing patients with liver disease whose disease is severe enough that they are eligible for transplant. A liver transplant is considered to be a curative treatment, but approximately 1 in 5 patients waiting for an organ will die each year, and many are de-listed as their health deteriorates and they become too unwell to undergo surgery. Many patients are not eligible for transplant assessment, for example, due to ongoing alcohol use. The importance of preparing patients and their families for the possibility that they may die without receiving an organ has been recognised (Poonja et al. 2014)

Key questions to answer to achieve optimum management

How advanced is the individual's liver disease?

Consider using a prognostic score (for example, Child–Pugh, Table 6.1) to identify risk of death at one year. The risk of death at one year is increased if a patient has Child–Pugh B or C cirrhosis and one or more of the following:

- Diuretic resistant ascites
- Hepatic encephalopathy
- Hepatorenal syndrome
- Bacterial peritonitis
- Variceal bleeding.

Table 6.1   Child–Pugh score.

Factor (units)	1	2	3
Bilirubin (mg/dL)	Under 2	2–3	Over 3
Serum albumin (g/dL)	>3.5	2.8–3.5	<2.8
Prothrombin time (seconds prolonged)	<4	4–6	>6
Ascites	None	Mild (or controlled with diuretics)	Mod–severe (diuretic refractory)
Hepatic encephalopathy	None	Grade I and II	Grade III and IV
	Class A	Class B	Class C
Total points	5–6	7–9	10–15
1-year survival (%)	100	80	45

Source: Adapted from Pugh et al. (1973) Transection of the oesophagus for bleeding oesophageal varices. British Journal of Surgery, 60(8): 646–649.

All of these complications are associated with a poor prognosis. This should trigger a conversation with a patient and their family to help plan the individual's care. It is often more straightforward to put plans in place when someone's wishes are identified in advance of a crisis or a deterioration, when it becomes more difficult to have meaningful conversations about the best management options.

Does the individual and their family understand their condition?

Many patients with decompensated cirrhosis are not aware that this may be a terminal illness. Cognitive impairment through alcohol-related brain injury or hepatic encephalopathy is not uncommon, and has a significant impact on both patient understanding and recall of discussions about their health. Having a carer or family member present is good practice whenever any significant discussions are taking place. Taking health literacy into account, and delivering information in a clear and understandable way, is critically important.

Some interventions which may offer benefit in an acute clinical situation (for example, oesophago-gastro-duodenoscopy (OGD), also known as gastroscopy, for a patient who is displaying signs of gastrointestinal bleeding) are perceived to be unpleasant, and are sometimes declined due to the discomfort that they cause. The decision not to have this procedure performed must be made in a fully informed way, with the individual being informed of the potentially life-shortening consequences of this decision. Having this discussion for the first time in an emergency situation is challenging, especially when cognitive function is impaired.

Hepatologists have identified that they do not feel confident in discussing the advanced nature of the illness with their patients and caregivers and, as a result, will sometimes avoid having these conversations (Low et al., 2016). However, it is hugely beneficial when the specialist team initiate these discussions, as they have the expertise to deliver key information to the patient and their family to allow informed treatment decisions to be made (refer to Chapter 3 – Communication, 'Sharing Bad News' on p. 61)

There is a clear benefit in involving the whole MDT in providing education and information for the individual with decompensated cirrhosis and their family. Advice about nutrition, hydration, exercise, weight and lifestyle management helps a person to understand their condition and take an active part in managing it.

Communicating the concept of uncertainty is an important part of addressing the care needs of someone with decompensated cirrhosis. It is difficult to be certain about the outcome when a patient is unwell with advanced liver disease. Being definite about outcomes, or timeframes for a person's prognosis, may cause distress for a patient or their family, especially if they are inaccurate. Addressing uncertainty may be achieved by speaking about hoping for some stability in the individual's clinical condition (and continuing the active treatments aimed at achieving this), whilst concurrently making a comprehensive plan of care in the event of a deterioration. It is important to emphasise the continued prioritisation of symptom management to ensure these are addressed regardless of the outcome of that illness episode, and that this approach is possible alongside active management. It is also imperative that this discussion is revisited when there is a change in that individual's clinical condition, so that goals of care may be reviewed and remain appropriate to the situation.

What is important for the person with advanced liver disease?

Patients with liver disease have identified that they value the opportunity to be involved in setting goals for their care (Hudson et al., 2018; Kimbell et al., 2015; Roth et al., 2000). This includes being given the information they need to express informed views about how and where they are cared for when they are unwell. For some people, their preference is for active treatment if there is the prospect of recovery, even if this is at the expense of comfort, especially in the context of invasive investigations and treatments. For other people with advanced disease, they may wish to prioritise comfort, good symptom control and quality of life, perhaps out of a hospital setting, though they are aware that this may be associated with a shorter life expectancy.

Is all of this important information recorded in an accessible place, and are the wider team aware of it?

A lot of care for patients with advanced liver disease is focused on their hospital admission. If an individual is able to be cared for at home, it is very important to transfer any key information to the community team (GP, district nursing team) about discussions that have taken place. Recording important decisions about plans of care in the event of a deterioration optimises the chances of management being in alignment with the patient's wishes (Standing et al., 2017).

Holistic assessment of the individual with decompensated cirrhosis

Proactive assessment of physical symptoms may improve quality of life but also enable people to tolerate active treatments alongside supportive management.

Physical symptoms

Guidelines are available to aid management of the main symptoms/complications of decompensated cirrhosis (European Association for the Study of the Liver, 2018; Scottish Palliative Care Guidelines, 2018). Each treatment is associated with relative benefits and drawbacks. These will be different for each individual (Table 6.2).

Psychological and spiritual assessment

The impact of an uncertain illness trajectory may be significant for the patient and those close to them. People with a history of alcohol or drug misuse may experience feelings of stigmatisation (Vaughn-Sandler, 2014), guilt and regret. Providing individuals and their families with support through this is a core part of good care.

Social assessment

There may be significant social stressors that are experienced by people who have advanced liver disease. For some people living in unpredictable circumstances this may make providing

Table 6.2   Management of physical symptoms in advanced liver disease.

Symptom/ problem	Treatment options	Potential benefits	Potential burdens
Ascites	Potassium-sparing diuretics	Reduction in ascites volume	Renal impairment Electrolyte derangement Polyuria/nocturia
	Large-volume paracentesis (LVP)	Rapid reduction in ascites volume Increased mobility	Needs inpatient setting Variable access to elective/ day case procedure Infection risk Procedure related complications
	Indwelling ascitic drain	Allows drainage of ascites in community	Procedure related complications Infection risk
Peripheral oedema	Potassium-sparing diuretics	Reduction in peripheral oedema Increased mobility	Renal impairment Electrolyte derangement Polyuria/nocturia
Pain	Non-pharmacological measures (for example, LVP if ascites causing discomfort) Analgesia	Improved pain	Side-effects from medications (need to counter constipating drugs)
Nausea	Non-pharmacological measures Anti-emetics	Improved appetite Improved nutritional intake	Side-effects from medications (caution with constipating drugs)
Itch	Non-pharmacological measures Medications (for example, to treat cholestasis)	Improved symptoms Improved sleep (itch often nocturnal)	Side-effects from medications (GI upset; sedation with some anti-histamines)
Confusion	Treatment of hepatic encephalopathy	Improved cognition Increased likelihood of care being delivered at home	If at end of life, invasive treatments (for example, enema, NG tube for lactulose) may not be appropriate
Bleeding	Endoscopy	Cessation of bleeding May be life-saving procedure	May not tolerate procedure well (pain, agitation) May not survive procedure if very unwell Increased likelihood of death in hospital

consistent care more complex. Social isolation may be significant. Addressing addictions to alcohol or drugs via specialist services, and ensuring social care teams are involved in optimising accommodation, are both important factors to consider, when required.

Individuals may have financial concerns which could be addressed through liaison with local health and social care organisations, who may be able to facilitate a review of the person's benefit entitlement, and access other associated support.

End stage liver disease is an illness that affects all aspects of an individual's life. Through recognition of the advanced stage of a person's illness, and pro-active discussion about what that means for the individual, it is possible to achieve good end-of-life care for that person, which has a significant impact on the bereavement response of family members and caregivers (Department of Health, 2012).

Kidney Failure

What is kidney failure?

Definitions

Kidney failure (previously known as end stage renal failure) is abnormal kidney function lasting more than 3 months with an estimated glomerular filtration rate (eGFR) of less than 15 ml/min/1.73 m^2. As eGFR declines, complications such as anaemia and acidosis occur and toxic molecules accumulate. Patients develop uraemic symptoms: nausea, pruritus, restless legs and sleep disturbances. Some individuals experience these symptoms when the urea level is greater than 20 mmol/l, while others remain asymptomatic even when the urea is greater than 40 mmol/l. Chronic kidney disease (CKD) is much more common than kidney failure, and many of the issues raised here are relevant to all patients with CKD. For example, care must be taken when prescribing medications for any individual with an eGFR of between 15 and 30 ml/min/1.73 m^2, particularly as they approach the end of their life.

Aetiology

The commonest causes of kidney failure in the UK are diabetes mellitus, glomerulonephritis and interstitial diseases such as polycystic kidney disease and pyelonephritis (Pyart et al., 2020). Several causes often contribute to abnormal kidney function, such as hypertension and vascular disease in older people.

Prevalence

Kidney failure affects approximately 0.1% of the population (Hill et al., 2016). A GP practice in the UK with 6,000 patients will have, on average, four kidney transplant patients, two patients on dialysis and many more with an eGFR below 30 ml/min/1.73 m^2 (Pyart et al., 2020; Hill et al., 2016). Black and Asian ethnic groups are disproportionately affected, largely due to high rates of hypertension and diabetes. As populations age and patients live longer with chronic diseases, the rates of kidney failure increase each year.

Common co-morbidities and their significance

Multi-morbidity and polypharmacy are universal amongst patients with kidney failure. Cardiovascular disease is the leading cause of morbidity and mortality, but investigations in these patients are often difficult. For example, coronary angiography can cause kidney damage. Over 40% of patients have diabetes, many with poor glycaemic control (Macdougall et al., 2018). The treatment options for diabetes have been revolutionised in recent years, but very few medications are licensed for patients with kidney failure. The investigation and treatment of co-morbidities in patients with kidney failure are therefore challenging. Co-morbid conditions in turn influence decisions around the treatment of kidney failure, such as if and when to start kidney replacement therapy (Fraser and Taal, 2016).

Treatment options

Kidney replacement therapy (KRT): choosing the right modality at the right time

A key function of the renal medicine team is to provide education and support to enable patients with progressive CKD to make informed choices about their future care. The education, decision-making and assessment process should begin at least one year prior to starting KRT, and it should be offered when the risk of developing kidney failure is 10–20% in one year (Stevens et al., 2013; NICE, 2018b).

This process should always be individualised and should involve the patient, their family or chosen support, and the multidisciplinary healthcare team. Each therapy for has to be considered in terms of the impact on a patient's quality of life, survival, personal preference and the wider context of their illness trajectory.

The decision about when to commence KRT must consider the burden of uraemic symptoms on the patient and the impact on their quality of life (NICE, 2018b). Other common indications to prompt initiation of KRT are hyperkalaemia, fluid overload which is refractory to medical therapies such as diuretics, and significant metabolic acidosis. Studies have suggested that starting haemodialysis early offers no advantage in terms of cardiovascular events or infection rates and therefore this decision should be centred on the patient's individual needs (Stevens et al., 2013).

Transplant

The optimum treatment for kidney failure is kidney transplantation before the need for dialysis, ideally from a living donor (Stevens et al., 2013). Patients with progressive CKD are often not eligible for kidney transplantation on the basis of age and co-morbidities, particularly cardiovascular disease, obesity and malignancy. The proportion of patients undergoing renal transplantation also reduces with advancing frailty (Alfaadhel et al., 2015). For a large group of patients, therefore, treatment with dialysis or comprehensive conservative care become the treatment options.

Dialysis

Peritoneal dialysis involves a plastic catheter being inserted into the abdomen and the movement in and out of fluid several times a day. It relies on an osmotic gradient to clear the blood of excess solute and fluid. This option is excellent for patients who desire autonomy and independence with their treatment. However, it requires good eyesight, manual dexterity and a suitable home environment for equipment. This therapy is generally not suitable for patients who have had significant previous abdominal surgery.

Haemodialysis is based on the diffusion of solutes across a semi-permeable membrane in order to clear toxins from the bloodstream. This process requires robust, long-term vascular access in order to facilitate the removal of blood for filtering and return of blood to the circulation. This is usually in the form of an arteriovenous fistula or a central venous dialysis catheter. Home haemodialysis is available to some patients, again requiring the skills to operate the machine independently and also a suitable home environment. For most patients, haemodialysis requires three sessions lasting around 4 hours each week, with additional time spent travelling to hospital. This can be burdensome for frail patients and for those with limited mobility. It can also prove challenging for people to maintain their other responsibilities such as employment and childcare. Both treatment modalities have similar survival rates.

Conservative care

Unfortunately, not all patients with kidney failure experience improvements in symptoms or quality of life as a result of KRT. For those patients with multiple co-morbidities, particularly cardiovascular disease, there is often no survival advantage to starting KRT. In addition, the initiation of KRT in frail elderly patients can prompt functional decline (Boyd et al., 2013).

Comprehensive conservative care strategies aim to manage kidney failure without the use of KRT. This typically involves optimisation of medical therapies to slow the rate of disease progression, and holistic patient-centred support to address symptoms. Studies comparing comprehensive conservative care approaches with haemodialysis have shown that patients often report better quality of life and preserved functional status with a conservative care approach (Alston et al., 2015).

Illness trajectories in kidney failure

Having open and informative discussions surrounding prognostication and future care planning can be particularly challenging in the context of progressive CKD. Patients with kidney failure are a diverse group, undergoing a variety of treatment modalities, and as a result can have many different illness trajectories.

Patients with kidney failure can experience periods of acute illness, most commonly attributed to infections or cardiovascular events, and often requiring hospital admission. For those who are undergoing dialysis, their illness trajectory is likely to be punctuated by adverse events related to their dialysis access modality. Most commonly this is a significant infection event related to the presence of synthetic material, for example dialysis lines.

Each acute event prompts a decline in baseline function and promotes frailty. In some circumstances, these events also create challenges around the ongoing delivery of dialysis. Typically, as patients approach the end of their lives with kidney failure, these acute declines become more frequent, result in longer hospital admissions, and become increasingly difficult to recover from (Murtagh et al., 2008).

A similar illness trajectory can be seen for patients who undergo kidney transplantation. Transplant recipients who are frail are more likely to have delayed transplant function, long hospital stays and hospital readmission following their transplant. An acute illness such as an infection results in similar losses of physiological reserve and decline in baseline function (Figure 6.2).

Dialysis withdrawal represents around a fifth of deaths from all causes in patients undergoing KRT (Scottish Renal Registry, 2020). Many patients will make the decision to withdraw from KRT as a result of progressive ill health and background functional decline. However, these patients are likely to have a much shorter terminal decline in the final days and weeks of life (Murtagh et al., 2008).

Unfortunately, some patients with kidney failure have sudden and unanticipated deaths. These events can have devastating long-lasting impact on patients' families, loved ones and the healthcare team providing their care.

Cardiovascular disease is the leading cause of death among patients undergoing KRT, accounting for around one third of deaths (Scottish Renal Registry, 2020). Sudden cardiac or arrhythmic death represents the majority of these deaths. A number of factors increase the likelihood of sudden cardiac death in kidney failure, including a vulnerable myocardium with vascular disease and remodelling; co-morbidities such as diabetes and hypertension; dialysis factors such as potassium shifts and hyperkalaemia (Makar et al., 2017).

As with other organ failure diagnoses, the population of patients with kidney failure is ageing. The average age at initiation of KRT is around 62 years, but one quarter of patients

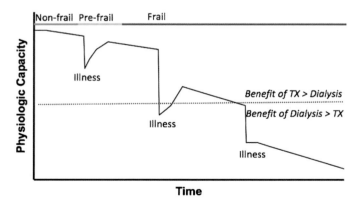

Figure 6.2 Functional trajectory of a patient on the transplant waiting list.
Source: Cheng et al., 2019.

Dyspnoea

(Treatment is as discussed in Chapter 4.3 – The Respiratory System.) In kidney failure there are often multifactorial causes of dyspnoea including renal anaemia, pulmonary oedema or from other co-morbidities such as COPD. Diuretics, fluid restriction and fluid removal by dialysis may be indicated. Renal anaemia can be reversed with erythropoietin or iron transfusions.

Restless legs

Restless legs syndrome is typically described as an urge to move the legs, usually with unpleasant sensations in the legs. It is often worse at night or when resting and can be relieved by physical activity. It can affect between 20 and 40% of people with kidney failure. It is thought to occur because the dopaminergic system in the central nervous system is disrupted. It can be made worse by anaemia, iron deficiency, low parathyroid hormone, hyperphosphataemia or hypercalcaemia. Initial management would be to try and correct any of these abnormalities (Douglas, 2014; Murtaugh, 2018; Wilcock et al., 2020; Garcia-Borreguero et al., 2017).

Pharmacological interventions include (Douglas, 2014; Murtaugh, 2018; Wilcock et al., 2020; Dunleavy et al., 2019; Garcia-Borreguero et al., 2017):

- Dopamine agonists (can accumulate in kidney failure)
  - Co-beneldopa 62.5–125 mg at night
  - Ropinirole 250 micrograms at night, increased according to tolerability up to 4 mg
- Low dose pregabalin or gabapentin
- There is no evidence for the use of quinine sulphate or clonazepam in the management of restless legs.

Nausea and vomiting

Uraemia and delayed gastric emptying (associated with diabetic neuropathy and uraemic neuropathy) are common causes of nausea and vomiting in kidney failure. A detailed assessment is required to help guide pharmacological management. Pharmacological interventions include (Douglas, 2014; Scottish Palliative Care Guidelines, 2021c; Wilcock et al., 2020; Dunleavy et al., 2019):

- Haloperidol
  Drug of choice for uraemia-induced nausea
  - 500 micrograms, twice daily
  - Reduced dose as can accumulate
- Domperidone
  Drug of choice for gastric paresis or delayed gastric emptying
  - 10–20 mg, up to 4 times a day
  - Reduce to 1–2 times a day with prolonged use

- o Metoclopramide is an alternative but caution with long-term use because of the risk of extra-pyramidal reactions
  - o 10 mg three times a day
- Levomepromazine
  A useful broad-spectrum anti-emetic for refractory nausea
  - o 3–6 mg orally, twice daily.

Anxiety and depression

The prevalence rates of depression and anxiety in patients with kidney failure are estimated to be between 20–30% and 12–52% respectively (Goh et al., 2018). There is an association between psychiatric illness and adverse clinical outcomes. This may be because there is decreased adherence to dialysis, medications and dietary limitations. Studies suggest that depression in kidney failure is under-recognised and under-treated. Treatment strategies can include cognitive behavioural therapy and antidepressant medication (Scottish Palliative Care Guidelines, 2020b). Selective serotonin reuptake inhibitors (SSRIs) can improve symptoms. However, dose reduction is often required and side-effects may limit their usefulness. Sertraline is considered generally safe as it does not accumulate in kidney failure (Wilcock et al., 2020) and therefore dose reduction is not required.

Anticipatory care planning

Ideally, conversations about planning for the future should start when patients are reaching kidney failure and are being informed about treatment options. For those patients who are on dialysis and subsequently deteriorate, they should gain access to the same level of ACP, symptom control and supportive services as may be offered to those patients managed conservatively.

ACP discussions for patients with kidney failure are hindered by lack of staff training, administrative complexities and the pressures of routine clinical care (O'Halloran, 2018). However, patients with kidney failure who are managed conservatively and have ACP conversations are more likely to avoid hospital admission towards the end of Life (Douglas et al., 2019).

Clinicians may avoid conversations as they are concerned that the patient may not *definitely* be deteriorating and dying. However, patients and families often find it difficult to initiate conversations about future care with professionals, and expect that the doctor should initiate the conversation (Luckett et al., 2014; Goff et al., 2015; Noble et al., 2008). (For more information on anticipatory care planning, see Chapter 1 – Principles of Palliative and End-of-Life Care (p. 8)).

How to identify those patients who may benefit from anticipatory care planning

Although prognostication can be very difficult and is variable in kidney failure (Murray, 2005), tools such as SPICT™ are helpful for the MDT in identifying those patients at risk of deteriorating and dying, therefore triggering the need for ACP conversations.

At a minimum, 'the surprise question' — 'Would you be surprised if your patient died in the next 6–12 months?' — should be used to identify those patients who may benefit from ACP and increased palliative and supportive care (Downar et al., 2017).

End-of-life care considerations in kidney failure

Patients with kidney failure are likely to be taking many drugs to manage their kidney disease and other co-morbidities. When it is recognised that a patient is deteriorating and approaching end of life there should be consideration as to how essential each drug is as the burden of taking tablets can be substantial. Some drugs if stopped abruptly could lead to significant symptoms, for example diuretics. Similarly, calcium and vitamin D preparations should be continued for as long as possible while on dialysis as there is a risk of symptomatic hypocalcaemia. However, drugs such as statins could be stopped early, and when food intake reduces or stops then there is no requirement for phosphate binders.

Patients may wish to relax their dietary restrictions, in particular potassium containing foods and drinks. Individualised discussion around risks of hyperkalaemia versus personal choice may be needed especially if there are patient or carer anxieties (Stevenson et al., 2017).

Withdrawal from dialysis

Although there are variable dying trajectories for patients with kidney failure, stopping dialysis requires further consideration. A fifth of deaths in patients receiving KRT is from dialysis withdrawal. Some of these patients may have been on a 'trial' of dialysis for a short period, but co-morbidity or quality of life has resulted in the wish to withdraw from dialysis. Others may have been on dialysis for many years, but have had a general deterioration through co-morbidity, frailty or another life-changing event. Often these patients will have had recurrent hospital admissions, and it is important that the MDT recognises that these patients may be approaching end of life and allow an opportunity for discussion and planning (Schmidt and Moss, 2014). These patients should be put on an 'at risk' register so that all professionals involved in the patient's care are aware that the patient may be in the last months of life. Some units offer 'palliative dialysis' which involves the patients spending less time on dialysis each week. Long-term dialysis patients often wish to die in the renal unit where they know staff and feel secure, therefore it is very important to discuss preferred place of care at end of life with the patient, family and healthcare professionals.

Life expectancy after stopping dialysis is likely to be measured in days to a short number of weeks. The median survival is around 9 days, with those who still pass urine or have underlying residual function more likely to live up to 6 weeks (Scottish Palliative Care Guidelines, 2020c). It is recommended that in the last days of life there should be good communication, symptom relief, psychological, spiritual and culturally sensitive care for the dying patient and their family followed by bereavement support.

Prescribing at the end of life

Prescribing of usual anticipatory drugs needs to take into account renal function. For opioid-naive patients, low dose alfentanil 100 micrograms hourly subcutaneously can be prescribed. However, as the duration of action is very short (about an hour), oxycodone 1 mg as required subcutaneous injection given less frequently (but with a longer duration of action) may be more practical in some settings, for example in the community. If a syringe pump is required then alfentanil would be the opioid of choice (Douglas, 2014; Wilcock et al., 2020).

Myoclonus can occur with rising urea. This can be managed with midazolam subcutaneous infusion 5–10 mg over 24 hours. Alternatively, clonazepam 500 micrograms orally or subcutaneous injection at night (Scottish Palliative Care Guidelines, 2020d).

Delirium commonly results from uraemia. The drug of choice is haloperidol 500 micrograms to 2 mg 8 hourly subcutaneous injection or infusion via a syringe pump. Levomepromazine can be used as an alternative if someone is very agitated (Scottish Palliative Care Guidelines, 2020d).

Nausea can be managed with haloperidol or levomepromazine (a broader spectrum anti-emetic) (Douglas, 2014; Scottish Palliative Care Guidelines, 2020d).

Dyspnoea can be relieved with opioids and/or midazolam (Douglas, 2014; Scottish Palliative Care Guidelines, 2020d; Wilcock et al., 2020). If fluid overload is a significant cause then dialysis may be offered at a reduced frequency and reduced duration to relieve symptoms.

Excess respiratory tract secretions may be managed in the usual way with either hyoscine butylbromide or glycopyrronium (Scottish Palliative Care Guidelines, 2020d). Hyoscine hydrobromide should be avoided as there is an increased risk of agitation (Wilcock et al., 2020).

References

Al-Chalabi A and Hardiman O (2013) The epidemiology of ALS: a conspiracy of genes, environment and time. *Nature Reviews Neurology*, 9(11): 617–628.

Al-Chalabi A et al. (2014) Analysis of amyotrophic lateral sclerosis as a multistep process: a population-based modelling study. *Lancet Neurology*, 13(11): 1108–1113.

Alfaadhel TA et al. (2015) Frailty and mortality in dialysis: evaluation of a clinical frailty scale. *Clinical Journal of the American Society of Nephrology*, 10(5): 832LP–840.

Alston H and Burns A (2015) Conservative care of the patient with end-stage renal disease. *Clinical Medicine (Northfield, IL)*, 15(6): 567LP–570.

Antman EM et al. (2016) Updated clinical practice guidelines on heart failure: an international alignment. *European Heart Journal*, 37(27): 2096.

Bak TH (2010) Motor neuron disease and frontotemporal dementia: one, two, or three diseases? *Annals of Indian Academy of Neurology*, 13(Suppl2): S81–S88.

Borasio GD and Voltz R (1997) Palliative care in amyotrophic lateral sclerosis. *Journal of Neurology*, 244: S11–S17.

Boyd J et al. (2013) The delivery of renal replacement therapy in Scotland – why the geographic variation? *QJM: An International Journal of Medicine*, 106(12): 1077–1085.

Cheng XS et al. (2019) Implications of frailty for peritransplant outcomes in kidney transplant recipients. *Current Transplant Reports*, 6(1): 16–25.

Cystic Fibrosis Trust (2019) Resources for cystic fibrosis clinicians: advance care planning for people with cystic fibrosis. Available at: https://www.cysticfibrosis.org.uk/the-work-we-do/resources-for-cf-professionals/supporting-clinicians/resources-for-clinicians

Department of Health (2012) *First National VOICES Survey of Bereaved People: Key Findings Report.* London: Department of Health.

Dharmadasa T and Kiernan MC (2018) Riluzole, disease stage and survival in ALS. *Lancet Neurology*, 17(5): 385–386.

Diabetes UK (2018) End of Life Diabetes Care: Clinical Care Recommendations, 3rd edition, March 2018. Available at: https://www.diabetes.org.uk/resources-s3/2018-03/EoL_Guidance_2018_Final.pdf

Douglas CA (2014) Palliative care for patients with advanced chronic kidney disease. *Journal of the Royal College of Physicians of Edinburgh*, 44(3): 224–231.

Douglas CA et al. (2019) The impact of a renal supportive care service on symptom control, advance care planning and place of death for patients with advance chronic kidney disease managed without dialysis. *British Journal of Renal Medicine*, 24(3): 60–65.

Downar J, Goldman R and Adhikari N (2017) The 'surprise question' for predicting death in seriously ill patients: a systematic review and meta-analysis. *Canadian Medical Association Journal*, 189(13): E484–E493.

Dunleavy A, and Ashley C (2019) *The Renal Drug Handbook*, 5th edition. Oxford: Radcliffe Medical Press.

Ekstrom MP et al. (2014) Safety of benzodiazepines and opioids in very severe respiratory disease: national prospective study. *BMJ*, 348: g455.

Elliott E et al. (2019) An epidemiological profile of dysarthria incidence and assistive technology use in the living population of people with MND in Scotland. *Amyotrophic Lateral Sclerosis and Frontotemporal Degeneration*. 21(1–2):116–122.

European Association for the Study of the Liver (2018). EASL Clinical Practice Guidelines for the management of patients with decompensated cirrhosis. *Journal of Hepatology*, https://doi.org/10.1016/j.jhep.2018.03.024

Exley C et al. (2005) Palliative care in the community for cancer and end-stage cardiorespiratory disease: the views of patients, lay-carers and healthcare professionals. *Palliative Medicine*, 19(1): 76–83.

Fraser SDS and Taal MW (2016) Multimorbidity in people with chronic kidney disease: implications for outcomes and treatment. *Current Opinion in Nephrology and Hypertension*, 25(6): 465–472.

Gadoud A et al. (2014) Palliative care among heart failure patients in primary care: a comparison to cancer patients using English family practice data. *PLoS One*, 9(11): e113188.

Garcia-Borreguero D and Cano-Pumarega I (2017) New concepts in the management of restless legs syndrome. *British Medical Journal*, 356: j104.

Goff SL et al. (2015) Advance care planning: a qualitative study of dialysis patients and families. *Clinical Journal of the American Society of Nephrology*, 10(3): 390–400.

Goh ZS and Griva K (2018) Anxiety and depression in patients with end-stage renal disease: impact and management challenges – a narrative review. *International Journal of Nephrology and Renovascular Disease*, 11: 93–102.

Gold Standards Framework (2016) The Gold Standards Framework Proactive Identification Guidance (PIG). Available at: https://www.goldstandardsframework.org.uk/cd-content/uploads/files/PIG/NEW%20PIG%20-%20%20%2020.1.17%20KT%20vs17.pdf

Gorrie GH et al. (2019) Improved survival and 30-day mortality after gastrostomy in Scottish motor neurone disease patients: evidence from a national retrospective cohort study using STROBE criteria. *Amyotrophic Lateral Sclerosis and Frontotemporal Degeneration*, 20(3–4): 165–171.

Hill NR et al. (2016) Global prevalence of chronic kidney disease – a systematic review and meta-analysis. *PLoS One*, 11(7): e0158765–e0158765.

Howard RS and Orrell RW (2002) Management of motor neurone disease. *Postgraduate Medical Journal*, 78(926): 736.

Hudson B et al. (2018) The incompatibility of healthcare services and end-of-life needs in advanced liver disease: a qualitative interview study of patients and bereaved carers. *Palliative Medicine*, 32(5): 908–918.

Kimbell B, Boyd K and Kendall M (2015) Managing uncertainty in advanced liver disease: a qualitative, multiperspective, serial interview study. *BMJ Open*, 5(11): e009241.

Kirker FJ and Oliver DJ (2003) The development and implementation of a standardized policy for the management of dysphagia in motor neurone disease. *Palliative Medicine*, 17(4): 322–326.

Leighton DJ et al. (2019) Changing epidemiology of motor neurone disease in Scotland. *Journal of Neurology*, 266(4): 817–825.

Low J, Vickerstaff V and Davis S (2016) Palliative care for cirrhosis: a UK survey of health professionals' perceptions, current practice and future needs. *Frontline Gastroenterology*, 7(1): 4–9.

Luckett T et al. (2014) Advance care planning for adults with CKD: a systematic integrative review. *American Journal of Kidney Diseases*, 63(5): 761–770.

Macdonald S et al. (2016) Illness identity as an important component of candidacy: contrasting experiences of help-seeking and access to care in cancer and heart disease. *Social Science and Medicine*, 168: 101–110.

Macdougall IC et al. (2018) Intravenous iron in patients undergoing maintenance hemodialysis. *New England Journal of Medicine*, 380(5): 447–458.

Maddocks M et al. (2017) Palliative care and management of troublesome symptoms for people with chronic obstructive pulmonary disease. *Lancet*, 390(10098): 988–1002.

Makar MS and Pun PH (2017) Sudden cardiac death among hemodialysis patients. *American Journal of Kidney Diseases*, 69(5): 684–695.

Mazzini L et al. (1995) Percutaneous endoscopic gastrostomy and enteral nutrition in amyotrophic lateral sclerosis. *Journal of Neurology*, 242(10): 695–698.

Miller RG et al. (1999) Practice parameter: the care of the patient with amyotrophic lateral sclerosis (an evidence-based review). *Neurology*, 52(7): 1311.

MND Scotland (2018) Figures show 'Aikman' impact on MND care. Available at: https://www.mndscotland.org.uk/latest/news/figures-show-aikman-impact-on-mnd-care/

Murray SA et al. (2002) Dying of lung cancer or cardiac failure: prospective qualitative interview study of patients and their carers in the community. *British Medical Journal*, 325(7370): 929.

Murray SA et al. (2005) Illness trajectories and palliative care. *BMJ*, 330(7498): 1007–1011.

Murtagh FE, Murphy E and Sheerin NS (2008) Illness trajectories: an important concept in the management of kidney failure. *Nephrology Dialysis Transplantation*, 23(12): 3746–3748.

Murtagh FE et al. (2010) Symptoms in the month before death for stage 5 chronic kidney disease patients managed without dialysis. *Journal of Pain and Symptom Management*, 40(3): 342–352.

Murtagh FE et al. (2011) Trajectories of illness in stage 5 chronic kidney disease: a longitudinal study of patient symptoms and concerns in the last year of life. *Clinical Journal of the American Society of Nephrology*, 6(7): 1580–1590.

Murtagh FE (2018) Palliative care in kidney disease. In MacLeod R and Van den Block L (eds) *Textbook of Palliative Care*. Champaign, IL: Springer.

Neudert C et al. (2001) The course of the terminal phase in patients with amyotrophic lateral sclerosis. *Journal of Neurology*, 248(7): 612–616.

Ng L et al. (2017) Symptomatic treatments for amyotrophic lateral sclerosis/motor neuron disease. *Cochrane Database Systematic Reviews*, 1(1): CD011776.

NICE (2017) Guideline cystic fibrosis: diagnosis and management. Available at: https://www.nice.org.uk/guidance/ng78

NICE (2018a) Chronic obstructive pulmonary disease in over 16s: diagnosis and management. Available at: https://www.nice.org.uk/guidance/NG115

NICE (2018b) renal replacement therapy and conservative management (NG 107). Available at: https://www.nice.org.uk/guidance/ng107

Noble H et al. (2008) Patient experience of dialysis refusal or withdrawal – a review of the literature. *Journal of Renal Care*, 34(2): 94–100.

O'Halloran P et al. (2018) Advance care planning with patients who have end-stage kidney disease: a systematic realist review. *Journal of Pain Symptom Management*, 56(5): 795–807.

Oliver D (1996) The quality of care and symptom control — the effects on the terminal phase of ALS/MND. *Journal of Neurological Science, Amyotrophic Lateral Sclerosis/Motor Neurone Disease*, 139: 134–136.

Oliver D (2002) Palliative care for motor neurone disease. *Practical Neurology*, 2(2): 68–79.

Poonja Z, Brisebois A and van Zanten SV (2014) Patients with cirrhosis and denied liver transplants rarely receive adequate palliative care or appropriate management. *Clinical Gastroenterology and Hepatology*, 12(4): 692–698.

Pugh RNH et al. (1973) Transection of the oesophagus for bleeding oesophageal varices. *British Journal of surgery*, 60(8):646–649.

Pyart R et al. (2020) The 21st UK Renal Registry Annual Report: a summary of analyses of adult data in 2017. *Nephron*, 144(2): 59–66.

Riva N et al. (2019) Safety and efficacy of nabiximols on spasticity symptoms in patients with motor neuron disease (CANALS): a multicentre, double-blind, randomised, placebo-controlled, phase 2 trial. *Lancet Neurology*, 18(2): 155–164.

Roth K, Lynn J and Zhong Z (2000) Dying with end stage liver disease with cirrhosis: insights from SUPPORT (Study to Understand Prognoses and Preferences for Outcomes and Risks of Treatment). *Journal of the American Geriatric Society*, 48(5 Suppl): S122–S130.

Schmidt RJ and Moss AH. (2014) Dying on dialysis: the case for a dignified withdrawal. *Clinical Journal of the American Society Nephrology*, 9(1): 174–180.

Scottish Renal Registry (2020) Scottish Renal Registry Report 2020. Available at: https://www.srr.scot.nhs.uk

Scottish Palliative Care Guidelines (2018) End Stage Liver Disease. Available at: https://www.palliativecareguidelines.scot.nhs.uk/guidelines/end-of-life-care/end-stage-liver-disease.aspx

Scottish Palliative Care Guidelines (2020a) Pruritis. Available at: https://www.palliativecareguidelines.scot.nhs.uk/guidelines/symptom-control/pruritis.aspx

Scottish Palliative Care Guidelines (2020b) Depression. Available at: https://www.palliativecareguidelines.scot.nhs.uk/guidelines/symptom-control/depression.aspx

Scottish Palliative Care Guidelines (2020c) Renal Disease in the Last Days of Life. Available at: https://www.palliativecareguidelines.scot.nhs.uk/guidelines/end-of-life-care/renal-disease-in-the-last-days-of-life.aspx

Scottish Palliative Care Guidelines (2020d) Care in the Last Days of Life. Available at: https://www.palliativecareguidelines.scot.nhs.uk/guidelines/end-of-life-care/care-in-the-last-days-of-life.aspx

Scottish Palliative Care Guidelines (2021a) Neuropathic Pain. Available at: https://www.palliativecareguidelines.scot.nhs.uk/guidelines/pain/neuropathic-pain.aspx

Scottish Palliative Care Guidelines (2021b) Hiccups. Available at: https://www.palliativecareguidelines.scot.nhs.uk/guidelines/symptom-control/hiccups.aspx

Scottish Palliative Care Guidelines (2021c) Nausea and Vomiting. Available at: https://www.palliativecareguidelines.scot.nhs.uk/guidelines/symptom-control/nausea-and-vomiting.aspx

Squires N et al. (2014) The use of botulinum toxin injections to manage drooling in amyotrophic lateral sclerosis/motor neurone disease: a systematic review. *Dysphagia*, 29: 500–508.

Standing H, Jarvis H and Orr J (2017) How can primary care enhance end-of-life care for liver disease? Qualitative study of general practitioners' perceptions and experiences. *BMJ Open*, 7(8): e017106.

Stevens PE, Levin A and Members for the Kidney Disease Improving Global Outcomes Chronic Kidney Disease Guideline Development Work Group (2013) Evaluation and management of chronic kidney disease: synopsis of the kidney disease: improving global outcomes 2012 clinical practice guideline. *Annals of Internal Medicine*, 158(11): 825–830.

Stevenson J et al. (2017) Nutrition in renal supportive care: patient-driven and flexible. *Nephrology*, 22(10): 739–747.

Turner MR et al. (2003) Prolonged survival in motor neuron disease: a descriptive study of the King's database 1990–2002. *Journal of Neurology, Neurosurgery and American Psychiatry*, 74(7): 995.

University of Edinburgh (2019) Supportive and Palliative Care Indicators Tool. Available at: https://www.spict.org.uk/

Vaughn-Sandler V, Sherman C and Aronsohn A (2014) Consequences of perceived stigma among patients with cirrhosis. *Digest Diseases and Sciences*, 59(3): 681–686.

Wilcock A, Howard P and Charlesworth S (2020) *Palliative Care Formulary* (PCF7). Nottingham: Palliativedrugs.com Ltd.

Williams R et al. (2014) Addressing liver disease in the UK: a blueprint for attaining excellence in health care and reducing premature mortality from lifestyle issues of excess consumption of alcohol, obesity, and viral hepatitis. *Lancet*, 384(9958): 1953–1997.

Chapter 7

Psychosocial and Spiritual Aspects of Palliative and End-of-Life Care

George Beuken and Mark R Evans

Learning Objectives

At the completion of this chapter you will be able to do the following:

- Understand the meaning and principals of spiritual care within a multi-faith and multicultural society

- Recognise patients as individuals with differing spiritual beliefs and psychosocial needs, and understand how these impact on their experience of palliative and end-of-life-care, and that of their families and carers

- Recognise transition loss and anticipatory grief and support the needs of people experiencing loss

- Support people to maintain their mental, spiritual and emotional well-being

- Understand how spiritual and psychosocial distress impacts on physical well-being

- Recognise your own spiritual and religious beliefs, if any, and be aware of how they affect your approach to caring for dying patients

- Recognise the impact on self of living and working with loss, death and bereavement, and support other members of the team in their roles as they deal with loss, death and bereavement.

Scenario

Background

Sean is a 52-year-old married man with two adult children in their mid to late twenties. He has recently had a diagnosis of advanced non-small cell lung cancer with liver and bone metastasis. Prior to his diagnosis Sean has enjoyed what he describes as good health.

Key points

- Sean was a high achiever, now limited by a terminal illness.
- Despite a marriage of 30 years the couple are struggling to communicate.
- The couple have different spiritual beliefs.

Timeline

Sean has been an achiever in life; he works as a civil engineer and has a senior position with his company. He has a variety of social and sporting interests. He is involved with his local community council. He and his wife Mary are due to celebrate their 30th wedding anniversary next month.

Sean's consultant has informed him that due to the advanced nature of his disease any treatment available to him will be palliative and that his prognosis is likely to be months rather than years.

Over the last few weeks Sean has become increasingly symptomatic: he is no longer able to get out and about and is rapidly losing weight. He is becoming more breathless with minimal exertion and is experiencing increasing levels of pain. He is becoming increasingly anxious especially around his family and his mood seems extremely low.

Understandably, his wife, Mary, is finding it very difficult to cope in the situation, saying that she feels as though she is treading on eggshells most of the time. She has also stated that she and Sean have enjoyed a close relationship throughout their married lives and have been able to share openly and honestly with one another; this is no longer the case. Mary states that a huge gulf has developed between her and Sean. She feels isolated and alone in dealing with the situation. Mary was brought up as a Roman Catholic and believes in life after death. Sean would describe himself as an atheist.

Key considerations

- Can you identify the areas of transition loss in Sean's life?
- As healthcare practitioners how do we know that we have the emotional maturity, skills and resilience to begin to engage with this couple in a meaningful way that might assist them to address the unspoken issues?
- What benefits and difficulties could Mary's faith present as her husband deteriorates?

Introduction

Though interconnected, there are distinctions between psychosocial and spiritual care that warrant separate attention. However, in this chapter we will integrate psychosocial and spiritual care to demonstrate a whole person approach rather than referring to them individually.

The practitioner's training in loss, grief and bereavement (See Chapter 14 – Bereavement) is integral to psychosocial care and spiritual care, as is the practitioners communication skills training (See Chapter 3 – Communication). For effective holistic care practitioners should be attentive to, and comfortable with, the patient/client, family or friend as they express their feelings of grief, loss and/or loneliness, isolation and distress.

Spiritual Care

In 2002 The Scottish Executive Health Department (SEHD, 2002) signalled a significant movement in the understanding and practice of spiritual care and chaplaincy. It recognised some of the major changes that had been taking place within Scottish society, and it described the essence and practice of spiritual care in ways which took account of such changes among people with and without any faith commitment. There are many with spiritual beliefs who do not belong to a particular faith or belief group. Some might call our age 'post-modern,' but all would recognise that we have a greater variety of faith, culture and belief throughout all our social institutions than ever before. Spirituality, in the early part of twenty-first-century Scotland, has many outlets.

It is widely recognised that spirituality is part of what it means to be human. This includes the awareness of self and of relationships with others and the natural world. The healthcare challenges faced by those people requiring palliative care may raise their need for spiritual or religious care (Scottish Government CEL, 2008).

Spiritual care is usually given in a one-to-one setting. It is completely person-centred and makes no assumptions about a patient's personal conviction or life orientation.

Religious care is given in the context of shared religious beliefs, values, liturgies and lifestyle of a faith community.

Spiritual care is not necessarily religious, while religious care should always be spiritual. Spiritual care might be said to be the umbrella term of which religious care is a part because it is the intention of religious care to meet spiritual need (Scottish Government CEL, 2008).

Spiritual care within healthcare

Among the basic spiritual needs that might be addressed within the normal daily activity of healthcare are (McSherry, 2006):

- The need to give and receive love
- The need to be understood
- The need to be valued as a human being
- The need for forgiveness, hope and trust
- The need to explore beliefs and values
- The need to express feelings honestly
- The need to find meaning and purpose in life.

The above principles should all be kept in mind during your work as a healthcare practitioner, as you may often be offering a form of spiritual care without even identifying it as such. The need for spiritual care demonstrates that people are not merely physical bodies requiring mechanical fixing. People find that their spirituality and the resilience it provides helps them maintain health and cope with illnesses, traumas, losses and life transitions by integrating body, mind and spirit. People, whether religious or not, share deep existential needs and concerns as they strive to make their lives meaningful and to maintain hope when illness or injury affects them.

Principles of spiritual care services

The principles of all spiritual care services provided by the NHS are that the service should:

- Be impartial and accessible to persons of all faith communities and those without a particular faith
- Facilitate spiritual and religious care of all kinds
- Respect the wide range of beliefs, lifestyles and backgrounds found within society today, particularly in relation to age, gender, ethnicity, sexual orientation, disability and religion/belief, and value this diversity
- Be a significant NHS resource in an increasingly multicultural society
- Be a unifying and encouraging presence in an NHS organisation
- Never be imposed or used to convert people religiously
- Be open, sensitive, compassionate and be characterised by the capacity to make and maintain attentive, helpful, supportive and caring relationships
- Affirm and secure the right of patients to be visited (or not visited) by a chaplain or their faith representative by incorporating flexibility into the means of obtaining informed consent for spiritual care, both at the time of admission and during a patient's time of treatment
- Be carried out in by a multidisciplinary team; and acknowledge that spiritual care in the NHS is given by many members of staff and by carers and patients.

(Scottish Government CEL, 2008)

Spiritual care competencies

Healthcare chaplaincy has achieved recognition as a healthcare profession with agreed standards of professional practice. In August 2017, the Professional Standards Authority (PSA) recognised the UK Board of Healthcare Chaplaincy (UKBHC) as an Accredited Register of healthcare chaplains in UK. The primary aim of UKBHC is the safety and well-being of the public, which it achieves by setting high standards for the professional practice of healthcare chaplains and the delivery of spiritual care within health and social care settings.

Established in 2009, the UKBHC agreed that there was a need to standardised titles and roles across the UK in a language and framework that employers and the public could understand. Following a consultation by the UKBHC, a Code of Conduct and Professional Standards & Competences for Healthcare Chaplains were agreed and published in June 2010 and subsequently revised in 2020 (UKBHC, 2021).

Total Pain

Dame Cicely Saunders coined the term 'total pain' and suggested that pain can be understood as having physical, psychological, social spiritual components. The total experience of pain is impacted by all of the elements both negatively and positively. An understanding of this allows for treatment beyond the use of analgesics. The combination of these elements is believed to result in a 'total pain' experience that is individualised and specific to each patient's particular situation (Mehta, 2008).

> 'The physical agony of an individual is normally compounded by fear of death, loss of independence, conflict with loved ones and a state of spiritual anguish in which faith is stretched to breaking point, and hope little more than a child's fantasy.'
>
> (Cicely Saunders, 1978)

Many examples demonstrate the 'total pain' experience, in which effective pain relief follows the acknowledgment and management of the physical, psychological, social and spiritual dimensions of the person. Spiritual needs may be met in a variety of ways such as practising and participating in a belief system, mindfulness, relaxation or simply listening to music or reading a book.

Pain control is a central component of symptom management for many patients in palliative care, and the assessment of pain is a critical part of this pain management. Without a clear conceptualisation of pain for the palliative patient population, it becomes difficult to assess patients' pain appropriately.

Understanding that people experience 'total pain' is critical for healthcare professionals. The physical, psychological, social and spiritual dimensions/causes may contribute to the patient's pain experience. Without a complete and thorough assessment of these dimensions, an accurate picture of the patient's situation cannot be obtained. The concept of 'total pain' may serve as the basis for pain assessment in order to intervene successfully when patients report pain, suffering or distress (see Figure 7.1).

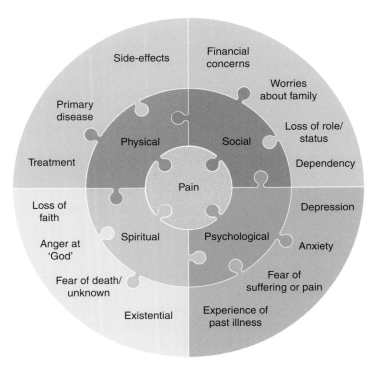

Figure 7.1 Elements of total pain.

Assessing Spiritual and Psychosocial Needs

The World Health Organization (WHO) definition of palliative care (World Health Organization, 2020) sets out our objectives admirably:

> *'Palliative care is an approach that improves the quality of life of patients (adults and children) and their families who are facing problems associated with life-threatening illness. It prevents and relieves suffering through the early identification, correct assessment and treatment of pain and other problems, whether physical, psychosocial or spiritual.'*

Very often it is the problems that are associated with life-threatening illness that present the biggest challenges to patients and their families.

The WHO speaks of 'impeccable assessment'. There is an abundance of assessment tools available for use with palliative and end-of-life care patients, but an impeccable assessment begins with listening attentively to the patient and family's story. To know a person is to know their story, their history and what is important to them. The challenge facing health and social care professionals is learning to be with people in their suffering and distress.

Effective psychosocial and spiritual care can go a long way in alleviating a patient and family's distress; this can only be achieved when we have established what matters to the patient and their family.

FICA spiritual history tool©*

This communication tool can be used as part of an assessment for treatment plans for palliative patients. It can be used to identify the patient's spirituality, sources of spiritual distress and existential thoughts and feelings (Puchalski and et al., 2000).

The acronym FICA can help to structure questions for healthcare professionals who are taking a spiritual history:

F – Faith, belief, meaning

- 'Do you consider yourself to be spiritual?' Or 'Is spirituality something important to you?'
- 'Do you have spiritual beliefs, practices or values that help you to cope with stress, difficult times, or what you are going through right now?'
- 'What gives your life meaning?'

I – Importance and influence

- 'What importance does spirituality have in your life?'
- 'Has your spirituality influenced how you take care of yourself, particularly regarding your health?'
- 'Does your spirituality affect your healthcare decision making?'

C – Community

- 'Are you part of a spiritual community?'
- 'Is your community a support to you and how?'
- For people who don't identify with a community consider asking 'Is there a group of people you really love or who are important to you?' (Communities such as churches, temples, mosques, family, groups of like-minded friends, or yoga or similar groups can serve as strong support systems for some patients).

A – Address/action in care

- 'How would you like me, as your healthcare provider, to address spiritual issues in your healthcare?'
- With newer models, including the diagnosis of spiritual distress, 'A' also refers to the 'Assessment and Plan' for patient spiritual distress, needs and/or resources within a treatment or care plan.

Source: © Copyright Christina Puchalski, MD, and The George Washington University 1996 (updated 2021). All rights reserved.

*Adapted from: Puchalski C and Romer AL (2000). Taking a spiritual history allows clinicians to understand patients more fully. *Journal of Palliative Medicine*, 3(1), 129-137. Reproduced in full with the kind permission of Christina Puchalski.

CARES tool

Another simple approach to spiritual assessment is the NHS Fife Spiritual CARES tool which:

- Can be used by anyone, for anyone, and in any context
- Ensures the continuous assessment of spiritual needs
- Places person-centred provision as its core value
- Develops confidence and skill as a listener and provider of (spiritual) care
- Is a clear, concise assessment tool which supports national and local delivery plans.

Use the CARES acronym to guide your assessment. When assessing patients for spiritual needs focus on the following aspects:

- Coping skills and strategies: enquire about how the individual is coping or coming to terms with their diagnosis/prognosis/illness/situation
- Assets: evaluate their means of support and help, for example self, family, community
- Role of faith/belief/culture: explore its influences on care plan/dietary requirements/ritual and practices
- Existential issues/crisis: enquire about feelings such as loneliness, isolation, fear or disengagement/meaning/purpose
- Signpost: extend additional support, for example healthcare chaplaincy.

What matters to you?

The 'What matters to you?' initiative is all about people and relationships and looks at five key must do with me areas:

1. What matters to you?
2. Who matters to you?
3. What information do you need?
4. Nothing about me without me.
5. Personalised contact.

Together these five 'Must do with me' areas will help to ensure that all of the interactions between people using services and the staff delivering them are characterised by listening, dignity, compassion and respect. Asking the question 'what matters to you?' can help to establish relationships between those giving and those receiving care. This question can be asked in many different ways:

- What things are most important to you at the moment?
- What would you like to achieve as a result of this support?
- When you have a good day, what are the things which make it good?

Having a conversation about the things which really matter to people can help you to do your job more effectively. It also helps the patient you are interacting with live a life which is fulfilling and meaningful to them (What matters to you, 2021).

The grief reaction in people experiencing transition loss can be tangible and resemble the grief reaction to all major losses in life. When Kübler-Ross published her theory of the stages of grief after first having completed her research with dying people, she was very careful to explain that these are normal reactions we have to tragic news. In fact, she called them defence mechanisms or coping mechanisms. This is exactly what they are when we apply the model to coping with change (Kübler-Ross, 1975). People need time to process and to come to terms with and accept the changed reality with which they live (Worden, 1991). Very often, what grieving people seem to need most is someone who will sit quietly with them in their suffering.

The fifth principle of 'must do with me' is personalised contact. Good palliative and end-of-life care is not achieved within a vacuum, it is achieved within the context of relationships. That is, the therapeutic relationship that is established between patient, family and caregiver when trust is established. Many of the skills required for this work will be addressed in the chapter on communication (Chapter 3 – Communication) in this book, but even the most skilled communicators can be reluctant to engage in conversations around dying, death and bereavement.

Faith, Culture and Religion

A multi-faith society

In a religiously and culturally diverse country it is important that staff are culturally sensitive and ensure that any specific spiritual, religious or cultural needs of patients are considered and met. Spiritual care is a core aspect of person-centred care and should be available to everyone regardless of their beliefs.

Everyone's spiritual care needs are different, so ask the patients what is important to them and what you can do to help meet such needs. Don't make assumptions about what you think patients spiritual care needs may be; even people from within the same belief group can have different perspectives. Failure to acknowledge such needs may contribute to a patient's distress and grief, especially if they feel that their spiritual care needs were not met.

A person's religion and culture is often central to their very being, and may have a direct effect on their needs, their care and often on their attitude to illness. At a time of crisis, such as illness and hospitalisation, a person may receive a great deal of comfort and benefit from their belief system and practising their faith, and from having their religious and cultural needs recognised and respected.

Spiritual care is rapidly moving into mainstream healthcare and it is incumbent on all healthcare professionals to know the reasons for integrating spirituality into patient care in a sensible and sensitive way, ensuring the health and well-being of our patients and their families in a holistic person-centred way.

Religious and cultural needs

Many people rely on their personal beliefs, religious practices or cultural heritage (and associated traditions) as a means of coping with illness and other stressful situations. During the last 20 years or so extensive research has shown that people who have faith/belief and regular religious practice have better mental health and adapt more quickly to health problems compared to other groups in society (Koening, 2012). The suggestion here is that these possible benefits to mental health and well-being can impact on physical health and influence the response to treatment. The vast majority of studies undertaken report significant relationships between religion/spirituality and better health (Koenig et al., 2012).

Although some people subscribe to a particular religious tradition, they are not always orthodox followers of that tradition. If a patient or family is established as having a particular religious tradition it is always better through conversation to establish the elements of that tradition that are important to them. As healthcare professionals it is important that we don't make assumptions about what we think patients' spiritual care needs may be; even people from within the same belief group can have different perspectives. Failure to acknowledge such needs may contribute to an individual's distress; especially if they feel that their spiritual care needs were not met. Table 7.1 gives a brief overview of particular end-of-life needs of the main faith groups.

Be mindful that not all individuals will necessarily adhere to established traditions and death customs. A useful resource which gives more detailed information and guidance about cultural and faith/religious traditions is 'A Multi-Faith Resource for Healthcare Staff' from NHS Education for Scotland (a link can be found in the resources section of this chapter).

Whatever the needs of the patient and/or family, practitioners must develop the ability to distinguish between what they, as non-specialists, can offer, and what a distressed person or family should seek from specialist resources. Each health board and hospice in Scotland provides a spiritual care service consisting of a team of specialised healthcare chaplains who can be a source of information and advice for community teams.

Our scenario gives no indication as to whether Sean and the extended family have any particular faith, culture or religious practice. Mary is, however, a Roman Catholic. We do well to remember that many people who do not have regular religious practice or belong to a particular religious group may nevertheless be people of faith.

Communication and translation

Within our multicultural society there is a diversity of languages. Patients and service users speak a wide range of languages and English may not be their 'main language'. It is important that healthcare professionals consider communication barriers and potential misunderstandings between professionals and patients with limited or no understanding of English.

Table 7.1 Overview of the main faith groups and cultures in relation to palliative care.

Faith	Practical care	Personal hygiene requirements	Language	Care of the dying
Baha'i	No special needs	Baha'is may wish to wash before praying	Various	As the vehicle of the soul, the body of the deceased is treated with great respect Baha'i law prescribes that the body be buried not more than one hour's journey from the place of death The body may not be cremated or embalmed.
Buddhist	Transplants may be an area of concern to patients	No special needs	Various	The patient may wish to have a quiet place in which to meditate and to light a candle or incense stick if possible.
Chinese	Reassurance and explanation about treatment is of great importance The use of a translator is often vital when caring for Chinese people. This will avoid unnecessary anxiety	No special needs	Hakka Cantonese Mandarin	There may be many different customs depending on the patient's cultural background
Christian	No special needs	No special needs	Various	The patient and/or family may request religious support from members of the clergy. In some branches of Christianity there are specific rituals and rites which may be requested prior to death or after death. There are no formal objections to postmortem or cremation
Hindu	Jewellery may have religious significance Hindu women prefer a female doctor for examination or treatment Sensitivity is essential	Water for hand washing before meals is essential. Water for washing is required in same room as WC or following the use of a bedpan Hindus prefer showers to baths	Punjabi Hindi Gujarati Urdu Bengali	If possible Hindu patients should be allowed to die at home. Prior to death a relative may bring money and clothes to touch for distribution to the needy Some may wish a holy book to be read to them. After death the body should be left covered Relatives may wish to wash the body and put on new clothes. Cremation is the tradition

(Continued)

303

Table 7.1 (Continued).

Faith	Practical care	Personal hygiene requirements	Language	Care of the dying
Jewish	Modesty is important in the Jewish culture; garments should ensure that dignity is preserved After giving birth 40 days of rest is required for the mother by custom If the child is still in hospital by the 8th day, the family may request the ritual of circumcision to be performed by a medically qualified religious functionary	Jews wash and say a brief blessing before eating Orthodox women keep their hair covered	English Hebrew Yiddish	Following death the body should be handled as little as possible by staff. Burial should take place within 24 hours of death if possible Burial is the custom rather than cremation
Sikh	Some female patients prefer to be examined by women doctors and men by male doctors Sensitivity is essential with regard to modesty Sikhs wear the '5 Ks' – symbols of their faith. Staff should be aware of the need for these to remain with the patient	Sikhs prefer to wash in free flowing water. They may wish to have a daily shower	Punjabi Hindi	Sikhs will accept postmortems if legally necessary. Following death the body is washed and white clothes put on (this is undertaken by the funeral director and the family) The Sikh priest can be contacted by the family. Cremation not burial is the custom
Muslim	It is preferable in most cases for Muslim women to be examined and treated by female members of staff. All Muslims dress with modesty and some women may cover their heads. A male Muslim baby is required to be circumcised	Muslims wash before eating and before prayer. They require a container of water after using the toilet and prefer free flowing water to a bath	Arabic Punjabi Bengali Hindi Urdu Gujarati	Following death, burial should take place as soon as possible. The next of kin will wish to arrange the washing of the body before burial Postmortems should be avoided unless legally necessary. All organs should be buried with the body Emotions may be expressed freely and consideration should be given to this

Whilst it is tempting to use family members to 'translate', it is good practice to use approved interpreters. Use of family members can, on occasions, cause further misunderstanding and distress. The patient may not wish the family member to know about their diagnosis, prognosis or treatment options. In some cultures talking about death with parents is seen as 'taboo', or the family member may simply decide that the patient cannot cope with the 'truth'. Such barriers can have a negative effect on symptom management, patient care and subsequently cause distress to all involved (Silva et al., 2016).

Use of approved interpreters can facilitate fewer communication errors, increased patient understanding, greater patient autonomy, and increased accessibility to health services (Karliner et al., 2007). As a result, appropriate use of professional interpreters will have a positive impact on the quality of care and positive effect on the health and well-being of the patient and the family. In addition, the use of interpreters will not only aid effective communication but can also ensure that such communication is culturally sensitive.

End-of-Life Anxieties

Money can't buy happiness, but it can give you more control, access to a greater choice of resources and reduce stress/anxiety due to financial concerns. It is now widely accepted that poverty, in all its forms, has an adverse effect on a person's health and well-being and is one of the main causes of poor health and health inequalities.

A source of anxiety and distress for patients and their families can be finance, whether that be financial difficulties in the present or impending financial difficulties that come about as the result of a loved one's death.

> 'End of life care is, sadly, a recurring and consistent theme in our casework... we see tragic cases where people's suffering could have been avoided or lessened with the right care and treatment as they approached the end of their lives. The anguish that this causes them and their loved ones is unimaginable.'
>
> (Parliamentary and Health Service Ombudsman, 2015)

As a patient nears the end of life there can be increased anxiety (for both the patient and the family) due to a decrease in income and increase in costs meaning it can be difficult for families to balance finances (for example, increased fuel bills with a decrease in income). As well as the patient being unable to work, partners or family members may also be unable to work due to caring for their loved one.

Many patients fear putting burdens on their families and loved ones. One area where anxiety can be alleviated is in relation to funeral arrangements. It is important to support patients and families to talk about their 'final wishes'. However, as we discussed earlier in this chapter, there can be a cultural resistance to this conversation. Very often family members have a fear of upsetting one another with a conversation of this nature. Once established that distress can be a natural and necessary part of this process, we can encourage people to engage with the conversation, often resulting in the relief of tension and anxiety for all concerned: 'Now we know what you want for your funeral we can go ahead and plan it.'

Funerals can be expensive, with families feeling pressured to spend more than they can afford. The average cost of a funeral in Scotland is just under £3,500 (Scottish Government, 2019). According to 'Fair Funerals' (Fair Funerals, 2020) in 2019, 12% of people faced with arranging a funeral struggled to pay for it. Fear of funeral poverty can be a real source of distress and anxiety and discussing the patient's wishes as a family can help alleviate such fears. It's worth remembering when planning a funeral that the cost of a basic or standard funeral can vary greatly depending on the funeral director you engage. Funeral poverty can have a negative impact on a person's emotional and mental well-being including affecting the grieving process.

Help with all these issues can be accessed through 'Money Matters', a one stop shop for help with all things financial, as well as Macmillan's Cancer Support advice on benefits and financial support (see resources at the end of the chapter).

Acceptance and commitment therapy

The BEACHeS (Brief Engagement and Acceptance Coaching in Community and Hospice Settings) Research Study is a project which develops our understanding that transition into palliative care results in loss, helplessness, uncertainty and fear that can lead to distress in many forms: psychological, emotional and existential (Hulbert-Williams et al., 2019). This study suggests that problematic symptoms and poor quality of life can inhibit planning for the future, and may be a barrier to anticipatory care planning. This study explores the use of 'Acceptance and Commitment Therapy' (ACT) (Hayes et al., 2003) with this patient group.

The aim of ACT is to normalise distress and suffering in challenging life situations and promote acceptance of, and resilience to, distress by increasing psychological flexibility (Hayes et al., 2016). Developing the ability to adapt, and to be able to 'sit with' unwanted experiences rather than try to change or alter them, it draws substantially on an already strong mindfulness evidence base.

The aim of spiritual care is not to fix things for people but to enable people to accept the reality with which they live.

Compassionate Care

When engaging with patients and families with palliative and end-of-life care needs, remember that you are the asset. You bring yourself with all your experience, knowledge, skills, talent and vulnerability to the situation and you meet people in their vulnerability. When we are able to recognise the humanity of one another our connectedness to the other brings with it a sense of understanding, compassion and hope. This is encapsulated by the ABCD of Dignity approach (see Chapter 1 – Principles of Palliative and End-of-Life Care (p. 4)).

Providing compassionate care may seem entirely reasonable to expect in palliative and end-of-life care but it can be incredibly hard work on the part of the individual providing the care. Good working environments have the right levels of staff with the right skills and support from colleagues and managers. If staff are to deliver good, compassionate care, it is critical to care for them too so that they can care properly for others. This is the foundation on which compassionate care must be built: it cannot be 'engineered in' through initiatives when this necessary condition does not apply (Department of Health, 2013).

Staff support

Delivering end-of-life care can be difficult for health and social care staff involved in this important aspect of care. Dr Rachel Naomi Remen stated that: *'the expectation that we can be immersed in suffering and loss daily and not be touched by it is as unrealistic as expecting to be able to walk through water without getting wet'* (Seltzer, 2018).

The invaluable role that a healthcare professional can provide at the end of life has at its heart comfort, dignity and peace for the patient, their family, and themselves on a journey of loss.

As healthcare staff, we can also experience grief at the death of a patient, and it may awaken in us our own feelings of grief and loss. In addition, you may be carrying the weight of issues and ethical dilemmas around withdrawal of active treatment. The weight can often seem too heavy to carry. It is crucial that we are all able to talk openly and honestly about our emotional and spiritual health and well-being.

Building resilience

You can help to build personal strength and resilience in the following ways:

- Recognise your strengths, limitations and vulnerabilities
- Care for yourself, and be aware of when support is needed (talk with the right people)
- Look out for other members of the team in dealing with dying, death and loss
- Know what triggers your emotions and what doesn't
- Know that your role and care is invaluable to others
- Remember, you're not alone – you're part of an amazing team – so work collaboratively.

We know that the building of good working environments and relationships are essential to influencing positive change, and key to fulfilling an individual's purpose in a role and workplace. Systematically creating an environment in which compassionate care is the norm requires imaginative commissioning, organisational commitment, planning, education and training, and above all reflection.

Reflective practice

Gibbs' (1988) reflective cycle is a popular model for reflection. The model includes 6 stages of reflection and is presented in Figure 7.2.

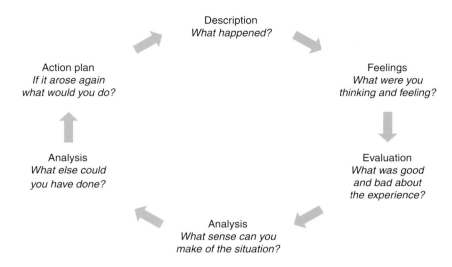

Figure 7.2 Gibbs' reflective cycle.

This is a simple model of reflective practice that will be familiar to many nurses from their time as students. Regular reflective practice promotes staff resilience, improves confidence and enhances patient and family care.

In concluding this chapter we can acknowledge that:

- The psychosocial and spiritual aspects of care with the focus on the patient's agenda is integral to effective palliative care and relieves suffering
- Open and honest communication between practitioners, patient and their significant others is imperative to minimise distress
- Analgesia is only one facet of 'total pain' control
- You only die once. We have one chance of getting it right.

Scenario Recap

When we reflect on this scenario, one of the first things that becomes apparent is the vast amount of loss that Sean has experienced in his life in the last weeks and months. Sean is a man who is essentially grieving. Whether he is conscious of this or not, of course, is another matter.

The second point that is apparent is contained in the second point of the 'must do with me' principles. That is, about the people who are important to Sean. We read that Sean 'is becoming increasingly anxious especially around his family and his mood is extremely low'. Is it possible that Sean's family are unwittingly triggering an anticipatory grief reaction for him simply by their presence? Might the very presence of close family members cause Sean to think about who and what he is about to leave behind? Is this too painful to even begin to contemplate, hence the gulf that is developing between him and his wife Mary? Might Sean require further information at this time?

The third 'must do with me' aspect is that Sean may have questions he needs to have answered in order for him to begin to have meaningful conversations with Mary. Sean, we read, is becoming increasingly symptomatic. Is it possible that the changes in condition that Sean is experiencing are generating fear in him? We know from Cicely Saunders' concept of 'total pain' that fear of death, loss of independence and conflict with loved ones are common sources of distress in palliative and end-of-life care patients.

From the scenario we can clearly recognise that Sean is a man who has always been in control of his life. Is there need for reassurance at this time, taking account of the fourth 'must do with me' principle, nothing about me without me? If Sean has a fear of loss of control, might a conversation around anticipatory care planning as a means of Sean maintaining control as his illness progresses be helpful? Anticipatory care planning is discussed in greater detail in the chapter on communication in this book (Chapter 3 – Communication (p. 64)).

We understand that Mary, Sean's wife, is finding it very difficult to cope in the situation. She has stated that she and Sean have enjoyed a close relationship throughout their married lives and have always been able to share openly and honestly with one another. Sadly, this is no longer the case. This highlights other areas of loss: the loss of intimacy and the loss of sexual intimacy, not only for Sean but also for Mary. The key to intimacy is open and honest communication. In this scenario the key has been lost.

Resources

Macmillan Cancer Support. Benefits and Financial Support: Available at: https://www.macmillan.org.uk/cancer-information-and-support/impacts-of-cancer/benefits-and-financial-support

Marie Curie and the Association of Hospice and Palliative Care Chaplains (AHPCC) Spiritual and Religious Care Competencies for Specialist Palliative Care. Available at: http://ahpcc.co.uk/wp-content/uploads/2014/07/spiritcomp.pdf

Money Matters; Money Advice Centre. Available at: http://www.moneymattersweb.co.uk/

NHS Education for Scotland. A Multi-faith Resource for Healthcare Staff. Available at: https://learn.nes.nhs.scot/50422/person-centred-care-zone/spiritual-care-and-healthcare-chaplaincy/resources/multi-faith-resource-for-healthcare-staff

NHS Education for Scotland. Palliative and End of Life Care: Enriching and improving experience. Available at: https://learn.nes.nhs.scot/2452/palliative-and-end-of-life-care-enriching-and-improving-experience/palliative-and-end-of-life-care-enriching-and-improving-experience

NHS Education for Scotland. Spiritual Care Matters: An introductory Resource for all NHS Scotland Staff. Available at: https://www.nes.scot.nhs.uk/media/23nphas3/spiritualcaremattersfinal.pdf

References

Department of Health (2013) *Patients First and Foremost: The Government Response to the Mid Staffordshire NHS Foundation Trust Public Inquiry.* London: HMSO.

Fair Funerals (2020) Fair Funerals pledge 2020: Guidelines & advice for funeral directors. Available at: https://fairfuneralscampaign.org.uk/sites/default/files/Fair%20Funerals%20pledge%20guidelines%20for%20FDs_2.pdf

Gibbs G (1988) *Learning by Doing: A Guide to Teaching and Learning Methods.* London: Further Education Unit.

Hayes SC, Strosahl KD and Wilson GK (2003) *Acceptance and Commitment Therapy: An Experiential Approach to Behaviour Change.* New York: Guilford Press.

Hayes SC, Strosahl KD and Wilson GK (2016) *Acceptance and Commitment Therapy: The Process and Practice of Mindful Change.* Second edition. New York: Guilford Press.

Hulbert-Williams NJ et al. (2019) Brief Engagement and Acceptance Coaching for Community and Hospice Settings (the BEACHeS Study): protocol for the development and pilot testing of an evidence-based psychological intervention to enhance wellbeing and aid transition into palliative care. *Pilot Feasibility Study*, 5: 104.

Karliner LS et al. (2007) Do professional interpreters improve clinical care for patients with limited English proficiency? A systematic review of the literature. *Health Services Research*, 42(2): 727–754.

Koenig HG, King DE and Carson VB (2012) *Handbook of Religion and Health.* Second edition. New York: Oxford University Press.

Kübler-Ross E (1975) *Death, the Final Stage of Growth.* Upper Saddle River, NJ: Prentice Hall.

McSherry W (2006) The principal components model: a model for advancing spirituality and spiritual care within nursing and health care practice. *Journal of Clinical Nursing*, 15(7): 905–917.

Mehta A (2008) Understanding of the concept of 'Total Pain': a prerequisite for pain control. *Journal of Hospice and Palliative Nursing*, 10(1): 26–32.

Parliamentary and Health Service Ombudsman (2015) Dying without Dignity. Available at: https://www.ombudsman.org.uk/sites/default/files/Dying_without_dignity.pdf

Puchalski C and Romer AL (2000) Taking a spiritual history allows clinicians to understand patients more fully. *Journal of Palliative Medicine*, 3(1): 129–137.

Saunders C (1978) *The Management of Terminal Disease.* London: Edward Arnold.

Scottish Government CEL (2008) 49: Guidance on spiritual care and chaplaincy in the NHS in Scotland. Available at: https://www.sehd.scot.nhs.uk/mels/cel2008_49.pdf

Scottish Government (2019) Funeral Costs Guidance: Fairer Scotland Duty Summary. Available at: https://www.gov.scot/publications/guidance-funeral-costs-fairer-scotland-duty-summary/ Scottish Executive Health Department (2002) Spiritual Care in NHS Scotland. Available at: https://www.sehd.scot.nhs.uk/mels/hdl2002_76.pdf

Seltzer L (2018) Why some people may simply run out of empathy. *Psychology Today.* Available at: https://www.psychologytoday.com/gb/blog/evolution-the-self/201808/why-some-people-may-simply-run-out-empathy

Silva MD et al. (2016) Interpreting at the end of life: a systematic review of the impact of interpreters on the delivery of palliative care services to cancer patients with limited English proficiency. *Journal of Pain and Symptom Management*, 51(3): 569–580.

UKBHC (2021) The UK Board of Healthcare Chaplaincy. Available at: https://www.ukbhc.org.uk/

What matters to you? (2021) Asking "what matters to you?" can make a real difference to health and care. Available at: https://www.whatmatterstoyou.scot/

Worden J W (1991) *Grief Counselling and Grief Therapy.* Second edition. New York: Springer Publishing.

World Health Organization (2020) Palliative Care. Available at: https://www.who.int/news-room/fact-sheets/detail/palliative-care

Palliative Care Emergencies

Kim Steel with Fiona McFatter

Learning Objectives

By the end of this chapter you should be able to:

- Demonstrate an understanding of the common palliative care emergencies including:
    - Hypercalcaemia of malignancy
    - Malignant spinal cord compression
    - Bleeding
    - Seizures
    - Superior vena cava obstruction (SVCO)
    - Bowel obstruction.
- Demonstrate an understanding of the context of a palliative care emergency for an individual patient
- Be able to discuss the common features of palliative care emergencies, including:
    - Clinical presentation
    - Assessment
    - Management.

Scenario

Background

You are the duty doctor in your practice. The son of 67-year-old Jean calls to say he is worried about his Mum. Jean usually takes care of his children one day a week but recently she has struggled because she is so tired. He arrived at her home today and his Mum was still in her pyjamas. The house was untidy, she seemed dazed and her conversation was muddled.

Key points

- You should have a low threshold for testing for hypercalcaemia. It can often mimic other problems or it can be very insidious.
- Management, depending on the patient's priorities, usually requires hospitalisation especially if it is associated with other red flags for malignancy.
- Lung cancer is one of the commonest causes of hypercalcaemia in a hospital setting.

Timeline

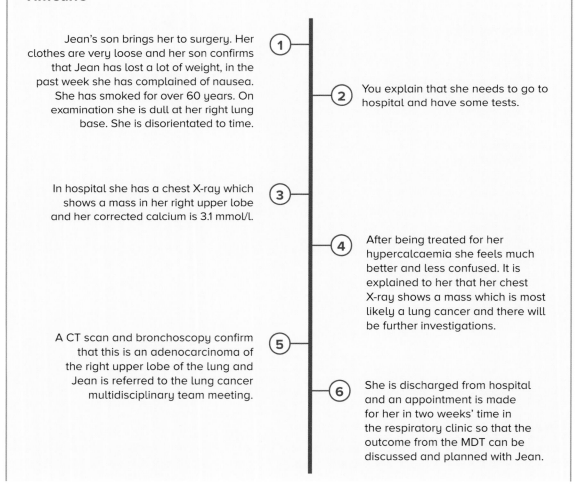

1 Jean's son brings her to surgery. Her clothes are very loose and her son confirms that Jean has lost a lot of weight, in the past week she has complained of nausea. She has smoked for over 60 years. On examination she is dull at her right lung base. She is disorientated to time.

2 You explain that she needs to go to hospital and have some tests.

3 In hospital she has a chest X-ray which shows a mass in her right upper lobe and her corrected calcium is 3.1 mmol/l.

4 After being treated for her hypercalcaemia she feels much better and less confused. It is explained to her that her chest X-ray shows a mass which is most likely a lung cancer and there will be further investigations.

5 A CT scan and bronchoscopy confirm that this is an adenocarcinoma of the right upper lobe of the lung and Jean is referred to the lung cancer multidisciplinary team meeting.

6 She is discharged from hospital and an appointment is made for her in two weeks' time in the respiratory clinic so that the outcome from the MDT can be discussed and planned with Jean.

Key considerations

- What are the key signs and symptoms that should make you consider hypercalcaemia?
- What would your priorities be in managing a patient with hypercalcaemia depending on which area you work in?

Introduction: What Is an Emergency?

An emergency is a serious, unexpected situation requiring an immediate response. In the setting of palliative care, emergencies may be sudden life-threatening changes in a patient's condition that, without an adequate response, will result in deterioration in that person's health or quality of life.

Some patients can be identified at higher risk because of the nature of their disease and emergency situations can be anticipated and planned for. In these circumstances the patient's wishes can be ascertained and discussions about the clinical response required to meet the patient's wishes can be established. It is important to discuss the benefits, burdens, harms and limits of acute treatments.

The palliative care emergencies which will be discussed in this chapter are:

1. Hypercalcaemia of malignancy
2. Malignant spinal cord compression
3. Bleeding
4. Seizures
5. Superior vena cava obstruction (SVCO)
6. Bowel obstruction.

Practice point

Often some of the most challenging decisions that we have to make include how to manage a person who has had an acute, unexpected deterioration in the context of a life-limiting illness, for example a hip fracture in someone who has advanced dementia.

In these circumstances always:

- Give immediate focus on symptoms while decision making is occurring – relieve pain/nausea/breathlessness as quickly as possible.
- Consider the person's baseline function. It is likely to deteriorate and if the person's functional status has been in decline (changing month on month

or week on week) then it is likely to accelerate, even if the best outcome is achieved from the acute issue.

- Talk to the person and their relatives about the uncertainty.
- After the immediate situation has been resolved, ensure that there is an advanced care planning discussion either for anticipated deterioration or, if the person stabilises, consider what should be done the next time if something similar happens.

Hypercalcaemia of Malignancy

Introduction

Hypercalcaemia is the commonest life-threatening metabolic disorder in cancer patients. It occurs in about 20–30% of patients with cancer (Lindner et al., 2013).

There are several pathological mechanisms whereby hypercalcaemia of malignancy can occur:

- Parathyroid hormone (PTH) related peptide released by tumour
- Osteolytic bone metastases
- Rarely, patients with cancer will present with primary hyperparathyroidism.

Eighty percent of hypercalaemia of malignancy is mediated by the production of recombinant parathyroid hormone, PTHrP (Stewart, 2005). PTHrP (PTH related peptide) is produced physiologically but some cancers produce this in large amounts. PTHrP causes osteoblasts to signal to osteoclasts to increase bone reabsorbtion which subsequently causes increases in the concentration of calcium in the blood.

Osteolytic metastatic bone disease can lead to excessive calcium release from the bone and an increase in serum calcium.

It is important to understand these mechanisms. It is a common misconception that a patient needs to have lytic bone lesions to develop hypercalcaemia and this is not the case. Conversely, an episode of hypercalcaemia does not always herald the presence of bone metastases; 20% of patients with hypercalcaemia do not have bone metastases (Jick et al., 2015).

Assessment

There are two main factors that determine how severe the symptoms of hypercalcaemia are:

1. The level of calcium
2. The rapidity of the rise in the calcium.

Symptoms

Common symptoms include:

- Malaise
- Weakness
- Anorexia
- Thirst
- Nausea
- Constipation
- Polyuria.

Severe symptoms include:

- Nausea
- Vomiting
- Ileus
- Seizures
- Drowsiness
- Coma.

Pain can be precipitated or exacerbated by hypercalcaemia. Low threshold for suspicion is key in detecting hypercalcaemia of malignancy.

Examination

- Can be normal
- Reduced skin turgor and dried mucus membranes
- Delirium
- Fatigue
- Signs associated with underlying malignancy.

Practice points

- It is important to explain to families about the signs and symptoms of hypercalcaemia.
- Sometimes, when patients are in the last hours and days of life, there may be little to be gained in treating the underlying hypercalcaemia.
- In patients who have had rapid deterioration in their functional capability, and it is the first episode of hypercalcaemia, then treatment can often result in significant benefit and therefore is strongly advised.

- In patients with recurrent hypercalaemia it is important to take into account the benefit of previous treatment in deciding on re-treating.
- Refractory or rapidly recurring hypercalcaemia can reflect advanced disease and poor prognosis.

Management

Initial management

- Stop calcium supplements
- To reduce risk of renal toxicity from bisphosphonate treatment, consider withholding medication that affects the renal function (for example non-steroidal anti-inflammatory drugs, diuretics, thiazide diuretics, angiotensin-converting-enzyme inhibitors).

Fluid

Intravenous fluids are the first component of therapy. This increases calciuresis and reverses the dehydration caused by the hypercalcaemia. Isotonic saline is the commonest choice of fluid and should be given at a rate of 200–250 ml per hour of fluid and the patient should receive 4–6 litres and at least 2 litres before bisphosphonate therapy.

Bisphosphonates

There is no evidence base for what level of calcium should necessitate what treatment. (please refer to local guidelines). However, there should be a low threshold for treating patients who feel non-specifically unwell. Because of the common mechanisms of hypercalcaemia of malignancy, if patients are not treated with bisphosphonates it is likely to recur, especially if there is no treatment of the underlying cancer. Bisphosphonates can cause flu-like symptoms and rarely cause symptomatic hypocalcaemia. Occasionally bisphosphonates can cause osteonecrosis of the jaw. This has a stronger association with poor dentition and often in the situation of hypercalcaemia the burden of the condition outweighs the risk of the treatment.

The main differences between the biphosphonates zoledronic acid and disodium pamidronate are outlined in Table 8.1.

Table 8.1 The main differences between zoledronic acid and disodium pamidronate.

	Zoledronic acid	Disodium pamidronate
Intravenous (IV) dose	4 mg	30 to 90 mg
Onset of effect	<4 days	<3 days
Maximum effect	4 to 7 days	5 to 7 days
Duration of effect	4 weeks	2.5 weeks

Source: Scottish Palliative Care Guidelines, 2019a.
Note: Local protocols should be followed to determine the dose.

Malignant Spinal Cord Compression (MSCC)

Practice points

- Early recognition and treatment improves outcomes
- Aim to diagnose MSCC when patients are still walking
- MRI whole spine is the investigation of choice
- High dose steroids should be started at the point of clinical suspicion of MSCC.

Scenario

Background

Pavel is a 70-year-old man with prostate cancer. He has developed bone metastases in the last year. He lives independently at home. He is widowed, his daughter and family live one hour away and he often takes the bus to visit them.

Key points

- Many patients presenting with spinal cord compression don't present with new back pain but a worsening of a chronic back pain.
- Classically, cancers which are associated with bone metastasis, and therefore spinal cord compression, are breast, lung, renal and prostate. However, bone metastasis can occur in any cancer and clinicians should have a low threshold of suspicion.
- Please see outcomes to illustrate how important it is to treat this as a time critical emergency.

Timeline

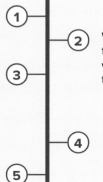

Pavel had been experiencing some mid back pain, worsening over the last month. **(1)**

(2) When he was on the bus this week he felt a band of pain round his middle when going over bumps and struggled to get off the bus in time at his stop.

He came to the surgery for his depot GnRH receptor/hormone antagonist. He mentions the pain to the practice nurse and tells her that his legs feel a bit funny and that his back pain has gotten a bit worse, but he is still walking unaided. **(3)**

(4) The practice nurse asks the GP for advice on what to do.

The GP is running late and has several patients waiting to be seen. **(5)**

Key considerations

- What else does the GP need to know in making decisions on what to do?
- What may they find if Pavel was examined?
- What are the management options?

Scenario 1	Scenario 2

You arrange to see Pavel before he leaves the practice.
 	
    What questions would you ask him?
 	
    What would you do next?
	You are unable to see Pavel before he leaves the practice. You ask the practice nurse to give him general advice about analgesia and to contact the practice if he gets worse.
	
	The next week there is a call from Pavel's neighbour, his back pain is much worse and he is unable to get out of bed this morning. You arrange an urgent house visit: Pavel has reduced power in his legs and on examination has a palpable bladder.
	
	You arrange urgent hospital admission.

Outcome 1	**Outcome 2**
You are concerned that Pavel may have spinal cord compression. You inform him of this and an urgent spine MRI is arranged via the local cord compression pathway. This shows thoracic cord compression. He receives high dose steroids followed by inpatient radiotherapy. He has MDT input and after a spell of rehabilitation he returns home.	Pavel is admitted to hospital and an MRI spine shows thoracic cord compression. He receives high dose steroids and radiotherapy. The power in his lower limbs does not improve, he has a urinary catheter and needs to be hoisted to sit in an adapted chair. He is transferred to a care home and his daughter visits him at weekends.

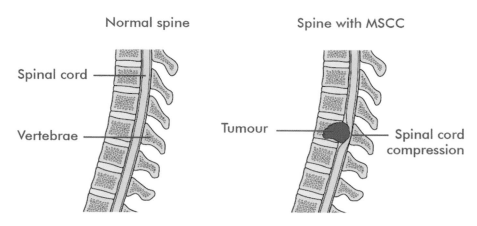

Figure 8.1 Malignant spinal cord compression (MSCC).

Source: This image was produced by Macmillan Cancer Support and is reused with permission.

What is malignant spinal cord compression?

Malignant spinal cord compression (MSCC) occurs when the dural sac and its contents are compressed at the level of the cord or cauda equina (Figure 8.1).

This can be caused by:

- Bone metastases to the spine causing vertebral collapse and compression (85% of cases of MSCC) (Loblaw et al., 2003)
- Direct extension of malignancy, for example peripheral posterior lung cancer
- Intradural masses causing MSCC are much less common.

It affects about 5 to 10% of patients with cancer (Nair, 2014). The most common cancer types affected are:

- Prostate
- Breast
- Lung
- Myeloma.

However, MSCC should be considered in any cancer, particularly with known bone metastases (note that MSCC can be the first presentation of cancer – this is the case in 20% of cases of MSCC).

After diagnosis of MSCC, mobility and bladder function at one month are determined by mobility and bladder function at diagnosis. Of those patients who could not walk at the time of diagnosis of MSCC only 7% regained full mobility (Prasad et al., 2005). Late diagnosis is common, causing permanent loss of function and significant morbidity. Rapid assessment, investigation and treatment may prevent or limit irreversible neurological damage. This means that education of patients, carers, and health and social care professionals is key to achieving early recognition. If you have a patient at risk of cord compression, warn them about early symptoms of MSCC.

The thoracic spine is the most common site for cord compression, seen in 60–80% of cases, however the site of pain does not always correlate with the level of compression. Less than 10% of patients present with MSCC in the cervical spine and 15–20% in the lumbosacral region. In addition 30–50% of patients have involvement at multiple levels (Al-Qurainy et al., 2016).

Presentation

Assessment – history and neurological examination

Back pain is the most common symptom, with limb weakness the second most common symptom.

- Pain:
  - Back pain is most common first symptom
  - Escalating pain
  - Pain may be localised to spine (15%) or radicular/nerve root (37%) or both (47%)
  - Patient may describe burning, shooting or band like pains
  - Pain can be worse on bending, straining, coughing and bilateral, radicular pain may present as abdominal pain
  - It can be difficult to distinguish between the pain from bone metastases alone and the pain from MSCC. Patients should be closely monitored with a low threshold for discussion of MRI spine.
- Loss of power:
  - Leg weakness affects 65–85% of patients at the time of diagnosis of MSCC
  - Patients may report new difficulty in walking or standing up
  - Neurological examination may be normal in evolving cord compression.
- Sensory impairment:
  - Less common. There may be radicular sensory loss and loss of tendon reflex (see Figure 8.2).
- Bladder or bowel dysfunction:
  - This is a late sign with a poor prognosis.
- Cauda equina syndrome (cauda equina from Latin for horse's tail):
  - This occurs if the lesion is below the level of the cord
  - This means a different presentation with reduced bladder and bowel sensation with most patients having urinary retention
  - There is reduced sensation in the saddle distribution and loss of anal tone on examination
  - Pain and motor weakness are less common.

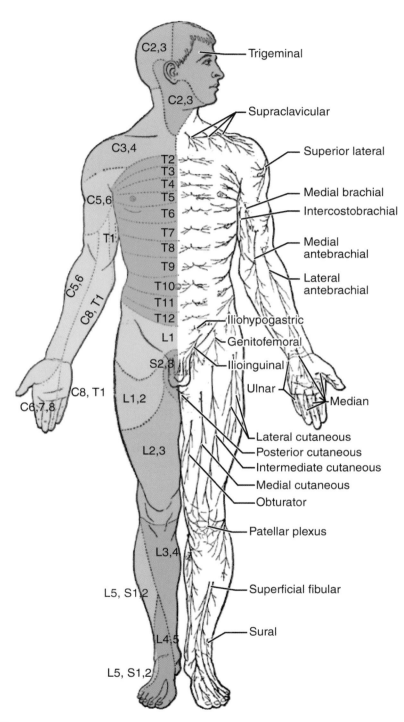

Figure 8.2 Dermatomes.

Investigation

The investigation of choice is an MRI of the whole spine within 24 hrs. There may be some circumstances where it is not appropriate to investigate or treat. This may be in patients with existing poor performance status with well-established paralysis and whose prognosis from their underlying cancer is very poor (days to weeks). Steroids may be used empirically, and pain and symptom control optimised.

Management

- Steroids – start promptly dexamethasone 8 mg twice daily
- Analgesia
- Consider stability and alignment – consider if severe pain on moving and immobilise until assessed if this is the case
- If this is first presentation of cancer then consider the feasibility of getting a tissue diagnosis and take advice from oncology promptly.

Definitive treatment

- Radiotherapy – generally first line treatment and usually delivered over 5 days:
  - Aims of treatment are (in order of likelihood of aim being achieved):
    - Pain relief
    - Prevention of neurological deterioration
    - Improvement in neurological function.
- Neurosurgical intervention:
  - Aims are to decompress spinal cord and stabilise spinal column
  - Patients with spinal instability, very good prognosis or tumours that respond poorly to radiotherapy may have better neurological outcomes with surgical intervention.
- Chemotherapy:
  - Usually has a limited role in MSCC unless the underlying malignancy is very chemosensitive, for example lymphoma.
- Support and rehabilitation:
  - MDT input for rehabilitation and to support patient and carers is vital
  - Focus should be the patient's wishes and goals
  - Discharge planning may be complex for patients with poor recovery of function.
- Taper steroids after treatment with aim of ceasing or to lowest maintenance dose.
- In patients whose bowel and bladder function have been affected it is important to consider how this will be managed early. In some cases a regime of catheterisation or drug-induced constipation with intermittent laxatives is required. If there are bladder and bowel issues please take advice from the palliative care or neurological rehabilitation unit early.

Bleeding

Introduction

Haemorrhage (frank or occult bleeding) occurs in 10 to 20% of patients with advanced cancer (Pereira et al., 2004). Acute massive haemorrhage, especially when it is visible, will cause distress to patient, family and staff. Bleeding can either occur because of damage or erosion of blood vessels or because of issues relating to clotting, such as bone-marrow infiltration from cancer.

Assessment

It is very important to know what the likelihood of controlling, stabilising or reversing the underlying disease is. Depending on the management plan for the underlying disease, or if the patient's overall function and quality of life is remarkably good, then management will involve full resuscitative measures and actions to identify and stop the bleeding.

The speed of bleeding is also important:

- For patients who are having a catastrophic haemorrhage then comfort and support is of the utmost importance.
- For patients who are suffering with slow oozing then there is more time to consider what the best course of action is.

Medication review

- Stop all anticoagulants and non-steroidal anti-inflammatory medication. However, other medications also have an anti-platelet effect such as antidepressants, so a thorough medication review is required. **Caution: If the patient has a stent or a metallic heart valve please discuss urgently with the appropriate specialist management of the patient's anticoagulant or anti-platelet therapy.**
- Steroids can cause gastritis and if bleeding is from the upper GI tract then they should be stopped; in other instances such as bone marrow failure, they may be helpful.

Management of acute severe bleeding

- Try to remain calm. Call for help. Talk to the patient and comfort them.
- If you're able to, apply direct pressure to the bleeding area; dark coloured towels are best.
- If the patient has a massive haemorrhage and is clearly dying, then trying to be calm and present are more important interventions than leaving the person to obtain sedative medication; the patient will usually lose consciousness rapidly and may be more frightened if left alone.

> ### Practice points
>
> If bleeding can be anticipated:
>
> - If significant bleeding can be anticipated, it is usually best to discuss the possibility with the patient and their family
> - Ensure carers at home have an emergency contact number
> - An anticipatory care plan is helpful. This includes having sedative medication prescribed for use if needed
> - Discuss resuscitation; document and communicate resuscitation status
> - Ensure a supply of dark sheets or towels along with other equipment: gloves, aprons, plastic sheets, and clinical waste bags
> - Fear of a major bleed may prevent ongoing care at home.

Sedative medication for use in massive terminal haemorrhage

If the patient is distressed, a rapidly acting benzodiazepine is indicated. The route of administration guides the choice of drug (Table 8.2).

After the event

It is important to recognise that this can be very traumatic for families and staff. Often people who have witnessed a massive haemorrhage need time to debrief and it would be important to signpost relatives to bereavement counselling.

Table 8.2   Route of administration of sedative medication.

	Intravenous	Intramuscular	Sublingual	Rectal/stoma
Midazolam	10 mg	10 mg	10 mg	
Diazepam	10 mg			10 mg

Source: Scottish Palliative Care Guidelines, 2019b.

Management of smaller level of bleeding

Smaller levels of bleeding are often distressing to the patient and family. The patient's condition can improve and worsen dramatically depending on whether the bleeding is active, whether their haemoglobin is stable or the bleeding can be controlled.

Blood products

Blood products can bring a lot of benefits, however in most patients their symptoms do become refractory to blood. By defining the severity of the patients prior to, and then after, a blood transfusion, we can begin to understand if any benefit is being achieved with blood transfusions. It is good practice to counsel the patient, in the beginning, that they will not continue to get blood once there is no clinical benefit.

Investigations

In patients who have a good performance status and who are fit enough for either surgical or radiological guided interventions, it may be appropriate to carry out endoscopies, bronchoscopies or CT angiograms. CT angiograms are particularly useful in those who have brisk bleeds as they can often pin-point the problem area.

Intervention

In some cases surgical or interventional radiology (IR) approaches may be appropriate. It is important to discuss cases with IR so information can be relayed to the patients about the risks and benefits and to help guide decision making.

Medication

Bleeding from skin (including fungating tumours) and mucous membranes (Scottish Palliative Care Guidelines, 2019b):

- Apply direct pressure if possible. This can be with gauze soaked in tranexamic acid (500 mg in 5 ml) or adrenaline (epinephrine) 1 in 1000.
- The tranexamic acid soaks can be left in situ with a dressing on top. Alternatively, a tranexamic acid paste (4 x 500 mg tablets crushed in 60 g base such as hydrophilic soft paraffin) can be applied twice daily under dressings.
- In the case of oral cavity bleeding, 10 ml four times daily of a 5% aqueous solution of tranexamic acid may be used as a mouth wash. (A 5% solution can be made by crushing and dispersing a 500 mg tranexamic tablet in 10 ml water or diluting the contents of one 500 mg/5 ml ampoule to a final volume of 10 ml. (If using the ampoules, the ampoule contents must be filtered before use to minimise risk of glass particles)).
- Silver nitrate sticks can be used to cauterise small bleeding points and surgical haemostatic sponges can be used at home by patients or families to control fast capillary bleeding.
- Nasal tampons or nasal packs can be used for epistaxis as available locally. Local A&E or ENT departments are able to advise.
- If bleeding not thought due to disseminated intravascular coagulation (DIC), consider systemic antifibrinolytics such as tranexamic acid:
  - Initial dose of 1.5 g orally followed thereafter by 1 g three times daily
  - If not settling after 3 days, increase to 1.5 g three times daily
  - Reduce or discontinue 1 week after bleeding stops; restart if recurs.
- If severe surface bleeding and above measures fail to control, take advice from the palliative care team.

Bleeding from respiratory tract

As with all episodes of haemorrhage the underlying cause and the rate of bleeding often determines the management of the patient. Massive bleeding from the respiratory tract is often fatal.

Management

In minor haemoptysis identify the underlying condition through normal investigation, and manage and treat accordingly.

In moderate haemoptysis try and maintain the patient's airway to reduce the sensation of choking. If the bleeding site is known, lay the patient on the bleeding side to reduce effect on the other lung.

- Use oxygen and suction as required
- If cough is an issue, then small dose opioids can be used
- Tranexamic acid can be used
- Radiotherapy can give full control of bleeding in 85% of patients with bleeding from lung cancer.

Bleeding from urinary tract

- Exclude or treat infection
- Consider tranexamic acid, although there is a risk of clot retention until the complete cessation of bleeding
- Bladder irrigation ± instillations with 0.9% sodium chloride or tranexamic acid (5 g in 50 ml water) can be tried once or twice daily if oral treatment is unsuccessful, or there are issues with absorption or the patient has no oral route.

Bleeding due to advanced haematological malignancy

- Platelet infusion may provide transient benefit in thrombocytopenia.
- A trial of steroids can be given but should be assessed: if the bone marrow has not stabilised or improved within a week it is unlikely to do so. If no other anti-cancer therapy is given then the thrombocytopenia is likely to reoccur.
- Sensitive discussions will be required regarding blood product support in bone marrow failure as often there will come a time where there is no benefit to be derived.

Terminal sedation

Irrespective of the cause of bleeding, sometimes there can be a large bleed from which the patient will not recover, but does not die immediately. Benzodiazepines can be helpful at this point, as patients are often active and describe a sensation of 'impending doom'. Midazolam is useful in this scenario as it causes amnesia.

Seizures

Introduction

Seizures are common with about 1 in 25 people having a seizure in their lifetime (Epilepsy Society, 2018). In patients with advanced disease the cause can be multifactorial:

- Primary brain tumours
- Brain metastasis
- Biochemical abnormalities (for example uraemia, hyponatraemia, hypoglycaemia)
- Drugs.

Seventy percent of patients with brain tumours have seizures during the course of their illness (Grewal et al., 2008).

Seizures can be very frightening for patients and their families. Often it precipitates time in acute hospital or heralds the progression of underlying disease. Care needs to be taken to acknowledge that seizures are distressing to experience and witness, to explain the reason for seizures, and to discuss management and the need for compliance with medication. It is good practice to discuss a plan with the caregiver should a seizure occur again.

Assessment

- Eliminate other causes of loss of consciousness or abnormal limb or facial movement (for example vasovagal episode, postural hypotension, arrhythmia, hypoglycaemia, extrapyramidal side effects from dopamine antagonists).
- Find out if there have been any previous seizures and establish what made the person vulnerable to a seizure — past medical history of epilepsy, previous secondary seizure, known cerebral disease, dementia. Investigate further if needed.
- Look for possible issues with pre-existing anti-epileptic drug therapy either from non-compliance or from drug interactions, both of which are quite common.
- If the patient has an underlying biochemical abnormality then it is important that this is corrected.
- If there is a space-occupying lesion then it is likely there will be further seizures if treatment is not initiated.

Management

Management of seizures (prognosis of years, months or weeks)

- Refer to local protocols and/or discuss with local neurology expert
- The adverse effects and interactions profiles of these medications should be key in deciding management of individuals
- Steroids can be useful in patients who have a space-occupying lesion, especially when there is known oedema; this can be helpful in the short term to let seizure medications get up to therapeutic level.

Management of seizures (last days of life *or* when oral route is unavailable *or* issues with gut absorption)

- For patients who are on anti-epileptic drugs, missing doses can precipitate seizures so it is important to maintain this in the last days of life or if there is severe nausea and vomiting or issues with absorption.
- Most anti-epileptics have a long half-life so although it is important to consider ongoing management, this can be done within 12 hours or so of the first missed dose.

Medication that can be given subcutaneously

- If the patient is already on levetiracetam this can be converted to a continuous subcutaneous infusion (CSCI) with a conversion from oral to subcutaneous of 1:1.
- Midazolam 20–30 mg via CSCI can be given over 24 hours as maintenance therapy if patients are taking other anti-epeleptics.

For seizures that are not self-terminating

- Midazolam 5 mg subcutaneously can be given or, if the patient is at home or in a care home, then buccal midazolam can be used.
- Buccolam 10 mg comes in a pre-filled syringe. Half the syringe should be put in the seizing person's mouth between their teeth and their gum on one side before putting the rest on the other side.

Superior Vena Cava Obstruction

Introduction

The superior vena cava (SVC) returns blood to the heart; when it is compressed by external compression, thrombosis or direct invasion superior vena cava obstruction occurs. Presentation is usually dependent on the rapidity of obstruction. If there is rapid obstruction there is no time for the collateral venous circulation to respond and the symptoms are sudden. Where compression happens slowly then often the collateral system can compensate so large obstructions can appear quite symptomless. Non-small cell lung cancer (NSCLC) accounts for about 50% of presentation, with small cell lung cancer (SCLC) accounting for a further 22%. Malignancy is the cause of 95% of superior vena cava obstruction (SVCO).

Assessment

Symptoms are caused by reduced blood flow from the head, neck and upper limbs. Sluggish flow through the vena cava can also cause clot formation.

Signs:

- Cyanosis – due to venous stasis rather arterial hypoxia
- Oedema of the arms, chest and face – usually starts periorbitally

- Papilloedema – late sign
- Dilated neck veins and dilated collateral veins on arms and anterior chest wall.

Symptoms

- Breathlessness
- Visual changes
- Dizziness
- Headache – worse on stooping
- Swelling of face, neck and arms
- Stridor.

Management

- Treatment is dependent on the cause of the obstruction; if this is a presenting complaint then histology is key to management.
- Consider the severity of the symptoms and the patient's prognosis to guide the urgency of management.
- The diagnosis of SVCO is often made on clinical grounds in patients with a history but a chest X-ray and CT scan may confirm the diagnosis and inform treatment.

Basic Measures

- Ensure restricting clothing is loosened and upper arms are supported on pillows
- Ensure head is raised to aid venous return
- A fan can make the patient more comfortable
- Benzodiazepines, opioids, oxygen and supportive care are helpful to most patients while waiting on a definitive management plan
- Discuss with or refer urgently to oncology, especially if the tumour is likely to be sensitive to anti-cancer therapies.

Referral for endovascular stenting

- Endovascular stenting provides rapid relief of symptoms in most patients (complications occur in about 6% of patients and failure is rare (Crowe et al., 1995)).

There is an absence of evidence to support steroid use (Rowell et al., 2002).

In patients who do not have anti-cancer therapies or the option of a stent then a therapeutic trial may be considered, and a trial of 16 mg of dexamethasone once a day may be considered *if* the syndrome is adding to the person's symptom burden.

In patients who do not have a histological diagnosis it is important to discuss this with clinicians involved in the diagnostic pathway, as some cancers will be highly responsive to steroids which would interfere with histological diagnosis.

Bowel Obstruction

Introduction

Bowel obstruction can be due to mechanical obstruction by, for example, a tumour in the bowel lumen. It can also be due to peristaltic failure which can occur for multiple reasons. It can be really difficult to manage the symptoms of bowel obstruction, especially when there is no definitive treatment option such as surgery or anti-cancer treatments.

Malignant bowel obstruction is common in patients with abdominal or pelvic cancers. Malignant bowel obstruction presents most frequently in advanced stage cancer patients although it can be a presenting feature. Bowel obstruction is often further classified depending on its anatomical site – gastric outlet, small bowel or large bowel (Cappell et al., 2008).

Assessment

Patients often present with large volume vomiting and abdominal pain. Nausea is often described as being present just before and being relieved by vomiting.

It is helpful to get a description of the content of the vomit as it gives some guidance on where the anatomical site of the obstruction is occurring, for example gastric outlet obstruction is often associated with undigested food while obstruction in the large bowel may result in infrequent but large volume feculent vomits.

It is important to exclude faecal impaction from history with all patients presenting with bowel obstruction requiring a PR examination.

An abdominal X-ray will in most cases give a definitive diagnosis of obstruction. Depending on patients fitness and preference a CT should considered. Patients with a localised obstruction even with advanced disease can benefit from surgery such as a palliative bypass procedure.

Symptoms

Presentation often depends on the level of obstruction, whether there is luminal obstruction or peristaltic failure and the length of time the obstruction has been present:

- Total constipation – the patient does not pass wind or faeces. In severe constipation which can often mimic obstruction there is often faeces in the rectum or 'over flow' flood. This is not present in obstruction.

- Nausea – initially in bowel obstruction the nausea is intense before vomiting and then fades after vomiting. If the bowel obstruction persists then the nausea can become persistent or worsen. This is thought to be due to colonisation of the small bowel by colonic bacteria.

- Vomiting – the frequency and content of the vomits depends on the level of obstruction. With gastric outlet obstruction vomits are small and frequent and contain undigested food. As there is also a lot of acid there is often heartburn-type symptoms. Small bowel obstruction results in less frequent vomiting as there is a bigger intestinal reservoir and more digested food is vomited, and large bowel obstruction results in infrequent vomiting but large volume and often feculent. If small bowel obstruction persists, then colonic bacteria spread means that the contents can often smell very feculent.

- Pain – direct pain from the tumour but the patient can also have colic-type pain (waves of pain that wax and wane, often associated with altered bowel sounds).

Examination

Typically, examination would show signs associated with dehydration. Abdominal palpation will reveal a distended, tympanic abdomen. Auscultation in patients with early obstruction reveals high-pitched bowel sounds. However, in proximal obstruction the abdomen can be less distended. In late obstruction the bowel has often become hypotonic and in many cases there are no bowel sounds.

Other findings could suggest the cause of the obstruction such as abdominal mass or ascites.

Management

Consider transfer to hospital if there may be a surgical option or further assessment is required.

Acute phase (first few days)

- Hydration is important in this first phase (Scottish Palliative Care Guidelines, 2019c).
- Conservative management and watchful waiting may be appropriate and enough to start the bowel moving – the bowel may be rested, nil by mouth +/- nasogastric (NG) tube.
- Mouth care is essential to protect dentition from stomach acid.
- During this time, after assessment with imaging consideration can be given to stenting, venting gastrostomy and surgery.
- Laxatives +/- rectal treatment should be considered if constipation might be contributing.

Post acute phase

If the bowel obstruction persists, and there is no surgery or procedural options, then consideration needs to be given to medical management:

- Fluids – hydration needs to be looked at on a case-by-case basis. Re-hydration often helps with nausea but can increase the amount of luminal fluid in the bowel leading to increased vomiting and reflux.

- Consider stopping medication reducing peristalsis (cyclizine, hyoscine, 5HT$_3$ antagonists, amitriptyline).
- Use a prokinetic anti-emetic, such as metoclopramide 30 mg, in a syringe pump. Instruction should be left to stop this if colic develops. Doses of up to 120 mg in 24 hours can be used if there is no colic.
- If there is colic consider using an alternative anti-emetic such as levomepromazine.
- Laxatives are often needed.
- Analgesia should be given through a syringe pump in the post acute phase. If the pain is stable then a fentanyl patch has less effect on peristalsis.
- Steroids (dexamethasone 4–8 mg) subcutaneously can help to reduce the oedema effect of tumours so can be effective when there is partial mechanical obstruction and when there is peristaltic failure (Feuer et al., 2000).
- For high volume vomiting consider an antisecretory such as hyoscine butylbromide (40–120 mg) or octreotide (200–500 mg). These can be titrated but at best will halve the volume of vomiting, so for patients who have very high-volume vomits consider an NG tube.

Scenario Recap

Jean is seen in the respiratory clinic the following week. She has a large tumour but has no distant metastasis. The option of radical radiotherapy is discussed with her. Three months later she comes to clinic for some analgesia. She is tired after the radiotherapy and looks thin but otherwise she feels well and the hypercalcaemia has not re-occurred.

References

Al-Qurainy R and Collis E (2016) Metastatic spinal cord compression: diagnosis and management. *British Medical Journal*, 353: i2539.

Cappell MS and Batke M (2008) Mechanical obstruction of the small bowel and colon. *Medical Clinics of North America*, 92(3): 575–597.

Crowe MTI, Davies CH and Gaines PA (1995) Percutaneous management of superior vena cava occlusions. *Cardiovascular and Interventional Radiology*, 18(6): 367–372.

Epilepsy Society (2018) Epilepsy facts and myths. Available at: https://www.epilepsysociety.org.uk/facts-and-statistics

Feuer DJ and Broadley KE (2000) Corticosteroids for the resolution of malignant bowel obstruction in advanced gynaecological and gastrointestinal cancer. *Cochrane Database Systematic Review*, 2000(2): CD001219.

Grewal J, Grewal HK and Forman AD (2008) Seizures and epilepsy in cancer: etiologies, evaluation, and management. *Current Oncology Reports,* 10(1): 63–71.

Jick S et al. (2015) Prevalence of hypercalcemia of malignancy among cancer patients in the UK: analysis of the Clinical Practice Research Datalink database. *Cancer Epidemiology*, 39(6): 901–907.

Lindner G et al. (2013) Hypercalcemia in the ED: prevalence, etiology, and outcome. *American Journal of Emergency Medicine*, 31(4): 657–660.

Loblaw DA, Laperriere NJ and Mackillop WJ (2003) A population based study of malignant spinal cord compression in Ontario. *Clinical Oncology*, 15(4): 472–480.

Nair C, Ranikkar S and Ray A (2014). How not to miss metastatic spinal cord compression. *British Journal of General Practice*, 64(626), e596-e598.

Pereira J and Phan T (2004) Management of bleeding in patients with advanced cancer. *The Oncologist*, 9(5): 561–570.

Prasad D and Schiff D (2005) Malignant spinal-cord compression. *Lancet Oncology,* 6(1): 15–24.

Rowell NP and Gleeson FV (2002) Steroids, radiotherapy, chemotherapy and stents for superior vena caval obstruction in carcinoma of the bronchus: a systematic review. *Clinical Oncology (Royal College of Radiologists (Great Britain))* 14(5): 338–51.

Scottish Palliative Care Guidelines (2019a) Hypercalcaemia. Available at: https://www.palliativecareguidelines.scot.nhs.uk/guidelines/palliative-emergencies/Hypercalcaemia.aspx

Scottish Palliative Care Guidelines (2019b) Bleeding. Available at: https://www.palliativecareguidelines.scot.nhs.uk/guidelines/palliative-emergencies/Bleeding.aspx

Scottish Palliative Care Guidelines (2019c) Bowel Obstruction. Available at: https://www.palliativecareguidelines.scot.nhs.uk/guidelines/symptom-control/bowel-obstruction.aspx

Stewart AF (2005) Clinical practice: hypercalcemia associated with cancer. *New England Journal of Medicine*, 352(4): 373–379.

Chapter 9

Rehabilitation

Charlie C Hall

> ### Learning Objectives
>
> This chapter will help you to understand:
>
> - The principles of rehabilitation and how this applies to palliative care
> - The different approaches to rehabilitation in patients with palliative care needs
> - The challenges and optimal approach to implementing rehabilitative palliative care.

Principles of Rehabilitation

The future of palliative care faces some significant challenges. People are living longer, with a greater number of co-morbidities. An ever-wider range of treatment options are becoming available for life-limiting diseases; indeed cancer is now in many cases morphing into a chronic condition (Salakari et al., 2015). While clearly a positive step, this has significant socioeconomic implications and represents a huge challenge for the delivery of palliative care.

There is frequently a misconception that palliative care involves focusing on death and dying. On the contrary, it is about helping patients to make the most of life, even when time is limited. Ask a person with life-limiting illness their priorities, and they often answer: aiming to maintain 'normality', preserving dignity and 'taking charge' of their condition (Carter et al., 2004). In her vision for modern palliative care, Dame Cicely Saunders said that we should

> *'enable the dying person to live until [they] die, at [their] own maximal potential performing to the limit of [their] physical and mental capacity with control and independence whenever possible.'*

(Saunders, 2006)

This fundamental tenet of palliative care shares many similarities with rehabilitation (Figure 9.1). Indeed, rehabilitation is now an 'essential component' of palliative care (Tiberini, 2015).

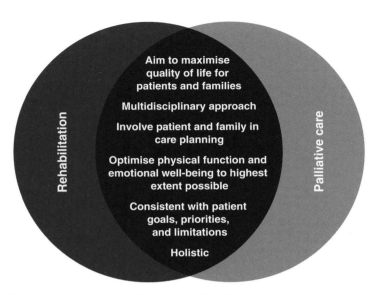

Figure 9.1   Interface between rehabilitation and palliative care.

Source: © Hospice UK, 2015. Charity registered in England and Wales No. 1014851, and in Scotland No. SC041112. Address: Hospice UK, Hospice House, 34–44 Britannia Street, London WC1X 9JG. Reused with permission.

What is meant by rehabilitation in the context of life-limiting disease?

To some, rehabilitation in the context of advanced, irreversible disease may sound paradoxical (Leslie et al., 2014). A common misperception is that rehabilitation relates only to recovery to a previous level of function. In fact, rehabilitation comes in many different forms, with varied goals according to the clinical context (Table 9.1).

Table 9.1   Goals of rehabilitation.

Rehabilitation goal	Context	Aim
Restorative	Patient has good potential to regain full function	To return patients to a previous level of function
Preventative	Patients at risk of deconditioning and weakness due to reduced activity	To prevent avoidable deterioration in patient's function due to disease or treatment
Supportive	Maximising function in the context of established impairment/disability	To maximise patient's functional independence and involvement in activities
Palliative	Adaptation and habituation with irreversible loss of function and new functional reality	Supporting patients to adapt to irreversible changes or loss of function

Source: Adapted from Tiberini, 2015, and Dietz, 1981.

The benefits of early palliative care are increasingly being recognised in terms of improving quality of life, symptom control and even survival (Smith et al., 2012; Temel et al., 2010). Rehabilitation goals in modern palliative care may therefore include any of those categories listed above.

Evidence of Benefit

Rehabilitation is a fundamental component of the management of chronic illnesses, including cardiac, neurological and respiratory disease. Such is the strength of evidence for pulmonary rehabilitation, a Cochrane review has stated it is now inappropriate to conduct further randomised controlled trials comparing it with standard care (Lacasse et al., 2015).

Rehabilitation for patients with cancer is a rapidly evolving area. It includes 'prehabilitation', optimising a patient's function between diagnosis and treatment (Silver, 2015) and 'habilitation', a term sometimes preferred to dispel expectations of a complete return to function. Rehabilitation has a wide range of benefits in multiple settings: it can improve activities of daily living (ADLs) in care home residents (Crocker et al., 2013), it has the potential to reduce hospital stays (Kelley et al., 2012) and can prevent hospital re-admissions (Maddocks et al., 2015). The benefit of rehabilitation interventions is that they are low cost and widely adaptable to different settings.

Interventions

Exercise

Exercise is one of the cornerstones of rehabilitation in non-malignant disease including pulmonary and cardiac rehabilitation (McCarthy et al., 2015; Jolliffe et al., 2001). Yet, in spite of growing evidence, rehabilitation has been slow to be incorporated into routine oncological care. Exercise in patients undergoing chemotherapy can improve fatigue, exercise capacity, muscle strength and physical activity levels (Adamsen et al., 2009). Exercise interventions are feasible in patients with incurable cancer and have multiple beneficial effects on physical well-being, functional mobility, fatigue, depression and overall quality of life (Litterini et al., 2013; Salakari et al., 2015; Oldervoll et al., 2011). There is a growing awareness of the benefits of exercise for cancer survivors, such that aerobic and resistance training is now recommended within international consensus guidelines (Schmitz et al., 2010; Arends et al., 2017).

Multi-modal interventions

Although exercise interventions have a strong evidence base, attention to nutrition is also vital. Cachexia is associated with chronic diseases including chronic obstructive pulmonary disease, congestive cardiac failure and cancer, where loss of muscle occurs most rapidly (Giordano et al., 2003). Cachexia is the 'multifactorial syndrome, defined by ongoing loss of skeletal muscle mass (with or without loss of fat mass) that can be partially but not fully reversed by conventional nutritional support, causing progressive functional impairment' (Fearon et al., 2011). As yet, there is no established treatment for cachexia. However, due to its multi-modal pathophysiology (including systemic inflammation, alterations in body metabolism and reduced caloric intake), multi-modal interventions have been proposed (Fearon, 2008). Interventions combining exercise and nutritional components have multiple benefits in patients with incurable cancer, the strongest evidence pertaining to improvements in mood and physical function (Hall et al., 2019). Trials are currently under way to evaluate the benefits of multi-modal interventions combining exercise, nutritional supplementation and anti-inflammatories for cancer cachexia (Solheim et al., 2018). Similar multi-modal interventions may in future be applicable to a general cancer rehabilitation model (Hall et al., 2018).

Delivering Rehabilitative Palliative Care

Although widely advocated, there are variations in the provision of rehabilitative palliative care in hospices throughout the UK (Wosahlo et al., 2015). Barriers to its provision include a lack of staff understanding of the definition and scope of rehabilitative palliative care (Runacres et al., 2017). Staff may not be aware of their own role in enabling patients due to a 'culture of care' and a belief that rehabilitation is only the domain of physiotherapists and occupational therapists. Lack of time and staffing levels are also cited as barriers to its provision (Harding et al., 2019). There may be concerns over the appropriateness of rehabilitation for patients who lack capacity, however evidence shows that rehabilitation is both feasible and beneficial for this group of patients (Bossers et al., 2014; Schwenk et al., 2014). There is a consensus among palliative care professionals, however, that rehabilitation involves maximising a person's quality of life, promoting independence and that it facilitates a shift away from dying towards living (Harding et al., 2019).

Summary

Rehabilitation should be individually tailored and incorporate patient goals (Boa et al., 2014). It involves fostering a culture of enablement and is the responsibility of all members of the care team (Tiberini, 2015). Helping patients with life-limiting illness to live to their maximum potential brings with it the potential to improve quality of life for patients and families and furthermore has potential economic benefits. Implementation of rehabilitation in palliative care presents challenges, which may be overcome by embedding it across three levels: from specialist interventions, to team-wide implementation and, furthermore, incorporating rehabilitation into the overarching values of an organisation (Figure 9.2).

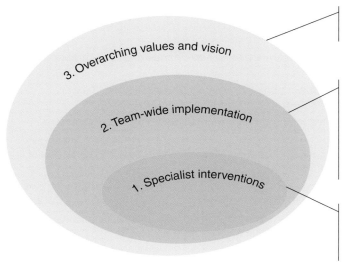

Values of rehabilitation – *e.g. autonomy, dignity, empowerment* – form the overarching vision at all levels of the organisation

Person-centre goal setting – working in partnership with an individual to identify their priorities and the steps to how these can be achieved

Supporting self-management – *e.g. giving people choice and control over the personal care they receive, supporting maximal participation in ADLs*

Input by physiotherapists, occupational therapists, dieticians etc. as required – *e.g. working with a physio to enable transfer from sit-to-stand, thus prevent a patient being bedbound*

Figure 9.2   Three levels of rehabilitation.

Source: Harding et al., 2019.

References

Adamsen et al. (2009) Effect of a multimodal high intensity exercise intervention in cancer patients undergoing chemotherapy: randomised controlled trial. *BMJ*, 339: b3410.

Arends J et al. (2017) ESPEN expert group recommendations for action against cancer-related malnutrition. *Clinical Nutrition*, 36(5): 1187–1196.

Boa S et al. (2014) Goal setting in palliative care: a structured review. *Progress in Palliative Care: Rehabilitation Guest Editors: Gail Eva and Cathy Payne*, 22(6): 326–333.

Bossers WJ et al. (2014) Feasibility of a combined aerobic and strength training program and its effects on cognitive and physical function in institutionalized dementia patients. A pilot study. *PLoS One*, 9: e97577.

Carter H et al. (2004) Living with a terminal illness: patients' priorities. *Journal of Advanced Nursing*, 45(6): 611–620.

Crocker T et al. (2013) The effect of physical rehabilitation on activities of daily living in older residents of long-term care facilities: systematic review with meta-analysis. *Age and Ageing*, 42(6): 682–688.

Dietz J (1981) *Rehabilitation Oncology*. Chichester: John Wiley and Sons.

Fearon KC (2008) Cancer cachexia: developing multimodal therapy for a multidimensional problem. *European Journal of Cancer*, 44(8): 1124–1132.

Fearon K et al. (2011) Definition and classification of cancer cachexia: an international consensus. *Lancet Oncology*, 12(50): 489–495.

Giordano A et al. (2003) Skeletal muscle metabolism in physiology and in cancer disease. *Journal of Cell Biochemistry*, 90(1): 170–186.

Hall CC et al. (2018) A randomised, phase II, unblinded trial of an Exercise and Nutrition-based Rehabilitation programme (ENeRgy) versus standard care in patients with cancer: feasibility trial protocol. *Pilot Feasibility Study*, 4: 192.

Hall CC et al. (2019) Combined exercise and nutritional rehabilitation in outpatients with incurable cancer: a systematic review. *Support Care Cancer*, 27(7): 2371–2384.

Harding Z, Hall C and Lloyd A (2019) Rehabilitation in palliative care: a qualitative study of team professionals. *BMJ Supportive and Palliative Care*, doi: 10.1136/bmjspcare-2019-002008.

Jolliffe JA et al. (2001) Exercise-based rehabilitation for coronary heart disease. *Cochrane Database Systematic Review*: CD001800.

Kelley AS et al. (2012) Disability and decline in physical function associated with hospital use at end of life. *Journal of General Internal Medicine*, 27(7): 794–800.

Lacasse Y et al. (2015) This Cochrane Review is closed: deciding what constitutes enough research and where next for pulmonary rehabilitation in COPD. *Cochrane Database Systematic Review*: ED000107.

Leslie P, Sandsund C and Roe J (2014) Researching the rehabilitation needs of patients with life-limiting disease: challenges and opportunities. *Progress in Palliative Care*, 22(6): 313–318.

Litterini AJ et al. (2013) Differential effects of cardiovascular and resistance exercise on functional mobility in individuals with advanced cancer: a randomized trial. *Archives of Physical Medicine and Rehabilitation*, 94(12): 2329–2335.

Maddocks M et al. (2015) Rehabilitation following hospitalization in patients with COPD: can it reduce readmissions? *Respirology*, 20(3): 395–404.

McCarthy B et al. (2015) Pulmonary rehabilitation for chronic obstructive pulmonary disease. *Cochrane Database Systematic Review*: CD003793.

Oldervoll LM et al. (2011) Physical exercise for cancer patients with advanced disease: a randomized controlled trial. *Oncologist*, 16(11): 1649–1657.

Runacres F, Gregory H and Ugalde A (2017) 'The horse has bolted I suspect': A qualitative study of clinicians' attitudes and perceptions regarding palliative rehabilitation. *Palliative Medicine*, 31(7): 642–650.

Salakari MR et al. (2015) Effects of rehabilitation among patients with advances cancer: a systematic review. *Acta Oncology*, 54(5): 618–628.

Saunders C (2006) *Cicely Saunders: Selected Writings 1958–2004*. Oxford: Oxford University Press.

Schmitz KH et al. (2010) American College of Sports Medicine roundtable on exercise guidelines for cancer survivors. *Medicine and Science in Sports Exercise*, 42(7): 1409–1426.

Schwenk M et al. (2014) Improvements in gait characteristics after intensive resistance and functional training in people with dementia: a randomised controlled trial. *BMC Geriatrics*, 14(73).

Silver JK (2015) Cancer prehabilitation and its role in improving health outcomes and reducing health care costs. *Seminars in Oncology Nursing*, 31(1): 13–30.

Smith TJ et al. (2012) American Society of Clinical Oncology provisional clinical opinion: the integration of palliative care into standard oncology care. *Journal of Clinical Oncology*, 30(8): 880–887.

Solheim TS et al. (2018) Cancer cachexia: rationale for the MENAC (Multimodal-Exercise, Nutrition and Anti-inflammatory medication for Cachexia) trial. *BMJ Supportive and Palliative Care*, 8(3): 258–265.

Temel JS et al. (2010) Early palliative care for patients with metastatic non-small-cell lung cancer. *New England Journal of Medicine*, 363(8): 733–742.

Tiberini RRH (2015) Rehabilitative palliative care enabling people to live fully until they die: a challenge for the 21st century. United Kingdom: Hospice UK, St Joseph's Hospice, St Christopher's, Burdett Trust for Nursing.

Wosahlo P and Maddocks M (2015) Benchmarking the provision of palliative rehabilitation within the hospice setting. *Palliatiative Medicine*, 29(5): 477–478.

Chapter 10

Complementary Resources

Trisha Hatt and Teri Perry

Learning Objectives

This chapter will help you:

- Understand how the third sector applies to palliative care
- Identify areas in which the third sector can help support patients and carers
- Understand the roles of volunteers within palliative and hospice care.

The Third and Independent Sectors

What is the third sector?

The third sector is diverse and can range from a very small group of people to large organisations such as registered charities and voluntary organisations. They are neither public nor private sector organisations, and are in the main (National Audit Office, 2010):

- Independent of government
- Value driven
- Not for profit.

What does the third sector bring to palliative care?

Third sector organisations (TSOs) have an important role in many areas of service provision including palliative and end-of-life care. The role of these organisations has been changing, and arguably is undergoing a further shift. There is a continuing imperative for closer integration between health and social care services (National Institute for Health Research, 2012). Yet, at the same time, the recent economic crisis and subsequent reductions in public expenditure are providing an environment of constrained financial resources. The impact of the COVID-19 pandemic has also added to the pressures on both the public and third sector.

How does the third sector apply to palliative care?

Public services can gain a lot from working with TSOs. Their involvement includes:

- Supporting the NHS and local authorities through various initiatives.
- Investment and assisting to maximise resources. This may include:
  - Funding numerous key roles (nurses/doctors/social care staff)
  - Providing grants for basic necessities (clothing/heating)
  - Delivering infrastructure: palliative care units/hospice/information and support hubs
  - Research.
- Delivering on stated strategy and outcomes. TSOs are often very influential and play a role in delivering on policy development.
- Developing and providing education and training.
- Acting as a bridge between statutory and not-for-profit organisations.
- Helping to understand the needs of the public – listening and understanding the experiences and views of people their spouses, partners, families and carers.
- Advocacy – providing an additional voice for people and carers.
- Providing carer education and support.
- Innovation – demonstrating 'proof of concept' and 'tests of change' initiatives in order to influence future direction and ways of working.
- Providing access for information and support. For example:
  - Drop-in centres
  - Volunteer structures
  - Assistance with access to financial benefits support
  - Telephone help/support lines
  - Bereavement support.
- Providing evidence and support for campaigns.

Some of the benefits and challenges of the TSOs are outlined in Table 10.1.

How does the third sector work with the NHS and social care?

The third sector is a key provider of palliative care, increasingly working in partnership with health and social care to plan and deliver services. Palliative and end-of-life care should be everyone's business. This includes the contribution of TSO providers who bring a wealth of knowledge and support to both the public and staff working in the health and care environment. Early involvement of palliative care can reduce the need for emergency admissions to hospital (Qureshi et al., 2019). TSOs contribute to systems that help people, family, carers and staff to care for and support a person with palliative or end-of-life needs.

In many areas charities provide funding for clinical and non-clinical posts and service infra-structure. This can be funding that is pump primed in order to set up new posts, test new ways

- o Roles and tasks associated with members of the palliative care team
- o Explanation of a holistic approach, definition of total pain and examples of total care.
- How to deal with the emotional care of patients and families:
  - o Grief and non-bereavement loss
  - o Life-shortening illness and examination of patient's anxieties
  - o Communication skills.
- Volunteer skills and self-care/improvement:
  - o Care of self
  - o Adopting a non-judgemental approach
  - o Equity and equality
  - o Prejudices and attitudes.

On suitable completion of the volunteer induction programme, volunteers commencing their role would be supported by a more experienced volunteer occupying the same role.

Volunteer roles

There are a variety of volunteer roles in the palliative care and hospice setting, each with its own responsibilities. The impact of some of the more typical volunteer roles are described below in Table 10.2.

Table 10.2   Volunteer activity and roles and their benefits and impacts.

Role	Outcomes	Impact
Drivers	Offer patients companionship and enable each patient to attend day hospice via the shortest possible route.	A firm trusting relationship is often formed with the driver and family members are able to gain respite.
Social support volunteers	Visit and offer patients companionship, for example they may have shared interests.	Patients may develop a role in bringing in material associated with personal interest, e.g. wildlife magazines or gardening information. This can have a knock-on effect with other patients as they also become interested and contribute.
Art and craft support and florists	Assist the art and craft worker in their role within the group, recognising the importance of group processes and patient empowerment. Florists may also facilitate workshops enabling patients to create floral displays.	Patients learn new skills, make items for their home and can feel a new sense of purpose and self-worth. This can also lead to a decrease in pain.

Table 10.2   (*Continued*).

Role	Outcomes	Impact
Receptionists	Meet and greet and offer support to family members and visitors.	Family members are reassured and enjoy the companionship this role brings.
General volunteer assistants	Make tea, coffee, toast and serve these to patients. Volunteers, patients and staff members sit round a large table and enjoy the companionship on offer whilst they have their hot drinks and toast.	Patients' visitors and family members are able to enjoy refreshments and companionship if they so wish. Private areas are available should individuals wish to have solitude and space to 'simply be.'

Source: Adapted from Lawrie, 1995.

Other roles include beauticians, hairdressers and activity leaders.

Benefits of volunteering

The work of volunteers is recognised as an important element contributing to an individual's sense of meaning and purpose. Actively volunteering may offer individuals the opportunity to have structure in their lives and may prove to be a fulfilling and rewarding experience (Watts, 2012).

Other reasons include the following:

- Volunteers enhance existing skills or learn new skills
- An increase in self-confidence
- A sense of achievement and belonging.

Further Reading

Third sector organisations in the UK

A small selection of TSOs that can support palliative care are listed below with links to more information. There are many other local support groups and charities that are a great resource for good quality care and management.

Macmillan Cancer Support is a charity that provides specialist healthcare, information and financial support to people affected by cancer. It also provides social, emotional and practical support. Macmillan is also a grant-giving organisation. It supports training, education and research. Macmillan's website has a wealth of free resources available to professionals.
www.macmillan.org.uk
Macmillan Support Line – 0800 8080000

Marie Curie is a charity that promotes and maintains the best quality of life and offers high-quality end-of-life care. It offers care and support for people living with a terminal illness. Marie Curie supports training and education and research.
https://www.mariecurie.org.uk/help/support

Maggie's is a charity providing free cancer support and information centres and online support. www.maggies.org

Hospice UK is the national charity for hospice care in the UK. They support and work for the benefit of people affected by death and dying, and collaborate with hospice members and other partners who work in end-of-life care.

Sue Ryder provides support for people living with a terminal illness or neurological condition as well as bereavement support. Palliative and neurological services are delivered at specialist centres across the country and in people's homes. www.sueryder.org

Compassion in Dying is a national charity providing information and resources to help you talk about and plan for the end of life. www.compassionindying.org.uk

The Health and Social Care Alliance is the national third sector for a range of health and social care organisations. www.alliance-scotland.org.uk

The Scottish Partnership for Palliative Care brings together health and social care professionals from hospital, social care services, primary care, hospices and other charities, to find ways of improving people's experiences of declining health, death, dying and bereavement. www.palliativecarescotland.org.uk

PATCH supports 24/7 specialist palliative care for patients in Scottish hospitals, providing resources such as dedicated beds, staff, advisory services and research. www.patchscotland.com

People with learning difficulties:

Beyond Words is a charity that provides books and training to support people who find pictures easier to understand than words. They have produced a booklet called *Jack Plans Ahead for Coronavirus*. www.booksbeyondwords.co.uk

Volunteering

Morris SM et al. (2015) *Hospice Volunteers: Bridging the gap to the community*. London: John Wiley and Sons Ltd.

Rogers CR (1990) *The Carl Rogers Reader*. London: Constable.

Stevens E and Edwards J (2008) *Palliative Care Learning in Practice*. Devon: Reflect Press Ltd.

Stevens E, Jackson S and Milligan S (2009) *Palliative Nursing Across the Spectrum of Care*. Oxford: Blackwell Publishing Ltd.

References

Cooper J (2008) *Stepping into Palliative Care Relationships and Responses*. Oxford: Radcliffe Publishing.

Doyle D (2002) *Volunteers in Hospice and Palliative Care. A handbook for volunteer service managers*. Oxford: Oxford University Press.

Dying Matters (2020) A Compassionate Country – A Charter for Wales. Available at: https://www.dyingmatters.org/blog/compassionate-country-%E2%80%93-charter-wales

Lawrie A (1995) *Managing Quality of Service*. London: The Directory of Social Change Publication.

McCurley S, Lynch R and Jackson R (2012) *The Complete Volunteer Management Handbook,* 3rd edition. London: The Directory of Social Change.

National Audit Office (2010) What are third sector organisations and their benefits for commissioners? Available at: https://www.nao.org.uk/successful-commissioning/introduction/what-are-civil-society-organisations-and-their-benefits-for-commissioners/

National Institute for Health Research (2012) The Role of the Third Sector in Delivering Social Care. Available at: http://eprints.lse.ac.uk/43538/1/The%20role%20of%20the%20third%20sector%20in%20delivering%20social%20care.pdf

Qureshi et al. (2019) Early initiation of palliative care is associated with reduced late-life acute hospital use: a population-based retrospective cohort study. *Palliative Medicine*, 33(2): 150–159.

Rochester C, Paine AE and Howlett S (2012) *Volunteering and Society in the 21st Century*. Hampshire: Palgrave MacMillan.

Scott R (2018) Volunteering in hospice and palliative care in the United Kingdom. *The changing Face of Volunteering in Hospice and Palliative Care*. Scott R and Howlett S eds. Oxford: Oxford university Press.

Scott R and Howlett S (2009) *Volunteers in Hospice and Palliative Care*. Oxford: Oxford University Press.

Scottish Government (2008) CEL 10 Refreshed Strategy for Volunteering in the NHS in Scotland. Available at: https://www.sehd.scot.nhs.uk/mels/CEL2008_10.pdf

Scottish Partnership for Palliative Care (2021) The truacanta project. Available at: https://www.goodlifedeathgrief.org.uk/content/thetruacantaproject

Third Sector: Dumfries and Galloway (2019) Invitation to help shape cancer and palliative care services. Available at: http://thirdsectordumgal.org.uk/invitation-to-help-shape-cancer-and-palliative-care-services/

Watts JH (2012) The Place of Volunteering in Palliative Care. *Contemporary and Innovative Practice in Palliative Care* ed. Esther Chang and Amanda Johnson. Rijeka: InTech Open.

Chapter 11

Complementary Therapies

Fiona Walker with Fiona Crowther, Denise Millar and Elaine Stevens

Learning Objectives

This chapter will help you to:

- Understand what different therapies are available and what they involve, including:
  - Mindfulness
  - Acupuncture
  - Reflexology
  - Reiki
  - Gentle touch massage
  - Aromatherapy
  - Visualisation – guided imagery and virtual reality
  - Hypnotherapy.
- Understand how they might help patients.
- Know when it might be appropriate to refer for complementary therapy.

Scenario

Background

Jack, a 62-year-old man with a history of chronic obstructive pulmonary disease (COPD) has now developed lung cancer. His disease is progressing rapidly and there are no oncological interventions available. He lives with his wife, Lorraine, who works during the week and keeps well. She cares for him where possible. Jack is having severe weekly panic attacks and feels unable to leave the house due to the fear of having an attack. There are frequent calls to the GP, district nurse and the out-of-hours service.

Key points

- Anxiety and panic can impact hugely on quality of life
- Impact on wider healthcare team
- Importance of including partner/family in therapy.

Timeline

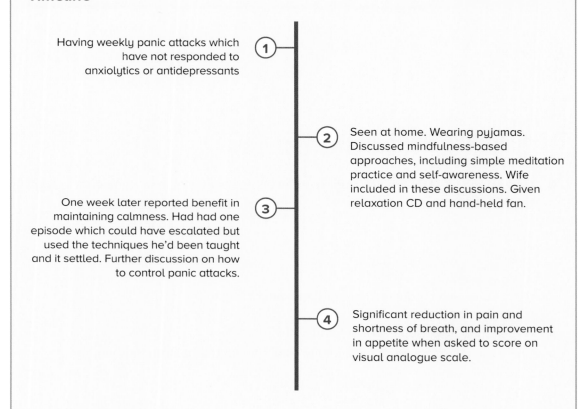

Having weekly panic attacks which have not responded to anxiolytics or antidepressants

1

2 Seen at home. Wearing pyjamas. Discussed mindfulness-based approaches, including simple meditation practice and self-awareness. Wife included in these discussions. Given relaxation CD and hand-held fan.

One week later reported benefit in maintaining calmness. Had had one episode which could have escalated but used the techniques he'd been taught and it settled. Further discussion on how to control panic attacks. **3**

4 Significant reduction in pain and shortness of breath, and improvement in appetite when asked to score on visual analogue scale.

Key considerations

- Why is it important to discuss techniques with the patient that they can implement themselves?
- Why is it important to consider non-pharmacological therapies to manage anxiety?
- What other therapies could be offered for anxiety?

Introduction

Complementary therapies are healthcare practices outside of the realms of mainstream medicine that are used for symptom management and to improve well-being alongside conventional treatments. It is important to stress that we are not discussing alternative medicines which are promoted for use instead of mainstream treatment. These therapies are often expensive and potentially harmful as they are untested and can encourage patients to avoid conventional treatments.

Many specialist palliative care services now offer a variety of complementary therapies. The role of complementary therapies is to enhance physical, mental and spiritual well-being. The evidence base for these treatments is not particularly strong in many cases, however it is generally accepted that the risk/benefit ratio is very favourable.

Many complementary therapies aim to help you relax and reduce stress. This chapter will explain a little about some of the most common therapies offered in the palliative care setting and give some examples of how they have been helpful. The therapies discussed are mindfulness, acupuncture, reflexology, reiki, gentle touch massage, aromatherapy, visualisation, virtual reality and hypnotherapy.

Mindfulness

Origin of mindfulness

In the West, mindfulness was introduced from Buddhist and Hindu traditions. Jon Kabat-Zinn in 1979 developed secular mindfulness meditation known as mindfulness-based stress reduction (MBSR) and applied it to those with significant medical conditions. This combines meditation with elements of yoga and education regarding stress alongside coping strategies (Zabat-Zinn, 2013). At the beginning of the twenty-first century, Zindel Segal, Mark Williams and John Teasdale built upon Kabat-Zinn's work to develop mindfulness-based cognitive therapy (MBCT). This is often used as part of the approach to helping with depression, anxiety and panic attacks (Segal et al., 2012).

Numerous studies have shown considerable evidence about the benefits of practising mindful meditation for those who face a range of health problems.

Mindfulness in palliative care

The significant impact of receiving a palliative diagnosis may be self-managed by avoidance of the reality which is faced. Moving to a position of acceptance can be an important element of an active coping process. With an attitude of acceptance, the person can embrace all aspects of experience, including the unpleasant. The concept of acceptance should not be confused with pessimism, giving-up or resignation. Zabat-Zinn described mindfulness as 'paying attention in a particular way, on purpose, in the present moment, without judgement' (Zabat-Zinn, 2013).

Awareness

A fundamental aspect of mindfulness meditation is the 'here and now' orientation – that is, paying attention to present moment reality. This enables better coping strategies and invites the ability to live one day at a time (Zabat-Zinn, 2013).

Perception

Through mindfulness practice, a decentered perspective is reinforced, where a shift is made from perceiving negative thoughts as distressing or dangerous to being seen as impersonal. Inviting curiosity around thoughts and not 'becoming' the thought brings an element of control enabling the ability to respond rather than react. From this, a balanced mind–body reconnection is established as the cycle of 'total pain' is broken.

Presence

This invites non-resistance towards difficulty and suffering with the ability to broaden awareness sensing all dimensions of experience. There can be co-existence of the often-subtle pleasant sensations alongside intense unpleasant experiences.

Self-compassion

Self-compassion provides a powerful tool for self-resilience. This is the ability to turn toward and acknowledge difficult thoughts and feelings with an attitude of openness and curiosity, responding to those difficulties with kindness and understanding.

Core mindfulness meditation practices

- Breathing anchor: a short meditation connecting to the movement of the breath. The breath becomes an anchor, a focus of attention.
- Three-minute breathing space: a breathing meditation providing structure for noticing experience, breathing, grounding and allowing.
- Body scan: this meditation focuses attention on physical sensations of the body. The purpose of this practice is to cultivate the ability to notice what is being experienced in the body. This is a useful practice to learn about how physical experience is tied to emotional experience, thus allowing and opening to what is felt within the body.
- Sitting practice: focuses initially on the movement of the breath then expands awareness to physical, emotional, mental, olfactory, visual and auditory senses. Allowing whatever is within oneself; to let it come, let it stay then let it go without the need to react, run away from, suppress or ignore. It develops an attitude of observing and accepting.
- Self-compassion: self-compassion develops kindness and care towards oneself as we would to others; it provides a tool for self-resilience and decreases depression, anxiety and stress. A variety of compassion practices are available.
- Mindful movement: invites being in the body through movement. This grounding practice develops focus and attention within movement and the breath.

Adapting mindfulness in palliative care

The format of mindfulness-based supportive therapy (MBST) or MBCT is delivered 2 hours a week for 8 weeks and one full day of practice (Cramer et al., 2019).

Palliative patients are often unable to sustain a regular mindfulness course due to fatigue, reduced concentration and cognition, and progression of disease. However, regular brief practice and an understanding of basic principles and attitudes of mindfulness, on a one to one basis, offer beneficial self-management strategies for pain, anxiety, breathlessness and insomnia. This increases enablement and encourages re-engagement with living (Beng et al., 2013; Zimmerman et al., 2018).

Acupuncture

Acupuncture originated in China more than 3,000 years ago, although there is some evidence of its use elsewhere from even earlier. It first came to prominence in the West in the 1970s following President Richard Nixon's visit to China when one of the press corps developed appendicitis and had acupuncture as part of his operative care (Lu et al., 2013).

Acupuncture is offered in many healthcare settings. It involves inserting sterile needles through the skin into specific points which vary depending on what you are treating. Single-use sterile stainless-steel needles are used and are usually inserted with the use of an introducer to a depth of 2–3 mm. Practice varies in how long the needles are left in, with a range of 2 to 30 minutes. Some practitioners stimulate the needles whilst they are in by rotating the needles. Electroacupuncture is offered by some practitioners and that involves passing a small current between two acupuncture needles.

Traditional Chinese medicine is based on the concept of meridians which are channels of energy flowing through the body. Each meridian has a name and points are numbered along it (Figure 11.1). A more Western medical approach is usually practised in a medical setting and this combines traditional Chinese teachings with a knowledge of anatomy and neurophysiological principles. This involves the use of trigger points – that is, a remote point that, when pressed, triggers the pain; tender points; and segmental needling – that is, insertion of needles in points along a meridian which share the same segmental nerve supply as the area of the complaint (Cancer Research UK, 2018). Research to prove the effectiveness of acupuncture is very difficult mainly due to it being impossible to have an effective placebo. It has been postulated that needling causes release of endorphins which results in the therapeutic effect and a general feeling of well-being. Some trials have attempted to use 'sham' acupuncture as a placebo. This involves either pretending to put needles in or inserting needles distant from the appropriate site, but both of these methods are difficult to conceal from the patient (Vickers et al., 2012). Another problem is that there is no funding available to conduct high quality trials. Despite this there are some trials which have had positive outcomes. At present the NICE guidelines recommend acupuncture for chronic tension-type headaches and migraines, and SIGN guidelines state it can be considered for chronic back pain or osteoarthritis as well as headaches (NICE, 2015; SIGN, 2013).

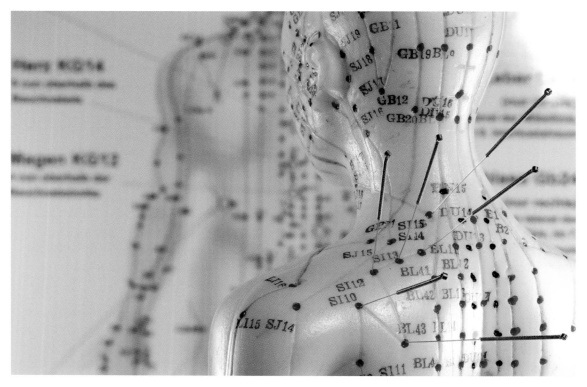

Figure 11.1 Acupuncture and meridians of the human body.

Acupuncture should be avoided in the immunocompromised due to the risk of introducing infection, and care should be taken in patients who are thrombocytopenic due to the bleeding risk (Cancer Research UK, 2018). You should avoid giving acupuncture in an area affected by lymphoedema due to the risk of lymphorrhoea and introducing infection (Bao et al., 2018). Care must also be taken when needling over the thorax in cachectic patients due to the small risk of causing a pneumothorax (Cancer Research UK, 2018).

In palliative care it can be helpful for pain, nausea, breathlessness, anxiety, sweats/hot flushes and dry mouth amongst other problems (Cancer Research UK, 2018).

Reflexology

Reflexology is a technique which applies gentle pressure to your feet or hands to aid relaxation, but also help the body's own healing process. It is believed that specific points on the feet or hands are related to organs, systems and glands within the body. Reflexology, like acupuncture, is based on the concept of energy pathways within the body which can become blocked (Cancer Research UK, 2019a) (Figure 11.2). By massaging the

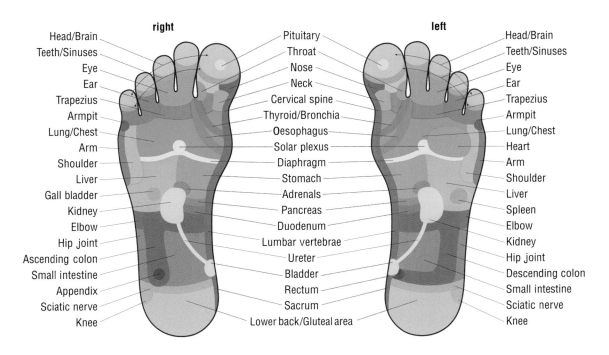

right

Head/Brain
Teeth/Sinuses
Eye
Ear
Trapezius
Armpit
Lung/Chest
Arm
Shoulder
Liver
Gall bladder
Kidney
Elbow
Hip joint
Ascending colon
Small intestine
Appendix
Sciatic nerve
Knee

Pituitary
Throat
Nose
Neck
Cervical spine
Thyroid/Bronchia
Oesophagus
Solar plexus
Diaphragm
Stomach
Adrenals
Pancreas
Duodenum
Lumbar vertebrae
Ureter
Bladder
Rectum
Sacrum
Lower back/Gluteal area

left

Head/Brain
Teeth/Sinuses
Eye
Ear
Trapezius
Armpit
Lung/Chest
Heart
Arm
Shoulder
Liver
Spleen
Elbow
Kidney
Hip joint
Descending colon
Small intestine
Sciatic nerve
Knee

Figure 11.2   Foot reflexology chart.

feet at certain points these pathways can be unblocked, allowing the energy to flow freely again and restoring balance to the body (Unlu et al., 2018).

Reflexology is generally well received by palliative care patients. Most patients have limited mobility and energy and spend a lot of their time lying in bed or sitting in a chair. Performing reflexology is easily done, accommodating them as they are. Patients are often open to trying this for the first time and then look forward to ongoing visits from the therapist. It brings a welcome distraction from the daily clinical routine they undergo. It offers a positive experience, taking their mind off any suffering and focusing it on the relaxation and feeling better.

The benefits of reflexology are numerous. In palliative care patients, the biggest benefit is reducing stress/anxiety and inducing deep relaxation (Cancer Research UK, 2019a). As a result, sleep patterns are often improved and patients report that they feel less fatigued. It can also be helpful in patients suffering from nausea and vomiting as well as dyspnoea. Some patients also report a reduction in pain levels (Lorence et al., 2019).

The warmth of a therapist's hands, the touch and attention given, make this a wonderful therapy to receive.

Reiki

Reiki is an energy-based healing system originating from Japan. It is carried out by placing hands on or over a person (who is always clothed) with the intent to channel reiki or 'universal energy'. Reiki practitioners believe that it heals on all levels, physically, mentally and spiritually, as well as supporting the body's natural ability to heal itself (Fernandez, 2003). The gentle nature of reiki is suited to palliative patients as there are relatively no risks involved in using it as a treatment (Cancer Research UK, 2019b). It is easy to administer whether a patient is supine or prone. The sensation of touch can bring comfort to a patient and in some patients can help alleviate pain. It is deeply relaxing, which in turn can promote good sleeping habits. Psychologically, it can help a patient cope with the difficulties that they are facing. It can relieve emotional stress and tension, helping to improve overall well-being (Burden et al., 2005).

On a spiritual level, when a patient is nearing end of life, it is said that reiki treatment can allow people to die at peace with themselves, without fear or struggle (Billot et al., 2019). Knowing this enables loved ones to be happy and at peace themselves, and helps with the grieving process. Relatives and friends can also benefit from receiving a reiki treatment during this time, helping their own state of mind.

Within a calm hospice environment, a therapist spending time with a patient can help them feel at ease and benefit from the relaxation that a reiki session provides. Anxiety is alleviated, giving the patient reassurance that their place of care takes a holistic approach in looking after them.

Gentle Touch Massage

Gentle touch massage is simple yet profound in its benefits. It combines a variety of techniques which calm, soothe and relax both physically and psychologically.

As the body prepares to die it becomes increasingly sensitive, and light gentle techniques as well as holding areas of the body instil the feeling of being held and cradled. Using this treatment for only a short period of time is appropriate; a delicate balance needs to be achieved, using experience and intuition for guidance, as patients are often quite frail and fatigued. Touch delivered sensitively with attentive, caring hands conveys understanding and support that invites the patient to feel safe and not alone on their journey.

Gentle touch massage can be delivered over bedclothes, clothing or directly onto the body in a non-invasive and non-obtrusive manner. Light flowing strokes over the body encourage muscles to relax, releasing tension and regulating the breath. The relaxation response can decrease activity of the sympathetic nervous system, releasing oxytocin and reducing cortisol, providing a sense of security, reducing blood pressure and encouraging rest. Overall it can promote an enriching sense of well-being, calm and peace (see Box 11.1).

Box 11.1 Benefits of gentle touch massage

- It provides relaxation and comfort
- Calms and regulates breathing/diaphragmatic breathing
- Enables the management of 'total pain'
- Relieves stress and anxiety
- Releases emotions
- Uplifts mood
- Tackles insomnia – invites a restful sleep
- Alleviates pain
- Eases terminal agitation
- Awakens the emotions and spirituality – touch may help a patient to 'let go' and die peacefully
- Brings relief to oedema
- Reduces anticipatory nausea response
- Maintains skin integrity
- Initiates a sense of well-being.

Patients who find relaxation difficult, perhaps due to a heightened state of anxiety, pain or agitation, respond well to a combination of gentle touch massage, aromatherapy, empathy and voice/music.

For some, the only touch that may be received is by medical or nursing intervention. Touch given in a positive and therapeutic way can offer deep relaxation, comfort and support, conveying respectful non-verbal messages of empathy, compassion and reassurance. There are however certain exclusions for safety reasons which apply to this particular therapy, such as:

- Pyrexia
- Infection
- Pulmonary embolism
- Deep vein thrombosis
- Superior vena cava obstruction
- Cellulitis
- Recent chemotherapy or radiotherapy
- Massaging over tumour, ascites, bowel obstruction and bony metastases should be avoided
- Pressure sore, fragile skin
- Seizure activity
- Spinal cord compression.

Gentle touch massage offers a way of reconnecting with the 'self', giving the person a feeling of being nurtured and cared for, providing a time for deep understanding and healing, for the release of emotions and fears, of letting go and being somewhere else... just for a time.

Aromatherapy

Aromatherapy is defined as the controlled use of essential oils that have been extracted from plants and trees using a process of distillation (Lai et al., 2011). Such oils are then diluted using a standard formula and are commonly administered in palliative care by applying them to the skin through massage carrier oils, creams and ointments, by adding them to bathwater or by inhaling them via burners/diffusers, incense sticks or personal vaporisers (Stringer and Donald, 2011; Boehm et al., 2012; Berger et al., 2013; Rose, 2017).

Table 11.1 identifies aromatherapy oils commonly used in cancer and palliative care and how they may potentially support quality of life and well-being.

Table 11.1   Aromatherapy oils commonly used in palliative care.

Types of oil	Benefits
Citrus oils: **Bergamot, grapefruit, mandarin, lime, orange, lemon**	Stimulates the mind and can uplift feelings. Lessens stress and anxiety. Can reduce/mask odour.
Floral oils: **Lavender, geranium, palma rosa, clary sage, ylang ylang, rose**	Lessens anxiety and irritability. Balances mood. Reduces sleep disturbance. Reduces fatigue levels. Promotes skin integrity.
Green and herbaceous oils: **Camomile, clary sage, marjoram, peppermint, thyme, lemongrass, rosemary, fennel**	Boosts the immune system. Lessens fatigue. Reduces gastrointestinal symptoms such as bloating, nausea and constipation.
Spice oils: **Black pepper, ginger**	Enhances the immune system. Promotes circulation. Reduces pain. Improves mood. Lessens nausea.
Root oils: **Spikenard, patchouli, vetiver**	Calms emotions. Grounds people.
Tree oils: **Eucalyptus, sandalwood, tea tree, pine/fir**	Uplifting and revitalising. Reduces anxiety. Relieves airway congestion and supports breathing. Reduces bloating/gas. Alleviates itch. Is antimicrobial and helpful in skin infections.
Resinous oils: **Frankincense, myrrh**	Consoling aroma. Reduces stress. Promotes sleep. Grounds people (roots them physically, emotionally, mentally, energetically and/or spiritually).

Source: Developed from Kyle, 2006; Lai et al., 2011; Stringer and Donald, 2011; Boehm et al., 2012; Berger et al., 2013; Pounds, 2012; Rose, 2016; Rose 2017; Simoes et al., 2018; National Cancer Institute, 2019.

While Table 11.1 identifies the potential benefits of aromatherapy, there is little robust research on which to support such claims and consequently more research is required (Shin et al., 2016). However the general consensus is that aromatherapy, while unlikely to cause harm, requires thoughtful consideration of the issues raised around its use (Boehm et al., 2012). For example, citrus oils can potentiate the activity of the sun, which may lead to phototoxicity (National Cancer Institute, 2019), while the oestrogenic and antiandrogenic activity of oils such as palma rosa, geranium, lavender, tea tree and clary sage may have an effect on hormone dependent tumours (Boehm et al., 2012; Simoes et al., 2018). It is therefore important that healthcare professionals and therapists understand the risks and benefits of all interventions a patient may receive (Rose, 2018).

For safe and effective care, aromatherapy should be provided by a qualified therapist who is able to conduct a thorough assessment of the patient's needs prior to the treatment. This should include their medical history as well as the identification of any issues that may contraindicate the use of essential oils (Berger et al., 2013). Following the assessment the therapist should provide the patient with enough information on the benefits, risks and outcomes of the proposed treatment to enable them to give informed consent (Dunning, 2005). Rose (2016) also suggests that the therapist should work with the patient to develop a personalised blend of oils that is not only suitable to treat the symptoms but generates an aroma the patient likes, as this may enhance and maintain the outcome of the treatment.

Dunning (2005) highlights that it is important to document the outcomes of treatments so that they can be reviewed against other interventions that may be taking place at the same time. This way it is more likely that the benefits of the aromatherapy are recognised as part of an integrated approach to care.

To maintain safe and effective aromatherapy practices the correct use of the oils is essential, and as with other active chemicals used in a patient's care, all oils should be purchased from a reputable source and diluted and mixed using current best practice guidance (Dunning, 2005). Once the oils are diluted and ready for use they should be clearly labelled to show the blend of oils being used, in what percentage and when they expire. This is especially important if the patient is to self-administer the treatment.

Visualisation

Guided imagery

Guided imagery is a non-pharmacological cognitive behavioural technique which uses multi-sensory cues and imagery (sight, sound and smells) to enable a person to believe they are in a peaceful place such as a garden, beach or forest (Schumacher et al., 2018; Adeola et al., 2015; Burnett, 2012). It is suggested that a guided imagery session generally has three stages: relaxation, which in palliative care should be relatively passive due to disease processes; visualisation, which uses imagery that is agreeable to the person; and positive suggestion, which is meaningful and allows a positive outcome (Burnett, 2012; Boog et al., 2008). However, in some guided imagery sessions music is also employed to aid relaxation and to enhance the guided imagery processes (Burns et al., 2018).

Adeola et al. (2015) proposed that guided imagery has a direct effect on brain activity, which leads to direct physiological effects. Coelho et al. (2018a) add to this by suggesting that guided imagery appears to induce neurochemical changes in the body that have an impact on psychological well-being and physical symptoms. This may be why Proud (2017) proposes that the care team should consider guided imagery as a concurrent intervention when managing complex symptoms. While guided imagery has been practised by a range of palliative care professionals and therapists there is little research evidence to prove this intervention has a positive impact on quality of life (Coelho et al., 2018b). However, reports that exist suggest that guided imagery can help in the holistic management of symptoms by reducing pain, insomnia, stress, fear, panic, anxiety and depression, as well as promoting control, coping skills, independence and comfort (Burnett, 2012; Coelho et al., 2018a; Galfin et al., 2011).

Guided imagery is used widely in occupational therapy and can be used by suitably trained nurses or other health professionals as well as qualified therapists (Burns et al., 2018; Adeola et al., 2015; Vadnais, 2013). This means that, as well as being an effective therapy, it may also be more cost effective than others that require a qualified therapist. However, if professionals are interested in delivering this therapy they must have relevant training (Proud, 2017). Patients can also be taught to practise guided imagery using recorded scenarios that reduce the need for attendance at a face-to-face session and which reduce the cost further. This approach can also promote self-management, which is an overarching goal of healthcare.

In practical terms the use of a robust delivery system and standard session guides ensure the person receives multi-sensory prompts that meet their needs (Coelho et al., 2018b; Burnett, 2012). Many such scripts are freely available on the internet, while Boog et al. (2008) also provide examples in their guidance on guided imagery. Guided imagery sessions can be conducted as a one-to-one therapy or in groups such as palliative day services where people come together for a period of time (Stevens et al., 2011). As such, the person delivering the session should ensure the environment is suitable for guided imagery, for example will people be sitting or lying down? Is there support available in case of distress? It is always important that the care team have the knowledge and skills to manage distress, and that when people have issues that are more complex they know how to refer them on to other more specialist services.

Virtual reality

A new concept that has recently been linked with guided imagery and relaxation is the use of VR. So while the benefits of virtual reality VR in palliative care have been known for over 20 years (Oyama, 1997), it is only recently that its use as a holistic intervention has come to the attention of palliative care services. VR uses computer-generated multi-sensory simulations of a wide variety of situations that people coming to the end of life may not be able to do in reality (Niki et al., 2019). It is suggested that people quickly become absorbed into the simulation which helps them to enjoy another environment in which to relax (Pabla et al., 2017). VR can also enable patients to achieve goals such as returning home, completing experiences from their 'bucket list' or enjoying an afternoon in the local park (Kazuyuki et al., 2019; Pabla et al., 2017). Enabling group VR sessions also allows patients to talk together and reminisce with each other about their experience, which promotes psychological well-being and self-worth (Pabla et al., 2017; Pinquart and Forstmeier, 2012).

As VR is a recent addition to the range of holistic interventions available in palliative care, there is little evidence of its impact on quality of life. However, a very recent study has shown VR has positive effects on a range of symptoms including pain, fatigue, drowsiness, dyspnoea, depression and anxiety, as well as overall well-being (Kazuyuki et al., 2019).

In summary, guided imagery has the potential to improve the quality of life of people who require palliative care. Guided imagery should be provided within a robust framework underpinned by best practice. Professionals who provide Guided imagery should be well trained and work within the standards of their professional body to ensure effective outcomes and promote patient safety. Virtual reality is a new intervention which can add to the holistic care of palliative care patients and only the future will tell if the provision of this new therapy will continue to blossom.

Hypnotherapy

Hypnosis is defined as 'a mental state usually induced by a procedure known as hypnotic induction' (Sharma et al., 2017). The process of induction commonly uses an instructional procedure which can include eye fixation and visualisation with or without purposeful muscle relaxation to induce a trance-like state (Plaskota et al., 2013). This procedure directs a person's awareness away from the current environment towards their inner experiences to generate modifications in perceptions and experiences through suggestion (Krouwel et al., 2017; Harlow et al., 2015).

Hypnotherapy is the therapeutic use of hypnosis in health and illness which has been utilised to enhance well-being for many centuries (Heap et al., 2001). Hypnotherapy enables people to manage a variety of physical and psychological issues as well as supporting them to change negative health behaviours and conquer addictions and phobias (Jain, 2006). However, while the benefits of hypnotherapy have been reported for many years, uncertainties and myths around how it works, who can be hypnotised and the role of the 'hypnotist' exist (Kihlstrom, 2012). This has resulted in a poor understanding of the therapy by professionals, patients and the general public and, as such, more information on its potential to improve health and well-being is required (Desai et al., 2011; Yeh et al., 2014; Krouwel et al., 2017).

The evidence base for the use of hypnotherapy in palliative care remains weak, although a number of reviews report that there is potential for this intervention to improve coping skills, physical symptoms and psychological and spiritual well-being (Zeng et al., 2018; Brugnoli, 2016;

Rajasekaran et al., 2005). More specifically, the use of hypnotherapy in palliative care has been considered to aid relaxation, improve pain and coping skills, as well as reducing nausea and vomiting, fatigue, insomnia, anxiety and depression (Sharma et al., 2017; Plaskota et al., 2012; Curtis, 2001; Finlay and Jones, 1996).

As in other therapies, using a qualified therapist who has an understanding of palliative care is essential to maintain effectiveness and safety (Tavares, 2003). Patients should also receive clear information on why they are being referred for this intervention to allow them to give informed consent (Harlow et al., 2015). There are a number of professional organisations who oversee best practice in hypnotherapy and often provide training to allow a person to become an accredited practitioner. NHS England (2018) provides guidance to people seeking to try hypnotherapy, which includes the following suggestions:

- Choose someone with a healthcare background – such as a doctor, psychologist or counsellor
- If you have mental ill health or a serious illness (such as cancer), make sure they're trained in working with your condition
- Check they're registered with an organisation that's accredited.

Supporting patients to follow such guidance helps ensure they understand how this intervention may benefit them.

As patients requiring palliative care may have a range of issues, the focus of individual hypnotherapy sessions will depend on the concerns they raise during their initial assessment by the therapist (Harlow et al., 2015). This assessment builds a relationship in which mutual trust and understanding emerge and lead effective deployment of the therapy (Fox, 2007). Once it is established that hypnotherapy may be of benefit, the patient will take part in a series of sessions where a hypnotic state will be induced, possibly using eye fixation and progressive relaxation (Jain, 2006). Whilst in this state patients are receptive to positive suggestions that may help them with their concerns, while visualisation may enable them to concentrate on how they may be in the future and may also help with intrusive thoughts (Plaskota et al., 2012 Jain, 2006). Patients may be taught to use an 'anchor', such as recalling a positive memory or being in a favourite place, to allow them to enter a more favourable mental state that has a positive effect on their situation (Hunter, 2010). This can be utilised alongside a 'trigger', such as taking a deep breath, which can be used by patients when faced with problematic events or negative emotions (Plaskota et al., 2012; Hunter, 2010). To end the hypnotic state the patient may be asked to gently open their eyes when the therapist counts from one to five (Jain, 2006).

In summary, it would appear that hypnotherapy has the potential to help in the holistic care of patients receiving palliative care. However, further research is required and, as such, professionals should provide each patient with enough information to allow them to make an informed choice as to whether this therapy may be beneficial to them.

Scenario Recap

One month later, Jack is now getting dressed and getting out of the house. There have been no calls to healthcare professionals. By discussing alternative therapies with the patient, a solution could be found which not only dealt with their symptoms but returned control to them which helped to improve their quality of life.

References

Adeola MT et al. (2015) Active despite pain: patient experiences with guided imagery with relaxation compared to planned rest. *Journal of Clinical Oncology Nursing*, 19(6): 649–652.

Bao T et al. (2018) Acupuncture versus medication for pain management: a cross-sectional study of breast cancer survivors. *Acupuncture in Medicine: Journal of the British Medical Acupuncture Society*, 36(2): 80–87.

Beng TS et al. (2013) Mindfulness-based supportive therapy (MBST): proposing a palliative psychotherapy from a conceptual perspective to address suffering in palliative care. *American Journal of Hospice and Palliative Medicine,* 32(2): 144–160.

Berger L, Tavares M and Berger B (2013) A Canadian experience of integrating complementary therapy into a hospital palliative care unit. *Journal of Palliative Medicine*, 16(10): 1294–1298.

Billot M et al. (2019) Reiki therapy for pain, anxiety and quality of life. *BMJ Supportive & Palliative Care*, 9(4): 434–438.

Boehm K, Bussing A and Ostermann T (2012) Aromatherapy as an adjuvant treatment in cancer care – a descriptive systematic review. *African Journal of Traditional, Complementary and Alternative Medicines*, 9(4): 503–518.

Boog K and Tester C (2008) *A Practical Guide to Working in Palliative Care: Finding Meaning and Purpose in Life*. London: Churchill Livingstone.

Brugnoli MP (2016) Clinical hypnosis for palliative care in severe chronic diseases: a review and the procedures for relieving physical, psychological and spiritual symptoms. *Annals of Palliative Medicine*, 5(4): 280–297.

Burden B, Herron-Marx S and Clifford C (2005) The increasing use of reiki as a complementary therapy in specialist palliative care. *International Journal of Palliative Nursing*, 11(5): 248–253.

Burnett J (2012) Guided imagery as an adjuvant to pharmacological pain control at the end of life. North American Association of Christians in Social Work. Available at: https://www.nacsw.org/Publications/Proceedings2012/BurnettJGuidedImagery.pdf

Burns DS et al. (2018) Differences between supportive music and imagery and music listening during outpatient chemotherapy and potential moderators of treatment effects. *Journal of Music Therapy*, 55(1): 83–108.

Cancer Research UK (2018) Acupuncture. Available at: https://www.cancerresearchuk.org/about-cancer/cancer-in-general/treatment/complementary-alternative-therapies/individual-therapies/acupuncture

Cancer Research UK (2019a) Reflexology. Available at: https://www.cancerresearchuk.org/about-cancer/cancer-in-general/treatment/complementary-alternative-therapies/individual-therapies/reflexology

Cancer Research UK (2019b) Reiki. Available at: https://www.cancerresearchuk.org/about-cancer/cancer-in-general/treatment/complementary-alternative-therapies/individual-therapies/reiki

Coelho A et al. (2018a) The effects of guided imagery on comfort in palliative care. *Journal of Hospice and Palliative Nursing*, 20(4): 393–399.

Coelho A et al. (2018b) Development of a guided imagery program for patients admitted to palliative care units. *Revista de Enfermagem Referência*, 4(17): 23–32.

Cramer H, Moenaert AC and the CAM Cancer Consortium (2019) Mindfulness. Available at: http://cam-cancer.org/en/mindfulness-cam

Curtis C (2001) Hypnotherapy in a specialist palliative care unit: evaluation of a pilot service. *International Journal of Palliative Nursing*, 7(12): 606–609.

Desai G, Chaturvedi SK and Ramachandra S (2011) Hypnotherapy: fact or fiction: a review in palliative care and opinions of healthcare professionals. *Indian Journal of Palliative Care*, 17(2): 146–149.

Dunning T (2005) Applying a quality use of medicines framework to using essential oils in nursing practice. *Complementary Therapies in Clinical Practice*, 11(3): 172–181.

Fernandez C (2003) *Step-by-Step Reiki*. London: Hermes House.

Finlay IG and Jones OL (1996) Hypnotherapy in palliative care. *Journal of the Royal Society of Medicine,* 89(9): 493–496.

Fox S (2007) *Relating to Clients: The Therapeutic Relationship for Complementary Therapists.* London: Jessica Kingsley Publishers.

Galfin JM, Watkins ER and Harlow T (2011) A brief guided self-help intervention for psychological distress in palliative care patients: a randomised controlled trial. *Palliative Medicine,* 36(3): 197–205.

Harlow T et al. (2015) Hypnotherapy for relief of pain and other symptoms in palliative care: a pilot study. *Contemporary Hypnosis and Integrative Therapy*, 30(4): 163–174.

Heap M and Aravind KK (2001) *Hartland's Medical and Dental Hypnosis,* 4th edition. Edinburgh: Churchill Livingstone.

Hunter (2010) *The Art of Hypnotherapy: Mastering Client Centred Techniques,* 4th edition. Carmarthen: Crown House Publishing.

Jain AK (2006) *Clinical and Meditative Hypnotherapy: A Spiritual and Quantum Approach.* New Jersey: Quantum Hypnotherapy.

Kazuyuki N et al. (2019) A novel palliative care approach using virtual reality for improving various symptoms of terminal cancer patients: a preliminary prospective, multicenter study. *Journal of Palliative Medicine*, 22(6): 702–707.

Kihlstrom JF (2012) The domain of hypnosis, revisited. In Nash MR and Barnier AJ (eds) *The Oxford Handbook of Hypnosis Theory, Research and Practice*. Oxford: Oxford University Press.

Krouwel M, Jolly K, Greenfield S (2017) What the public think about hypnosis and hypnotherapy: a narrative review of literature covering opinions and attitudes of the general public 1996–2016. *Complementary Therapies in Medicine*, 32: 75–84.

Kyle G (2006) Evaluating the effectiveness of aromatherapy in reducing levels of anxiety in palliative care patients: results of a pilot study. *Complementary Therapies in Clinical Practice*, 12(2): 148–155.

Lai TKT et al. (2011) Effectiveness of aroma massage on advanced cancer patients with constipation: a pilot study. *Complementary Therapies in Clinical Practice*, 17(1): 37–43.

Lorence A, Cooke H and the CAM Cancer Consortium (2019) Reflexology. Available at: http://cam-cancer.org/en/reflexology

Lu D and Lu G (2013) An historical review and perspective on the impact of acupuncture on U.S. medicine and society. *Medical Acupuncture*, 25(5): 311–316.

National Cancer Institute (2019) Aromatherapy with essential oils. Available at: https://www.cancer.gov/about-cancer/treatment/cam/hp/aromatherapy-pdq#_1

NHS England (2018) Hypnotherapy. Available at: https://www.nhs.uk/conditions/hypnotherapy/

NICE (National Institute for Health and Care Excellence) (2015) Headaches in over 12s: diagnosis and management (NICE guideline 150). London: NICE.

Niki K et al. (2019) A novel palliative care approach using virtual reality for improving various symptoms of terminal cancer patients: A preliminary prospective, multicenter study. *Journal of Palliative Medicine*, 22(6):702–707.

Oyama H (1997) Virtual reality for palliative care in cancer. *Virtual Reality in Neuro-Psycho-Physiology*, 44: 87–94.

Pabla K, Knight J and Morley M (2017) Virtual reality transforming the lives of terminally ill patients. *BMJ Supportive and Palliative Care,* 7(Suppl 2): A9.

Pinquart M and Forstmeier S (2012) Effects of reminiscence on psychosocial outcomes: a meta-analysis. *Aging & Mental Health*, 16(5): 541–558.

Plaskota M et al. (2012) A hypnotherapy intervention for the treatment of anxiety in patients with cancer receiving palliative care. *International Journal of Palliative Nursing*, 18(2) 69–75.

Pounds LK (2012) Art of aromatherapy for end-of-life care. *Beginnings, Journal of American Holistic Nurse Association*, 32(4): 20–23.

Proud J (2017) The use of relaxation, guided imagery and visualisation techniques to help relieve anxiety and pain in palliative care. *BMJ Supportive and Palliative Care,* 7(Suppl 2): A55.

Rajasekaran M, Edmonds PM and Higginson IJ (2005) Systematic review of hypnotherapy for treating symptoms in terminally ill adult cancer patients. *Palliative Medicine*, 19(5): 418–426.

Rose C (2016) Cancer related fatigue: the potential of aromatherapy. *International Journal of Clinical Aromatherapy*, 11(2): 39–47.

Rose C (2017) Spiritual distress in patients with cancer: the potential of aromatherapy. *International Journal of Clinical Aromatherapy*, 12(1): 19–25.

Rose C (2018) Aromatherapy in palliative care aids relaxation and improves quality of life for patients with life-limiting illness. *Kai Tiaki Nursing New Zealand*, 24(3): 38–39.

Schumacher S, Kemps E and Tiggemann M (2018) Cognitive defusion and guided imagery tasks reduce naturalistic food cravings and consumption: a field study. *Appetite*, 127: 393–399.

Segal ZV, Williams JMG and Teasdale JD (2012) *Mindfulness-Based Cognitive Therapy for Depression*. New York: Guilford Press.

Sharma VK (2017) Hypnotherapy in cancer care: clinical benefits and prospective implications. Journal of Health Research & Reviews, 4(3): 96–103.

Shin ES et al. (2016) Massage with or without aromatherapy for symptom relief in people with cancer. *Cochrane Database of Systematic Reviews*, (6): CD009873.

SIGN (Scottish Intercollegiate Guidelines Network) (2013) Management of chronic pain (SIGN publication no 136). Edinburgh: SIGN.

Simoes BM et al. (2018) Estrogenicity of essential oils is not required to relieve symptoms of urogenital atrophy in breast cancer survivors. *Therapeutic Advances in Medical Oncology*, 10: 1–11.

Stevens E, Martin CR and White CA (2011) The outcomes of palliative day services: a systematic review. *Palliative Medicine*, 25(2): 153–169.

Stringer J and Donald G (2011) Aromasticks in cancer care: an innovation not to be sniffed at. *Complementary Therapies in Clinical Practice*, 17(2): 116–121.

Tavares M (2003) *National Guidelines for the Use of Complementary Therapies in Supportive and Palliative Care*. London: Prince of Wales Foundation for Integrated Health.

Unlu A, Kirka O and Ozdogan M (2018) Reflexology and cancer. *Journal of Oncological Sciences*, 4(2): 96–101.

Vadnais E (2013) What is guided imagery? OTs can tap a person's inner wisdom for health, healing and wellness. *ADVANCE Magazine*, July: 1–4. Available at: http://holisticot.org/wp-content/uploads/2014/09/What-is-Guided-Imagery.pdf

Vickers AJ et al. (2012) Acupuncture for chronic pain: individual patient data meta-analysis. *Archives of Internal Medicine,* 172(19): 1444–1453.

Yeh VM, Schnur JB and Montgomery GH (2014) Disseminating hypnosis to health care settings: applying the RE-AIM framework. *Psychology of Consciousness*, 1(2): 213–228.

Zabat-Zinn J (2013) *Full Catastrophe Living: How to Cope with Stress, Pain and Illness Using Mindfulness Meditation*. Revised edition. London: Piatkus.

Zeng YS et al. (2018) Complementary and alternative medicine in hospice and palliative care: a systematic review. *Journal of Pain and Symptom Management*, 56(5): 781–794.

Zimmermann FF, Burnell B and Jordan J (2018) The acceptability and potential benefits of mindfulness-based interventions in improving psychological well-being for adults with advanced cancer: a systematic review. *Complementary Therapies in Clinical Practice*, 30: 68–78.

Chapter 12

Specific Populations

James Neil with Gail Allan, Scott Jamieson,
Holly McGuigan, Allison O'Donnell,
Joy Rafferty, Liz Smith
and Paul Watson

Learning Objectives

This chapter will help you to:

- Recognise that there are certain unmet needs for specific populations who require palliative care and identify ways in which their needs can be met. Specific populations covered here include:
  - LGBTQ+
  - The learning disabled
  - Frail adults
  - Care home residents
  - Remote and rural populations
  - People experiencing homelessness
  - Those living in poverty
  - Prison inmates.
- Understand the challenges which these populations may face when trying to access palliative care
- Understand the importance of communication and the language used when communicating with specific groups with particular needs
- Identify the need for a multidisciplinary approach and cross-sector communication in order to provide the best care for the palliative care patient, including out-of-hours considerations
- Define specific conditions and other social and psychological issues associated with these specific groups and how to manage them, pharmacologically and non-pharmacologically
- Describe certain management strategies used in dealing with specific populations.

Scenario

Background

Bob is a 71-year-old man with metastatic lung cancer who has presented to hospital with increasing shortness of breath. Bob's main carer is his husband Michael. Bob has never been admitted to hospital before and doesn't know what to expect. He is too embarrassed to correct the doctor in the emergency department who assumes that Michael is his brother.

Key points

- Bob may be worried that he will face stigma or discrimination from healthcare professionals when in hospital.
- Bob's experience of professionals making incorrect assumptions about his partner's identity is a common one.
- There may be increased pressure on Michael here as a carer. Bob and Michael are less likely than a straight couple of their age to have children and more likely to be estranged from their families of origin.

Timeline

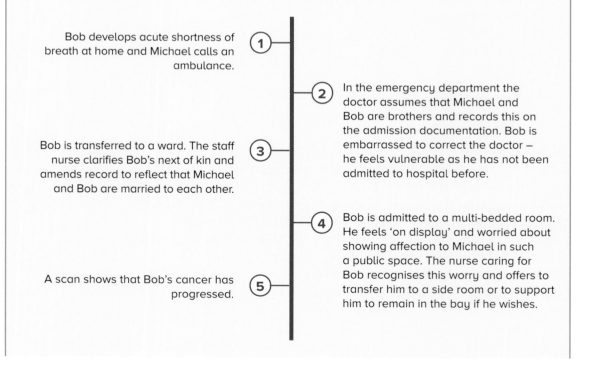

Bob develops acute shortness of breath at home and Michael calls an ambulance. **(1)**

(2) In the emergency department the doctor assumes that Michael and Bob are brothers and records this on the admission documentation. Bob is embarrassed to correct the doctor – he feels vulnerable as he has not been admitted to hospital before.

Bob is transferred to a ward. The staff nurse clarifies Bob's next of kin and amends record to reflect that Michael and Bob are married to each other. **(3)**

(4) Bob is admitted to a multi-bedded room. He feels 'on display' and worried about showing affection to Michael in such a public space. The nurse caring for Bob recognises this worry and offers to transfer him to a side room or to support him to remain in the bay if he wishes.

A scan shows that Bob's cancer has progressed. **(5)**

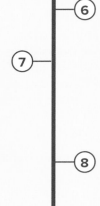

6 The ward team spend time with Bob and Michael discussing anticipatory care planning (ACP). Bob wishes to be cared for at home at the end of his life but recognises that this may be challenging because Bob and Michael do not have any children and Bob doesn't have any contact with his family of origin.

7 Bob is discharged home for end-of-life care with Michael as his main carer. They are supported by Michael's sister and her son. Bob is reluctant to accept a package of care as he is worried about welcoming strangers into their home. Michael discusses this concern with friends who also require carers and is reassured by them and by the care agency's anti-discrimination policies.

8 Bob dies at home supported by friends, family, a care package and his local hospice. Michael is offered bereavement support from the hospice after Bob's death.

Key considerations

- What worries might Bob have about coming into hospital?
- What barriers might Bob experience to appropriate care?
- What particular pressures might the couple be facing because they are gay?
- What challenges may face Bob and Michael as Bob is cared for at home at the end of life?

Palliative Care for LGBTQ+ Individuals

LGBTQ+ people have an increased risk of some life-limiting illnesses (Harding et al., 2012) but may struggle to access the care that they need. Dying and bereaved LGBTQ+ individuals face additional stressors including the failure of others to acknowledge their relationship, complex financial and legal barriers, and homophobia (Bristowe et al., 2016).

Glossary

- **LGBTQ**: Lesbian, Gay, Bisexual, Trans and Queer or questioning.
- **Lesbian**: Refers to a woman who has a romantic and/or sexual orientation towards women.
- **Gay**: Refers to a man who has a romantic and/or sexual orientation towards men. Also a generic term for lesbian and gay sexuality.
- **Bisexual**: Bisexual or Bi is a term used to describe a romantic and/or sexual orientation towards more than one gender.

- **Trans**: Describes people whose gender is not the same as, or does not sit comfortably with, the sex they were assigned at birth.

- **Queer**: Queer is a term used by those wanting to reject specific labels of romantic orientation, sexual orientation and/or gender identity. It can also be a way of rejecting the perceived norms of the LGBTQ+ community (racism, sizeism, ableism, etc.). Although some LGBTQ+ people view the word as a slur, it was reclaimed in the late 1980s by the queer community, who have embraced it.

Other useful terms

- **Cis/Cisgender**: Someone whose gender identity is the same as the sex they were assigned at birth.

- **Deadnaming**: Calling someone by their birth name after they have changed their name. This term is often associated with trans people who have changed their name as part of their transition.

- **Gender**: Often expressed in terms of masculinity and femininity, gender is largely culturally determined and is assumed from the sex assigned at birth.

- **Gender identity**: A person's innate sense of their own gender, whether masculine, feminine or something else which may or may not correspond to the sex assigned at birth.

- **Gender dysphoria**: Used to describe when a person experiences discomfort or distress because there is a mismatch between their sex assigned at birth and their gender identity. This is also the clinical diagnosis for someone who doesn't feel comfortable with the sex they were assigned at birth.

- **Non-binary**: A term for people whose gender identity doesn't sit comfortably with 'man' or 'woman'. Non-binary identities are varied and can include people who identify with some aspects of binary identities, while others reject them entirely.

- **Pansexual/Pan**: Refers to a person whose romantic and/or sexual attraction towards others is not limited by sex or gender.

- **Transgender man**: A term used to describe someone who is assigned female at birth but identifies and lives as a man. This may be shortened to trans man, or FTM, an abbreviation for female-to-male.

- **Transgender woman**: A term used to describe someone who is assigned male at birth but identifies and lives as a woman. This may be shortened to trans woman, or MTF, an abbreviation for male-to-female.

- **Transitioning**: The steps a trans person may take to live in the gender with which they identify. Each person's transition will involve different things. For some this involves medical intervention, such as hormone therapy and surgeries, but not all trans people want or are able to have this. Transitioning also might involve things such as telling friends and family, dressing differently and changing official documents.

(Stonewall, 2019) Reproduced with the kind permission of Stonewall.

Inequalities

LGBTQ+ people are:

- More likely to be single than non-LGBTQ+ people
- Less likely to have children than non-LGBTQ+ people
- Much more likely to be estranged from their birth families (though many LGBTQ+ people will have alternative family structures in place)
- More likely to have worse general health outcomes when compared to heterosexual people, including higher rates of mental health problems, attempted suicide, self-harm, anxiety and depression.

(LGBT Foundation, 2020; Government Equalities Office, 2018)

These issues can impact patients and carers in several ways, including increased pressure on carers toward the end of life due to the increased likelihood of care being provided by a small network of people rather than an extended family group. There is also increased risk of unsupported bereavement (Marie Curie, 2016).

Many older LGBTQ+ people have lived through a period of intense social change regarding acceptance of their identities and relationships. Whilst the law may have changed, society remains not completely accepting of LGBTQ+ identities or relationships. Some LGBTQ+ people remain reluctant to come out to a healthcare professional they have just met as they anticipate discrimination (Marie Curie, 2016).

Practice Points

It is important that organisations include LGBTQ+ people in equality and diversity training, have clear anti-discrimination policies and consider displaying visible symbols of inclusion, for example rainbow lanyards or pin badges. This creates a culture of inclusion and can go some way to removing the fear of discrimination that those in the LGBTQ+ community often face (Marie Curie, 2019).

Aim not to make assumptions, but instead to carefully explore which relationships are important to patients. You could consider using questions such as, 'who's at home with you?' or 'who is important to you?'. Partners should be included in discussions in accordance with the patient's wishes. Actively invite the patient to suggest who else they would like to be involved in discussions – to make clear that you welcome their partner or family of choice to the discussions but also that their autonomy is paramount.

Table 12.1 shows ten straightforward recommendations from the ACCESSCare study to improve health and social care for LGBTQ+ people.

Table 12.1   Improving health and social care for LGBTQ+ people.

For individuals	1. Avoid using heterosexually framed or assumption-laden language
	2. Demonstrate sensitivity in exploration of sexual orientation in history
	3. Respect individuals' preferences regarding disclosure of sexual identity or gender history
	4. Carefully explore intimate relationships and significant others, including biological and chosen family (friends)
	5. Explicitly include partners and/or significant others in discussions
For services and institutions	6. Make clear statements of policies and procedures related to discrimination
	7. Include content regarding LGBTQ+ communities in training on diversity and discrimination
	8. Increase LGBTQ+ visibility in materials (in written content and images)
	9. Provide explicit markers of inclusion (e.g. rainbow lanyards or pin badges)
	10. Initiate partnerships and/or engagement with LGBTQ+ community groups

Source: Bristowe et al., 2018.

Specific practice points related to trans people

- Ask don't assume:
  - If you are not sure about someone's gender identity ask them and don't attempt to guess. Remember that some people identify as non-binary.
  - Ask the patient before placing them in a single gender multi-bedded room and take their preferences into account where possible.
- Language matters:
  - Use your patient's preferred name and pronouns at all times when talking to them or about them. Some people may wish not to use the binary pronouns he/she, they may prefer others to refer to them in gender neutral language and use pronouns such as they/their and ze/zir.

- Confidentiality:
  - Respect your patient's confidentiality and do not inappropriately disclose any information about yours patient's trans status or gender history without their consent.
- Record keeping:
  - If a patient asks for medical records to be updated with a new name or gender this can and should be done. You do not need to wait for a new birth certificate, for example.
- Not everything's about gender:
  - Gender identity and trans status is not relevant to many aspects of healthcare. 'Diagnostic overshadowing' can occur when we wrongly assume that a patient's problem is related to their transition or to transition-related healthcare. If a patient presents with a broken leg, we don't need information about their gender identity or sexuality to treat it.
- Be aware of mental health problems:
  - Being trans is not a symptom of mental illness but it is a risk factor for mental health problems, which should be considered. Be aware of the patient's increased risk of suicide or self-harm and discuss support where appropriate.

(General Medical Council, 2021)

Scenario recap

When Bob was admitted to hospital he was concerned about facing stigma due to his sexuality. Despite a rocky start to his admission, good communication from the ward team allowed him to open up about his concerns regarding end-of-life care at home and discuss ACP with the team.

This open communication allowed Bob and Michael to access the support that they needed to care for Bob at home at the end of his life and to ensure that Michael was able to access the bereavement support that he needed.

Learning Disabilities

It is estimated that there are 1.5 million people with learning disabilities living in the UK (NHS, 2018). The increase in the number of people living with learning disabilities runs parallel to improvements in both health and social care. Nevertheless, people with learning disabilities continue to experience poorer health than those without and face various barriers in accessing effective and appropriate healthcare, which leads to poorer outcomes (University of Bristol Norah Fry Centre for Disability Studies, 2017; Heslop et al., 2013).

Different malignant and non-malignant disease profiles, as well as increasing numbers of people with learning disabilities living at both ends of the age spectrum with co-morbid conditions and complex health needs mean that there is a growing need for palliative care provision for this population. People with learning disabilities who have life-limiting illness require coordinated, skilled support from their core healthcare teams, with equitable access to specialist palliative care services as required.

The role of the learning disability nurse

The learning disability nurse has a key role in supporting people with learning disabilities who have a palliative care need.

In partnership they can support the generalist or specialist healthcare role by:

- Effectively identifying and meeting health needs, including palliative care needs
- Reducing health inequalities through the promotion and implementation of reasonable adjustments supporting the patient's journey
- Promoting improved health outcomes and increasing access to general health services
- Safeguarding and supporting decision making around capacity to consent and best interests.

The learning disability nurse's role is an enablement role and does not replace the role of either generalist or specialist services.

Multidisciplinary team-working

People with a learning disability may require additional support accessing health services. When a person with a learning disability goes to their GP or is admitted to hospital, it is understood that it is important to look after both their general health and learning disability needs. Good communication between primary and acute care services and the local learning disability team is essential. Acute care liaison can ensure individuals with learning disability get additional support prior to admission, on admission or as part of the discharge process. This improves communication and supports better outcomes.

Specialist learning disability team

Learning disability nurses usually work within the wider specialist learning disability team, which is made up of a range of other professionals and may include:

- Psychiatrists
- Psychologists
- Occupational therapists
- Speech and language therapists
- Team assistants
- Administration staff
- Social workers.

Teams also work in partnership with a range of professionals, including dieticians, podiatrists and other specialist services, including mental health and palliative care.

The role of the GP

People with a learning disability often have unmet health needs. Studies have shown that they are less likely to access health screening, consult their GP or tell someone if they are feeling unwell (Help the Hospices, 2013), potentially because they do not know that they are unwell or find it difficult to communicate this.

The GP has a crucial role as the gatekeeper to other health services, ensuring diagnostic assessment as well as timely and appropriate interventions are in place to achieve good outcomes. Good outcomes for people with learning disability are achieved through collaborative and partnership working between the patient, carer, specialist learning disability services and other health and social care partners.

Diagnostic overshadowing

Diagnostic overshadowing can delay diagnosis and prevent appropriate interventions being considered, and occurs when a person's symptoms are associated with their learning disability rather than a treatable cause (Help the Hospices, 2013). Diagnostic overshadowing is especially significant when new behaviours develop, or existing ones increase. It is vital that physiological and physical changes are explored in the context of behaviour change, given the high risk of poor health in this population.

All health services have a duty to provide people with learning disability the same opportunity to services as those without. Reasonable adjustments mean that services must anticipate and be responsive and flexible so that diagnosis or treatment takes into account both the learning disability and the needs of the individual, to ensure the best health outcomes for that person are achieved. Health services must be aware that equal treatment does not mean that treatment should be the same but that it needs to be adapted or enhanced to meet the individual's needs.

Communication

Communication plays a central part in everyone's life. Most people learn to communicate as part of their natural development, but people with learning disability often need specialist help and support in order to communicate effectively with others. Health passports or communication passports may give you information to support the individual better when accessing services. It is useful to get information from the carer as well as the person with the learning disability as there may be differences in the information that you get, and it is good to hear both points of view (Sheehan et al. 2016).

It is important that we do not assume that the person with a learning disability would not understand the 'bad news' associated with palliative care and take every opportunity to engage with them in a person-centred way to support their understanding of events. Remember that, even when bad news has not been discussed, the individual will experience changes taking place, and that this can lead to stress and distress

(See Chapter 3 – Communication for more information). Often people with learning disability will be supported by a number of agencies and carers and it is important to consider coordinated, planned communication with all partners in care.

People with learning disability should be involved in decisions around their care and every opportunity should be taken to apply the principles of anticipatory care planning at every stage of the patient journey involving those that are close to them.

Frailty

Frailty is a syndrome which is related to the ageing process. Multiple body systems lose their in-built reserves, causing a progressive physiological decline, particularly characterised by sarcopenia (loss of skeletal muscle function). Patients living with frailty are at increased risk of adverse outcomes, from stressors which can be apparently minor such as an infection or new medication. Frail older people are an increasingly important group due to demographic change, but it is important to note that frailty is not an inevitable consequence of ageing and not all older people are frail (British Geriatrics Society, 2014).

Frailty can be quantified by calculating the accumulation of deficits into a frailty index. The deficits are wide ranging, from symptoms such as incontinence or hearing loss, signs such as shuffling gait, and diseases such as dementia. The frailty index correlates to a clinical frailty scale which defines patients as mildly, moderately or severely frail. Frailty can also be defined by the presence of three or more of the following criteria: involuntary weight loss, exhaustion, slow gait speed, poor handgrip strength, and sedentary behaviour (Clegg et al., 2013; Koller et al., 2013).

Frailty is dynamic, and can improve, but transition to a level of worse frailty is more common. Increased frailty is strongly correlated with risk of death and has a greater correlation with death than does chronological age (Kulminski et al., 2008). Frailty can therefore be used to aid prognostication and help align medical decision making with predicted prognosis, particularly in the absence of cancer or severe single-system pathology.

The end-of-life trajectory of the frail shows slowly progressive functional decline, often with intermittent episodes of sharper decline, then acceleration in decline as death approaches (Bone et al., 2016). This means that identifying the start of a terminal phase is challenging (Covinsky et al., 2003) and may contribute to the finding that although people with frailty have physical, psychosocial and support needs that are amenable to palliative intervention, they are less likely to have these needs assessed (Stow et al., 2019).

There is much a generalist can do – not least to introduce a palliative care approach early in frail patients, and then naturally increase the emphasis on this approach as frailty advances. Within this approach, end-of-life care can include curative treatments of some episodes with a more pragmatic approach to other problems (Koller et al., 2013). Communicating about such choices with patients and carers takes considerable skill.

Pain in people with frailty is similar in prevalence to pain in people with cancer (Stow et al., 2019), but despite this, pain is widely under-assessed and undertreated in older patients, especially those with cognitive impairment (Pal et al., 2014). Further to this is the theory that the presence of persistent pain further reduces physiological reserve and therefore worsens frailty itself (Shega et al., 2012).

Many of the commonly used symptom control drugs in palliative care are associated with increased risk of adverse drug reactions and side effects in the frail elderly. This often results in the drugs being prescribed inappropriately, particularly not to therapeutic levels. Drugs such as opioids and benzodiazepines should be started at low doses, with regular review and upward titration to monitor for side effects and ensure therapeutic levels are reached. Adjunctive therapies can also be useful in this drug-sensitive population and topical preparations are often well tolerated (Koller et al., 2013; Pal et al., 2014).

Polypharmacy is independently associated with frailty, and active de-prescribing should be considered in this population. Specific guidelines such as STOPP/START criteria are available and emphasise the need to keep medications which still contribute to quality of life and stop drugs which have little meaningful benefit in patients with limited life expectancy (O'Mahony et al., 2014). Frailty is specifically associated with weight loss, reduced mobility, falls and incontinence. These problems should be screened for and treatment plans included as part of frailty palliative care reviews.

It can be difficult for a generalist to know if and when to involve specialist palliative care services. Bone et al. (2016) recommend indications for referral to specialist palliative care such as complex symptoms, readiness to discuss future care, increased health service utilisation and unmet carer needs. Using a short-term integrated approach of one to three visits was found to have improved symptom management, carer well-being and reduced hospital admission, but the authors note that timing of intervention must 'balance the possible benefits of early intervention with the reality of finite specialist resource'. In reality, specialist services are often best involved for persistent or refractory symptoms (Pal et al., 2014).

Care Homes

Care homes provide a place for people to live in a homely setting. Their personal, social and nursing care needs are met by suitably trained staff. In Scotland these are residential or nursing homes run by the local authority or private providers.

Of the 34,101 long-stay residents in care homes in Scotland in 2017, 33% died within that same year (NHS National Services Scotland, 2018). Comparative data shows that in a similar community dwelling population, the annual mortality rate is on average only 3.3% (Shah et al., 2013). Although the total number of residents has fallen slightly between 2007 and 2017, there has been a significant shift in the demographic distribution, with an increase of 85–94-year-olds by 4% and a 19% increase of those aged over 95 years. The number of people admitted for respite/short-stay admissions over the same time period also increased by 96%. This data affirms the need for proactive palliative and end-of-life care to be embedded in care home healthcare provision.

Realistic anticipatory care planning is critically important and needs to begin at the time of admission to the care home, if not before. A formalised admission process should include gathering information beyond registration details, including:

- Welfare guardian/power of attorney status
- Whether an *Adults with Incapacity Act* Section 47 certificate of incapacity (in Scotland, or equivalent in other areas) and treatment plan is in place, or required, and when it should be reviewed
- Whether there is a 'Do not attempt cardiopulmonary resuscitation' (DNACPR) form and when it should be reviewed
- Weight, height and blood pressure (to support a polypharmacy review)
- Consideration of renal function assessment if medications taken require monitoring or dose adjustments for creatinine clearance
- Documentation of baseline mobility, continence, cognition and communication.

Additionally, and just as important, there should be a discussion with the next of kin and/ or their legally appointed representative regarding anticipatory care planning. This should document considerations such as:

- What would the person like to happen if they suddenly became unwell?
- What would the person like to happen if they gradually deteriorate and stop eating and drinking?
- What would the person like to happen if they don't improve after starting oral antibiotics?

Options could include:

- Being kept comfortable in the care home setting
- Having a discussion with relatives/nominated person at the time
- Going to hospital if the clinician feels this is likely to be in the person's best interests.

Planning allows the patient and family to consider realistic options, but rigid adherence may not be in their best interests and a degree of flexibility should be expected, and discussed.

With the significant mortality rate in care homes, all patients should be considered for inclusion in the Palliative Care Scheme Direct Enhanced Service (Scottish Government, Population Health Directorate, Primary Care Division, 2019), or similar assessment and review model, if available. Admission to a care home should also include a polypharmacy review (Scottish Government Polypharmacy Model of Care Group, 2018) with consideration for the individual's predicted life expectancy, to ensure all medicines are necessary and reflect Realistic Medicine principals (Calderwood, 2014–15). When deterioration is noted, medications should be further reviewed.

Pertinent information should be included in shared notes, physical or electronic, such as the Key Information Summary (KIS, e-Kis). Care can be improved in an anticipated deterioration by signposting care homes to seek suitable support in line with the patient's wishes. Moreover, when over two-thirds of the hours of the week are in the out-of-hours period, deterioration in a care home patient will often be managed by clinicians meeting the patient for the first time. Good planning will support better care.

Care homes can each stock a supply of consumables to support administration of medication for end-of-life care and these can be ordered with their other stock items such as gloves. However, medication must be on a named patient basis and there is no legal way to keep an unnamed stock supply for a prescription-only medicine in a care home setting. When syringe pumps are required these are usually provided by the local community nurse teams. Obtaining medications, in particular during the out-of-hours period, can be difficult. As such, provision during normal working hours of sufficient quantities of the right medications will avert delay. The provision of a 'just in case' box should be considered.

Taking these measures proactively does take time but allows the wishes of patients to be actively incorporated into their care and averts uncertainty at the time of any deterioration.

Remote and Rural Populations

Delivering palliative care in a remote and rural setting poses similar challenges to other care situations but can often be more exposed. This means that remote and rural clinicians have to be flexible, multi-skilled generalists.

Planning and communication

Careful planning is even more important in this setting and the need to collect as much information as possible prior to reviewing a palliative patient is essential as the distances involved can be considerably different to the more usual urban GP practice. The reviewing of hospital letters, the Key Information Summary, discussion with community staff and family, as well as the patient, prior to making a preliminary plan will ensure you have gathered whatever equipment, forms and medications you might need.

The same GP team may be providing both the in- and out-of-hours care and they must ensure communication is maintained and up to date with the wider team. In some areas, GPs work singlehandedly and provide the care with support from home care, community nurses and the family. This type of work is well deserving of the title of expert medical generalists.

Data and mobile telephone blackspots can hamper communications. Careful planning reduces the risks of delay to symptom control posed by the challenges of distance, access to medications, equipment and specialist support.

Team approach

Remote and rural areas may pose significant challenges to caring for patients with palliative and end-of-life needs due to having less access to hospitals, hospice and nursing homes (Rainsford et al., 2016). Solutions to these challenges are very much dependent on the locality and availability of the services within your area. An example of good practice to address some of those challenges is by promoting greater working partnerships between local GPs, district nurses and ambulance clinicians. A close working partnership along with timely recognition of transition to end-of-life care will facilitate suitable preparations to avoid crisis.

Following recognition of a patient requiring end-of-life care, and again once anticipatory medications have been supplied, the full team should be made aware of the patient's circumstance, history and wishes. In addition, joint training sessions may cover education in the context of anticipatory care planning, common presentations, symptom management and communication skills. This collaborative approach may facilitate the prevention of crisis before it occurs.

Transfers

Transferring patients near end of life can bring many challenges both for the crew and patient. It may be particularly challenging to find a comfortable position in which to transfer patients who may be at great risk of developing sores but need to be kept in a particular position to help their symptoms. Patients may also require continuous treatment during the transfer which could include humidified oxygen and the use of syringe pumps. With proper planning before the transfer, these issues can be identified and addressed early on.

Ambulance crews may feel apprehensive transferring such unwell patients, particularly final journeys to home/home setting. This type of journey will often be undertaken by non-clinical ambulance care assistants who may benefit from reassurance from the clinical team. A plan should be in place if the patient deteriorates during the journey: should the crew continue to the destination or divert? Is there a contact number available to the crew for support? When appropriate a family member should be encouraged to accompany the patient during transfer at the end of life.

Paramedic drug intervention

Paramedics are increasingly using anticipatory medications in the community in and out of hours (Brady, 2014). Anticipatory medications may have been prescribed in advance and available in their 'just in case' box, along with a patient specific direction (PSD) to administer as appropriate. Paramedics may use these medications legally (Department of Health, 2006), however they will need to ensure they are working in line with their trust's own clinical guidelines (JRCALC and AACE, 2019). In the absence of anticipatory medications, paramedics can still provide symptom control via their own supply of medications in line with JRCALC Clinical Guidelines – End of Life Care (JRCALC, 2019).

Roos L et al. (2013) Relationship between adverse childhood experiences and homelessness and the impact of Axis I and II disorders. *American Journal of Public Health*, 103(S2): s275–s281.

Scottish Government Polypharmacy Model of Care Group (2018) Polypharmacy Guidance Realistic Prescribing 3rd Edition. *Scottish Government*. Available at: https://www.therapeutics.scot.nhs.uk/wp-content/uploads/2018/04/Polypharmacy-Guidance-2018.pdf

Scottish Government, Population Health Directorate, Primary Care Division (2019) The Primary Medical Services Directed Enhanced Services (Scotland) 2019 Palliative Care Scheme. Available at: https://www.sehd.scot.nhs.uk/pca/PCA2019(M)06.pdf

Scottish Palliative Care Guidelines (2021). Choosing and Changing Opioids. Available at: https://www.palliativecareguidelines.scot.nhs.uk/guidelines/pain/choosing-and-changing-opioids.aspx

Shah S et al. (2013) Mortality in older care home residents in England and Wales. *Age and Ageing*, 42(2): 209–215.

Sheehan R et al. (2016) An audit of the quality of inpatient care for adults with learning disability in the UK. *BMJ Open*, 6: e010480.

Shega JW et al. (2012) Persistent pain and frailty: a case for homeostenosis. *Journal of the American Geriatric Society*, 60(1): 113–117.

Shulman C et al. (2018) End-of-life care for homeless people: a qualitative analysis exploring the challenges to access and provision of palliative care. *Palliative Medicine*, 32(1): 36–45.

Song J et al. (2007a) Dying on the streets: homeless persons' concerns and desires about end of life care. *Journal of General Internal Medicine*, 22(4): 435–441.

Song J et al. (2007b) Experiences with and attitudes towards death and dying among homeless persons. *Journal of General Internal Medicine*, 22(4): 427–434.

Stonewall (2019) Glossary of terms. Available at: https://www.stonewall.org.uk/help-advice/faqs-and-glossary/glossary-terms

Stow D et al. (2019) What is the evidence that people with frailty have need for palliative care at the end of life? A systematic review and narrative synthesis. *Palliative Medicine*, 33(4): 399–414.

Tobey M et al. (2017) Homeless individuals approaching the end of life: symptoms and attitudes. *Journal of Pain and Symptom Management*, 53(4): 738–744.

Turner M et al. (2018) Ageing and dying in the contemporary neoliberal prison system: exploring the 'double burden' for older prisoners. *Social Science and Medicine*, 212: 161–167.

University of Bristol Norah Fry Centre for Disability Studies (2017) The Learning Disabilities Mortality Review (LeDeR) Programme: Annual Report. Bristol: Norah Fry Centre for Disability Studies, University of Bristol.

World Prison Brief (2019) World prison population lists. Available at: http://www.prisonstudies.org/highest-to-lowest/prison-population-total

Chapter 13

Caring for People in the Last Days and Hours of Life

Sandra Campbell with Jane Boyden, Emma Dymond, Nicola Lewthwaite, Lesley Middleton and Elaine Stevens

Learning Objectives

At the completion of this chapter, you will be able to do the following:

- Describe the value of applying the four key principles defined in the guidance from the Scottish Government (2014), *Caring for People in the Last Days and Hours of Life*
- Discuss the complexity of recognising the dying phase and the importance of performing a holistic assessment
- Discuss the importance of open and honest communication in the provision of care in the last days of life
- Discuss how to manage care of the dying in different care settings
- Describe the procedure for the confirmation of death and provide care of the person after death as well as the bereaved.

Scenarios

The scenarios presented below provide a discussion point to highlight the application of the key principles with reference made to particular nuances depending upon care setting. They highlight the need for and demonstrate the value of ongoing assessment.

Scenario 1

Background

Seamus is a 60-year-old man with locally advanced tonsillar cancer and learning difficulties. A multidisciplinary decision was reached to treat with palliative intent from the outset with a focus on a person-centred approach as he would not tolerate complex interventions, for example the use of a feeding tube. He has a team of carers and nurses in his nursing home, but no remaining family. He is unable to swallow, so oral route medicines cannot be used. A fentanyl patch is used for analgesia.

Key points

- Capacity issues
- No family or next of kin to offer him support
- Overwhelming fear
- Applying four key principles
- Recognising the dying phase
- Managing terminal agitation in the community
- Support for nursing home team.

Timeline

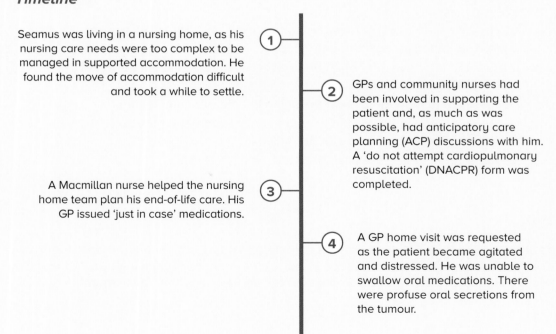

Seamus was living in a nursing home, as his nursing care needs were too complex to be managed in supported accommodation. He found the move of accommodation difficult and took a while to settle.

1

2 GPs and community nurses had been involved in supporting the patient and, as much as was possible, had anticipatory care planning (ACP) discussions with him. A 'do not attempt cardiopulmonary resuscitation' (DNACPR) form was completed.

A Macmillan nurse helped the nursing home team plan his end-of-life care. His GP issued 'just in case' medications.

3

4 A GP home visit was requested as the patient became agitated and distressed. He was unable to swallow oral medications. There were profuse oral secretions from the tumour.

Reversible causes of agitation and deterioration were excluded. Review of GP and multidisciplinary team (MDT) discussions. **(5)**

(6) A difficult decision regarding place of care was settled in the nursing home and well supported by staff.

Key considerations

- What process would the care home staff have gone through to get support and advice regarding the initial challenge of feeding?
- Are we always responsive in a timely manner?
- Can we consider the relationship between the carers and the person in the care home?

Scenario 2

Background

Preeta is a 62-year-old woman who was admitted to hospital with dyspnoea, lethargy and collapse. A CT scan shows pneumonia, bilateral pulmonary emboli and lung mass with liver mediastinal lymphadenopathy; bloods show hypercalcaemia. Initial treatment improves her condition, but then there is a sudden decline. Her husband is her next of kin.

Key points

- Prioritising patients' wishes when they lack capacity; using adults with incapacity legislation as well as principles of the Act
- In last days of life discontinue bloods, observations, unnecessary interventions and review medications
- New diagnosis and time for patient and significant other to come to terms with this
- Impact on her husband and the rest of the staff caring for her.

Timeline

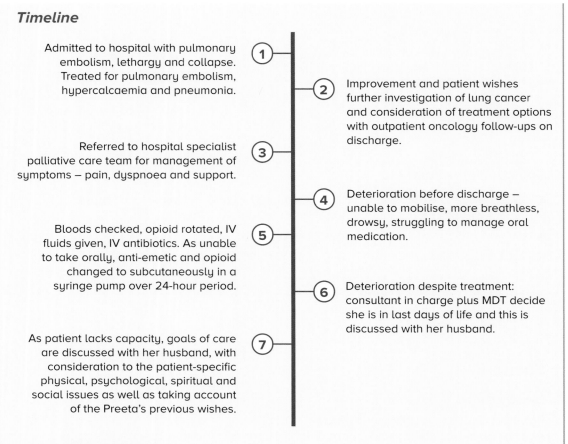

① Admitted to hospital with pulmonary embolism, lethargy and collapse. Treated for pulmonary embolism, hypercalcaemia and pneumonia.

② Improvement and patient wishes further investigation of lung cancer and consideration of treatment options with outpatient oncology follow-ups on discharge.

③ Referred to hospital specialist palliative care team for management of symptoms – pain, dyspnoea and support.

④ Deterioration before discharge – unable to mobilise, more breathless, drowsy, struggling to manage oral medication.

⑤ Bloods checked, opioid rotated, IV fluids given, IV antibiotics. As unable to take orally, anti-emetic and opioid changed to subcutaneously in a syringe pump over 24-hour period.

⑥ Deterioration despite treatment: consultant in charge plus MDT decide she is in last days of life and this is discussed with her husband.

⑦ As patient lacks capacity, goals of care are discussed with her husband, with consideration to the patient-specific physical, psychological, spiritual and social issues as well as taking account of the Preeta's previous wishes.

Key considerations

- How do we facilitate conversations with families when the patient lacks capacity?
- How do we support families when dying is so rapid from the onset of illness?
- What factors influence remaining in hospital?

Key Principles

In response to the withdrawal of the Liverpool Care Pathway, the Scottish Government developed guidance for caring for people in the last days and hours of life (Scottish Government, 2014). This guidance suggests compliance with four key principles (see Table 13.1) relating to communication and care planning according to individual needs and including caring for those who are bereaved. The information within this chapter will support application of these key principles.

Table 13.1   The four key principles.

No.	Key principle
1	Informative, timely and sensitive communication is an essential component of each individual person's care.
2	Significant decisions about a person's care, including diagnosing dying, are made on the basis of multidisciplinary discussion.
3	Each individual person's physical, psychological, social and spiritual needs are addressed as far as is possible.
4	Consideration is given to the well-being of relatives or carers attending the person.

Source: Scottish Government, 2014.

Recognition of the Dying Phase

It can be challenging to identify when someone is entering the dying phase. At times it can be unclear if a patient will respond to treatment, however there are some indicators that will help to allow the team looking after a patient to review the appropriateness of ongoing treatment. This is a crucial time for sensitive communication with patients and significant others around changing the focus of care. Staff in various care settings, including prison staff and those working in homeless shelters, also require education and knowledge to recognise deterioration in a person's condition that may signify the dying phase. Failure to act on these changes may also result in missed opportunities for family reconciliation (Jones, 2011) (see Chapter 12 – Specific Populations for more information on palliative care for the homeless and those in prison, as well as other communities and groups).

All patients should be assessed individually but if there is an ongoing deterioration despite treating reversible causes, then some signs in someone with a life-limiting condition that might indicate a patient's prognosis is short include:

- Reduced consciousness
- Reduced oral intake
- Inability to take oral medication
- Significant change in usual mobility – bed-bound.

Preferred Place of Care

In Scotland in 2018/19, there were 53,168 deaths recorded. For these people, 89.2% of their last six months of life was spent either at home or in the community setting, with the remaining 10.8% spent in hospital (Information Services Division Scotland, 2019). This is equivalent to each individual spending an average of 20 days in hospital in the 6 months prior to their death.

In England and Wales in 2016, 46.9% of people died in hospital, 21.8% in care homes, 23.5% at home and 5.7% in hospices (Figure 13.1).

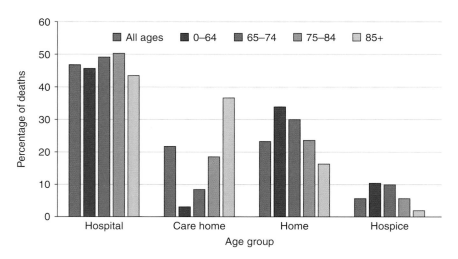

Figure 13.1 Percentage of deaths (persons, all ages) in hospital, care homes, home and hospices, England, 2016.

Source: Public Health England, 2018.

For people approaching the end of life, being cared for and dying at home surrounded by loved ones is often the preferred choice. However, we also know that currently too many people's preferences are not being met. For example, 64% of people with cancer would prefer to die at home with the right support (Macmillan, 2018), yet less than a third (30%) do so (Office for National Statistics, 2016). Macmillan estimates that every year in the UK 62,000 people die of cancer in hospital, despite the majority of people with cancer stating that they would like to die at home (Macmillan, 2017). The numbers above show that a significant group of people are not where they would prefer to be at the end of their life.

Finding out a person's preferred place for end-of-life care, and death, should be part of good anticipatory care planning and documented in the person's record. However, people can change their minds and it is therefore important to revisit the preferred place of care at different points in their illness, including when they are approaching the last days of life. Clarifying the person's wishes by facilitating open conversations about the realistic options in their individual situation is paramount to achieving the best outcome. It is important to be open and honest about the complexity of managing beds in a hospice, for instance, and to communicate sensitively but effectively that beds are allocated according to priority of need.

Considerations for patients in hospital

For some patients, hospital is their preferred place of care, with some patients having established trust in their relationships with hospital teams. Other patients may find themselves deteriorating and require hospital admission, and at this point a careful discussion around the preferred place of death may be necessary. There needs to be careful consideration given to realistic options to meet the patient's care needs and if it is decided that they should remain in the environment of an acute medical ward, then the goals of care – prioritising the patient's comfort and supporting their next of kin – should be clear to the medical and nursing teams involved in their care.

Should a rapid discharge home be decided upon at the end of life, there is a robust framework in the Scottish Palliative Care Guidelines to support the objective that everyone involved in the patient's care is aware of their role in making the discharge to home as successful as possible (Scottish Palliative Care Guidelines, 2020a).

For many patients, dying at home is their final wish. To achieve this effectively, care coordination between all professionals is vital. Collaborative working between health and social care, acute and community, as well as third sector organisations, is central to ensuring a high standard of patient care with the community nurse being the main link between them all.

One vital aspect of care of the dying is the level of support in place for family and informal carers whilst the person is at home. Informal carers play a significant role in the person being able to remain in the home safely. It is also crucial that the carer receives the support they require to enable them to continue caring. It can be challenging to balance support and the necessary care provision with the intrusion on family life. When care is being coordinated, careful consideration should be given to what services are commissioned, with the minimum number of different people being involved.

Goals of Care and Holistic Assessment of Needs

Considerations irrespective of care setting

When meeting a new patient, consider adopting the use of the Patient Dignity Question (PDQ) by Professor Harvey Chochinov (Chochinov et al., 2005): 'What do I need to know about you as a person to provide the best care possible?'.

Research in Scotland demonstrates that dignity therapy improves the perception of care by patients and carers (Johnston et al., 2015).

Discuss with the patient and their significant others (as much as is desired by the patient) the current situation, likely changes over time and what their priorities of care are, given the deterioration in their condition.

Common considerations in this context are:

- Continue holistic assessment in the four domains: physical, psychological, social and spiritual
- Discontinue medications that are not providing symptom benefit
- Establish an individual care plan to reflect the patient's priorities

- Ensure regular reassessment for effective ongoing care and timely symptom management
- If the patient is unable to communicate their wishes, take into account any previous wishes, anticipatory care plans and consult their power of attorney, welfare guardian or next of kin
- A DNACPR decision should be part of discussions and decisions documented in the patient's notes
- Consider the environment, guided by patient's individual needs
- Provide support for the carer
- Ensure that the patient's and family's wishes are met regarding who is present at the time of death; this is important although not always possible.

These common considerations are fundamental to providing excellent end-of-life care.

Specific considerations for patients in hospital

When a decision has been made by the consultant in charge of a patient's care, their MDT and the patient and significant others that the patient is deteriorating and further treatment/ escalation of care is not appropriate, then the focus of care changes to include all of the common considerations above as well as the following:

- Avoid unnecessary investigations – discontinue blood tests and observations
- Consider the environment guided by the patient's individual needs, for example a single side room and removing unneeded medical equipment from the room
- Open visiting for significant others whilst balancing the needs of the person who is imminently dying and those important to them, but with respect for the privacy of the other patients in the hospital.

Specific considerations in the community

- Avoid admission to hospital if that would not be purposeful or effective nor in the person's best interests
- It is essential to ensure that the relevant equipment is available at short notice, that is, systems that are responsive and can provide what is required in a timely manner.

Managing Symptoms

Regular assessment is required to identify changing needs with regard to symptom control. It is important to consider whether any oral medication that the patient may no longer be able to manage needs to be converted to a syringe pump. There should be anticipatory medication prescribed for pain, anxiety, agitation, nausea and vomiting, respiratory secretions and any other anticipated problem in each individual. Consideration should be given to whether a patient is at risk of a significant event such as terminal hemorrhage, airway obstruction or seizure. Sensitive communication with informal carers is essential, especially if the person is in their own home, to prepare them should any of these situations arise.

Since the COVID-19 pandemic, the number of deaths has increased significantly within the palliative care setting. This has had a serious impact on services and staff. Patients dying from COVID-19 often deteriorate rapidly and require more timely access to as-required medication. Systems must be in place, especially in care homes, to ensure drugs may be administered every 15 minutes if necessary. Current advice is available from the Scottish Palliative Care Guidelines. However, these guidelines are in constant flux as our understanding of COVID-19 evolves.

'Just in case' boxes

When someone is in their own home, a lack of breakthrough symptom control and anticipatory palliative care medication is a factor in contributing to unnecessary hospital admissions at end of life. Palliative care 'just in case' boxes within the community setting are one solution to this. If it is anticipated that the patient's medical condition may deteriorate into the terminal phase of illness, and with consent from the patient and/or carer, the community team can initiate and prescribe a palliative care 'just in case' emergency medicines box. The community pharmacy will receive the prescription and supply the emergency medicines box. The box will be kept in the patient's home for rapid administration of medicines commonly prescribed for breakthrough symptom control.

All medicines need to be prescribed with doses, indication and directions for administration then signed and dated as usual in the patient's community nursing notes. This then enables a community nurse to administer the prescribed medication in a timely manner. The community nurse records the use of any medications in the patient's notes and arranges for the box to be restocked. If symptoms persist, a review of continuous medications should be carried out to ensure patient comfort. If a 'just in case' box is being considered, sensitive communication to explain what this is for and how to store drugs/box is required. It may be appropriate for the family to administer breakthrough medication, but this will depend upon local policies. Community teams should follow local policy/guidance on this practice, which should comply with the Scottish Palliative Care Guidelines (2020b).

Nutrition and Hydration

In the last days of life patients may be unconscious or be unable to swallow. It is important to make sure that if patients are able to take food/fluid orally that this is supported and offered. When patients can no longer swallow then good mouth care is essential. The goals of care and overall benefit versus burden of artificial hydration/nutrition should always be considered in discussion with the patient (where possible) and their significant others.

Subcutaneous fluids may be considered in certain situations for patients in their last days of life if it is felt that this would alleviate particular symptoms such as thirst or thick secretions, but should be reviewed regularly. However, subcutaneous fluids may not be possible in every care setting and therefore careful consideration of the burden versus benefit of using them in individual cases should be discussed between the clinical team involved in care, the patient (where possible) and their significant others. It is important to have sensitive communication with families about the reduced need for food and fluids when natural dying is occurring. See Chapter 4.2 – The Gastrointestinal System 'Nutrition' (p. 123) and 'Mouth Care' (p. 129) for more information.

Communication

Communication with those important to the person who is dying is pivotal in supporting them to cope with what is for most a highly emotional time. It is also essential that staff communicate effectively with the person who is dying if they are conscious and able to communicate. If the person is not conscious, staff should continue to communicate, for example explaining what care is being given. It is therefore important that teams communicate with each other and ensure that any staff caring for people who are dying are made aware of the situation before they enter a room in a ward or arrive at the place of care. Training appropriate to their role should be available to staff at all levels.

Please refer to Chapter 3 – Communication, for detailed information regarding communication and further information on the importance of anticipatory care planning. Additional helpful hints for consideration are suggested below to support staff with communication when caring for someone in the dying phase.

Communicating with the person who is dying

'Truth hurts but deceit hurts more', Fallowfield et al. (2004). Always answer honestly!

If asked 'Am I dying?' – rather than a direct 'yes' use a gentle response such as: 'You must be feeling really poorly to ask me that?' or 'Has anyone talked to you about dying'? 'Are you able to tell me what the doctor said?' Try to facilitate open conversation that is person-led before saying that they are dying. Consider using a model to establish what level of perception the person has before responding.

Continue talking to the person even when they lose consciousness, gently explaining what care is being provided.

Consider the importance of the environment, perhaps music that the person liked playing quietly in the background and perfume that is familiar to the person. Minimise the medicalisation of death by removing unnecessary equipment.

Communicating with those important to the person who is dying

It can be very alarming for families when they know their loved one is dying and they do not know what to expect. It is helpful to provide gentle explanations as families do want to know what to expect (Mannix, 2017).

Below are some useful phrases:

Do not resuscitate does not mean no care.

By not performing CPR we allow a natural death that ensures respect and dignity for...

Can you tell me how you think mum is doing ... and how were they a few weeks ago?

Can you help me understand...

I can see this is really difficult for you...

Would it be helpful if I explained what to expect?

Supporting significant others

It can be an unpredictable and extremely upsetting time for the significant others of a patient who is in the last days of life. It is important to include them in discussion (with the patient's permission, where possible) around how the patient's current care needs are being met, and allow time for any concerns or questions to be addressed. It may be important to consider giving further information about local bereavement support or signpost to helpful information for specific issues.

Not all deaths are 'expected' and for the more traumatic situations, such as experienced in an intensive care unit when a person has perhaps only had a short illness, or has had an accident resulting in brain injury requiring a ventilator to be switched off, it is important that staff are familiar with local policy and practices to provide as much support as possible to those important to the person dying. Sensitive communication with those close to the person regarding the practical process of withdrawal of treatment and what to expect is critical. White et al. (2019) identified three main areas of distress for nursing staff in providing end-of-life care in an acute setting:

- Moral distress: when there is perceived over-treatment
- Managing pain: when there is uncertainty regarding effective pain control
- Care/cure dichotomy: when working in an area where there is a cure-focused approach for some patients and a comfort approach for others.

(See Chapter 2 – Ethical and Legal Considerations.)

Where death is imminent and perhaps in such cases as mentioned above where young children or babies are bereaved, staff can take handprints of the person who is dying alongside handprints of the child, which is almost a gift for the child as they grow up without their parent or grandparent.

What to do after death

Please refer to Chapter 14 – Bereavement for more detailed information on bereavement care, but it is very helpful for families if the practical aspect of care around the actual time of death is managed well. It is also important to support families after the death of their loved one. There are practical considerations after death that are important to communicate to families and next of kin, as well as practical considerations for healthcare professionals.

Practical considerations for healthcare professionals

For confirmation of death, and certification, it is important to be aware of local policies in line with national guidance (NES, 2020). A consistent approach to the actual procedure of confirming the death is advocated (See Box 13.1).

- Last offices: nursing care continues after the death has occurred, however, there is limited evidence base to this practice. A crucial component of end-of-life care is to have an awareness of any religious or cultural preferences before performing last offices. Consider involving the family with the care of the person at this time, being respectful when removing any devices. (Royal Marsden NHS Foundation Trust, 2011). If the person dies at home, the community nurse may be called to confirm the death and can perform last offices at this time if the family wish this to be done.

- Make sure appropriate people are notified of the patient's death:
  - Family/next of kin/guardian/power of attorney
  - Use clear language, for example 'I'm really sorry but mum has died'. Avoid phrases such as 'passed away' or 'gone'
  - If having to inform by telephone, check when they last saw the person and gently inform them of the death.

Box 13.1   Clinical signs to confirm death

- Absence of carotid pulse over one minute confirmed AND
- Absence of heart sounds over one minute confirmed AND
- Absence of respiratory sounds over one minute confirmed AND
- No response to painful stimuli (for example trapezius squeeze) confirmed AND
- Fixed dilated pupils (unresponsive to bright light) confirmed
- Time and date clinical signs noted to be absent.

- Follow local communication systems to inform community teams (GP, district nurse, etc.):
  - It is particularly important to inform external agencies who may have been involved and may arrive at the home to perform care
  - Secondary care teams (clinics attended as outpatients, etc).
- When issuing the death certificate, do so in privacy and in as timely a manner as possible, and explain the content of the death certificate.
- Consider if there is a requirement for a post-mortem, if death is reportable to the procurator fiscal/coroner or if the patient has a previously explicit wish for organ donation/donation of body to medical science.
- When all reversible causes of deterioration have been ruled out, and where dying is possible, it is important that communication occurs between medical/nursing teams and patients and their families about clinical decisions, and that there is patient and family agreement and understanding wherever possible. Ensuring the family and significant others are aware not to call an ambulance is important to avoid unnecessary distress. It is also important they know who to phone when the death occurs.

It is important to acknowledge the potential emotional impact of caring for dying patients and for staff to be supported. Creating a culture of kindness to staff within teams is as important as kindness to patients and carers (Ballatt et al., 2015). It is also important to provide a supportive environment so staff may thrive and are able to continue to provide care. If staff are not supported with bereavement care, there is a risk they will not perform to their best, and may even be driven to leave their roles.

Practical considerations for families

- Written information such as the Scottish Government booklet 'What to do after death in Scotland – practical advice for times of bereavement' (2016) or other regional information is useful to give to next of kin, as well as advice on the death certification review service, including advance registration.
- Advice should be given on how and when to collect the death certificate, how to register a death, and the need for the family to arrange a funeral director, as well as discussing their role in arranging transfer of the patient's body and liaising with the next of kin.

Summary

It can be concluded that recognition of the dying phase and management of care in the last few days of life can be highly complex, but is viewed as a core aspect of care and at the heart of care delivery. This phase of someone's life can be managed in a more seamless manner when good communication and anticipatory care planning has facilitated conversations earlier on the journey of illness. This will support an understanding of what to expect by the patient and those important to them. Education of staff in the core domains of care as defined by NHS Education for Scotland (NES, 2017), developing skills of holistic assessment, and symptom control, as well as good communication, is vital to enable staff to provide the highest standard of care possible at, what can be for some, a most traumatic time. Compliance with the four key principles relating to communication, assessment and care planning, and care of the relatives will facilitate the optimum outcome.

Scenario Recap

Scenario 1

When death was imminent, Seamus was too distressed to be transferred to a hospice. Terminal agitation was managed in the community. 'Just in case' medication use was reviewed and a syringe pump was prescribed as a backup for symptom control. The GP communicated with the local palliative care team on medicines and doses to use. Good symptom control was achieved and the GP visited regularly to review the patient and completed a palliative care summary for the out of hours teams. The district nurses offered support to the nursing home team. The patient died peacefully two days later. The GP checked in with nursing home team after the event.

Scenario 2

It was decided that Preeta would remain in a side room on the ward for end-of-life care with treatment of symptoms and comfort prioritised. Observations, antibiotics, IV fluids and bloods, were all stopped as she approached the end of her life. Support was offered to her husband and regular updates were given to him on Preeta's condition, as well as information of what to expect as the patient deteriorated. When Preeta's condition began to deteriorate rapidly her husband was informed and was by her side when she died in hospital.

References

Chochinov H et al. (2005) Dignity therapy: a novel psychotherapeutic intervention for patients near the end of life. *Journal of Clinical Oncology*, 23(24): 5520–5525.

Ballatt J and Campling P (2015) *Intelligent Kindness, Reforming the Culture of Healthcare*. London: Royal College of Psychiatrists Publications.

Fallowfield L and Jenkins V (2004) Communicating sad, bad, and difficult news in medicine. *Lancet*, 363(9405): 312–319.

Information Services Division Scotland (2019) Percentage of End of Life Spent at Home or in a Community Setting. An Official Statistics Publication for Scotland. Available at: https://www.isdscotland.org/Health-Topics/Health-and-Social-Community-Care/Publications/2019-05-28/2019-05-28-End-of-Life-Report.pdf?20408266783

Johnston B et al. (2015) The person behind the patient: a feasibility study using the PDQ for patients with palliative care needs. *International Journal of Palliative Nursing*, 21(2): 71–77.

Jones L (2011) Homeless people. In Oliverie D, Monroe B and Payne S (2011) *Death, Dying, and Social Differences*, 2nd edition. Oxford: Oxford University Press.

Macmillan (2017). The final injustice: variation in end of life care in England. Available from: https://www.macmillan.org.uk/_images/MAC16904-end-of-life-policy-report_tcm9-321025.pdf

Macmillan (2018) Missed opportunities. Advanced care planning report. Available at: https://www. macmillan.org.uk/_images/missed-opportunities-end-of-life-advance-care-planning_tcm9-326204.pdf

Mannix K (2017) *With the End in Mind: Dying, Death and Wisdom in an Age of Denial.* London: William Collins.

NHS Education for Scotland (NES) (2017) Palliative and end of life care: a framework to support learning and development needs of the health and social service workforce in Scotland. Edinburgh: NHS Education Scotland.

NHS Education for Scotland (2020) Guidance and supporting resources for practitioners undertaking the Confirmation of Death procedure in Scotland. Available at: https://policyonline.nhslothian.scot/Policies/ Guideline/NES%20Guidance%20and%20supporting%20resources%20re%20Confirmation%20of%20 Death%20Procedure%20in%20Scotland.pdf

Office for National Statistics (2016) Deaths registered in England and Wales in 2015. Available at: https://www.ons.gov.uk/peoplepopulationandcommunity/birthsdeathsandmarriages/deaths/bulletins/ deathsregistrationsummarytables/2015

Public Health England (2018) Statistical commentary: end of life care profiles, February 2018 update. Available at: https://www.gov.uk/government/statistics/end-of-life-care-profiles-february-2018-update/ statistical-commentary-end-of-life-care-profiles-february-2018-update

Royal Marsden NHS Foundation Trust (2011) *The Royal Marsden Hospital Manual of Clinical Nursing Procedures*, 8th edition. London: Wiley-Blackwell.

Scottish Government (2014) Caring for people in the last days and hours of life – guidance. Available at: https://www.gov.scot/publications/caring-people-last-days-hours-life-guidance/

Scottish Government (2017) What to do after a death in Scotland – practical advice for times of bereavement: revised 11th edition 2016 (web only). Available at: https://www.gov.scot/publications/ death-scotland-practical-advice-times-bereavement-revised-11th-edition-2016-9781786522726/

Scottish Palliative Care Guidelines (2020a) Rapid Transfer Home in the Last Days of Life. Available at: https://www.palliativecareguidelines.scot.nhs.uk/guidelines/end-of-life-care/rapid-transfer-home-in-the- last-days-of-life.aspx

Scottish Palliative Care Guidelines (2020b). Anticipatory Prescribing. Available at: https://www. palliativecareguidelines.scot.nhs.uk/guidelines/pain/anticipatory-prescribing.aspx

White D and Meeker MA (2019) Guiding the process of dying: the personal impact on nurses. *Journal of Hospice and Palliative Nursing*, 21(5): 390–396.

Chapter 14

Bereavement

Mark R Evans with Alison Allan, Sharon Dick,
Liz Henderson and Catriona Macpherson

Learning Objectives

At the completion of this chapter you should be able to:

- Understand that grief is a normal emotional response experienced by an individual following the death of a significant person
- Identify the different types of grief responses
- Understand the principles of bereavement care.

Scenario

Background

Betty is a 73-year-old woman being cared for at home with end stage heart failure. Betty has been offered a bed in the local hospice, but she wants to die at home surrounded by her family. Betty's husband, Sam, died suddenly in the local hospital 5 years previously. Betty wasn't present when Sam died and she regrets this, feeling that she let Sam and Gemma, her daughter, down. She is terrified that she may be taken into the hospice or the hospital and die surrounded by strangers.

Key points

- For many patients and carers the processes around death can be frightening and isolating
- For family and carers, the grief journey can start long before the death of the patient. However, it is important to remember that the patient may also experience a grief reaction

- Healthcare professionals should recognise the specific needs of the various members of the family and give appropriate information and support

- Terminal patients and the wider family can experience intense emotions before the death (for example regret, fear) and after the death (for example anger, guilt)

Timeline

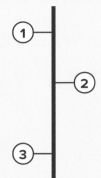

Betty lives with her daughter Gemma and grandchildren (Laura, 7 years old, and Peter, 14 years old, who suffers from anxiety and depression). Betty has expressed that her preferred place of care and death is at home surrounded by her family.

② Betty's daughter Gemma, while wanting to carry out Betty's wishes, is anxious about how Betty's dying at home may affect her children. Gemma is struggling to support both Betty and her children whilst caring for herself.

Betty's symptoms are well managed by the community team. She often speaks to the district nurses about her fears and concerns for her daughter and her grandchildren and how they will cope following her death.

Key considerations

- What preparation/support may Betty and the family need prior to death?

- How can the healthcare team support Gemma and her children after Betty's death?

- What possible complications/difficulties may Gemma and her family face following Betty's death?

Introduction to Bereavement and Grief

In 2020 there were 62,415 deaths in Scotland (Scottish Government, 2021). On average, for each death four people will experience some form of grief. As such, it is important that healthcare professionals have some understanding of what is meant by grief and bereavement and how to provide appropriate support.

The Oxford English Dictionary describes 'grief' as 'a feeling of great sadness, especially when someone dies'. It also defines 'bereavement' as 'the action or condition of being bereaved' (Stevension A, 2010). It is important to remember that grief is not a condition or an illness but a normal emotional reaction to the death of a significant person. Death, grief and bereavement are all normal experiences of life.

Stages, phases and theories

It was Freud who first sought to describe grief as a condition, suggesting that for the bereaved to recover they had to break the emotional ties with the deceased. Since the 1950s a number of models have been developed (for example Kübler-Ross's '5 Stages of Grief') that have sought to theorise the experience of grief (Buglass, 2010). Such theories have shaped our understanding of grief and have influenced bereavement care. In the past there has been a tendency to medicalise and pathologise grief and bereavement. Whilst such models can be helpful in supporting our understanding of the processes, they should not be used as 'tick lists'. It is important to remember that, when talking about grief, we are not talking about a condition or a process but an experience, an experience that is unique to each individual. Rather than a process, grief should be seen as a journey, a journey on which people may need support to adapt to life without the deceased (Dyregrov et al., 2008).

A pill for all ills

Whilst there is evidence that the bereaved can be at a greater risk of developing physical and mental health issues, it is important to remember that grief, in itself, is not an illness and should not be treated as such (Stroebe et al., 2017). Those experiencing grief will often experience intense and prolonged emotions such as sadness, guilt, regret, anger and betrayal. In addition, the bereaved may also experience low mood, a change in dietary habits and a general loss of interest in life.

Due to the intensity of the emotions and the unfamiliar experience as a whole, it is common for the bereaved to seek help from healthcare professionals. The bereaved often come seeking 'something' to 'make it better' and take away the pain. When faced with the raw pain of grief, healthcare professionals can feel powerless. In trying to help it can be tempting to provide medication to alleviate the intense feelings experienced by the bereaved, especially in the initial stages.

Antidepressants

The difference between the manifestations of grief and the symptoms of clinical depression or mental illness can, at times, be tissue thin. However, established symptomatic criteria should be used where there is concern about the presence of depression. It is therefore important that a full assessment is carried out to rule out depression, underlying health issues or the presence of unresolved or complex grief. Whilst unresolved grief can lead to depression and mental health issues, grief is not an illness and is unlikely to respond to medication such as antidepressants (Royal College of Psychiatrists, 2015). Antidepressants should only be considered if there are indications that the grief is deepening or contributing to the development of clinical depression (Tol et al., 2014).

Sleeping tablets

Those experiencing bereavement will often complain of poor or broken sleep and may seek 'something' to help them sleep. It is important that the healthcare professional discusses good sleep hygiene with the bereaved. Individuals may find complementary therapies such as aromatherapy (e.g. lavender oil) or relaxation techniques such as mindfulness and relaxation useful (see Chapter 11 – Complementary Therapies, for further information on this). Caution should be taken before prescribing barbiturates and other medications to help sleep, especially in the first few days following a death, depending on the client's needs. If problems with sleeping continue for a prolonged period of time it may be appropriate to consider offering the bereaved a short course (2–3 days) of sleeping tablets (Royal College of Psychiatrists, 2015).

Sick leave

Doctors will frequently be asked for a 'sick note' as the bereaved person feels unable to attend their work. Careful consideration should be given to the length of time that the bereaved are perceived as being 'unfit' for work. Whilst some bereaved people may be unable or, depending on their job, unsafe to return to work (especially in the initial stages), returning to work on a phased/part-time basis within a supportive environment can provide structure, routine and companionship to those who feel lost, alone and out of control.

Counselling

The experience of grief can be very unsettling and the bereaved may report 'feeling out of control'. Due to the intense emotional response the bereaved may report seeing the deceased or experiencing noises or smells associated with the deceased. Such experiences may cause the bereaved to think that they are 'not coping' or are 'going crazy'. As such, the bereaved, their family and friends may seek counselling to help them cope.

Only 10–20% of those who are bereaved will develop complex or unresolved grief that will require some form of therapy or counselling (Dyregrov et al., 2008). In most cases referral to psychology or mental health teams is inappropriate. In addition, some research questions the benefits of referring those with noncomplex (normal) grief. That being said, most bereaved people will benefit from bereavement support. It is therefore advisable that healthcare professionals are aware of local and national organisations and groups providing bereavement support.

The doctor will see you now...

There is no magical anaesthetic or medication for the pain of grief and bereavement. However, Healthcare professionals have a vital role in 'normalising' the experience of grief and supporting the bereaved as they adjust to life without the deceased.

Listening is the essence of bereavement care. In caring for the bereaved we need to listen and hear their story; a listening ear is the most important therapeutic intervention which can be offered. When healthcare professionals get it right (showing empathy and providing compassionate care), those who are experiencing grief can be supported to adapt and re-establish meaning, purpose and hope (see Chapter 3 – Communication, for more information). Table 14.1 also gives some recommendations on providing bereavement care as a healthcare professional.

Table 14.1   Tips on bereavement care.

Try to:	Try not to:
• Encourage the bereaved to share their story at their pace	• Avoid those who are experiencing grief
• Tolerate silences and emotions; don't take anger and other emotions personally	• Use platitudes such as 'time heals' or 'I know how you feel'
• Offer reassurance and support and 'normalise'	• Use euphemisms such as 'passed' or 'lost'
• Accept that you cannot make things better or take away their pain	• Assume that you know what the person is feeling/experiencing
• Know your limitations and know when to refer	• Speak about your own experience or beliefs
• Have a multicultural understanding of/ approach to death	• Make the client feel rushed
• Be familiar with the developmental stages of understanding around death	• Appear abrupt when using words such as death or dead
• Be aware of other significant points such as adolescence, familial relationships, that could impact the grieving process	• Assume all is well. Very seldom will a death not generate strong feelings, even if the event might seem to generate 'happy' feelings (for example when a perpetrator of abuse has died).
• Gently use the correct terminology such as dying, died and dead	
• Read between the lines – what you see might not be what is really presenting	
• Help the client know that, if you are not the right person, a referral has been sent to the appropriate provider to help him/ her know they are not left unsupported.	

Preparation

Death remains one of the few great taboos, with the process surrounding it shrouded in myth and mystery. Whilst care of the dying and the death of patients is a regular occurrence for most healthcare professionals, for family and carers the death of a loved one is a unique event and is only witnessed and experienced a few times in life. Those who care for a dying loved one are frequently unprepared for the last few days and hours. Changes in the patient's symptoms and overall condition, whilst normal and expected in a clinical sense, can be frightening and distressing for the patient, their loved ones and those caring for them.

Dame Cicely Saunders, the founder of the modern palliative care movement, said: 'How people die remains in the memory of those who live on.' Whilst we can never be fully prepared for the death of a loved one, timely, sensitive and clear communication from healthcare professionals about possible events and changes to an individual's condition when they are dying can reduce fear and distress. It is therefore essential that when healthcare staff recognise that a patient has entered the 'dying phase', discussions take place between the healthcare team and those caring for the patient to ensure that a care plan is in place to meet the needs of the patient and support relatives (Scottish Palliative Care Guidelines, 2019).

It is important that the family are aware of which interventions can be offered by the healthcare team and which interventions would be inappropriate, for example the decision not to carry out cardiopulmonary resuscitation or provide IV fluids. It is vital that loved ones and family understand the rationale for such clinical decisions. If there is not a shared understanding, or if the family do not fully understand why clinicians made certain decisions, this can add to guilt and distress following the death of a patient, especially if the bereaved feel that they did not speak up or ensure that the person who died got the 'proper care'.

Many of the changes which occur when patients are approaching death can be very distressing for family and loved ones. As a patient once commented, 'No one gives you a Haynes Manual on death and dying.' Taking time to explain some of the changes which may occur before the event will not only reduce the anxiety and distress of those concerned, but can also reduce contacts and calls to the healthcare team (especially out of hours). Table 14.2 explores some of the areas and issues which can be useful to discuss with the family.

Table 14.2   Issues that may be discussed with the family.

Issues/areas of concern	Considerations
Agreed anticipatory care	Has a DNACPR been discussed and signed? Do the family/carers understand that the patient is dying? Do the family understand the rationale for stopping certain medication? Do they understand what interventions are now appropriate/inappropriate and why?
Decreased appetite	A lack of dietary and fluid intake can be very distressing for the family, who may be concerned that the patient is being 'starved'. Explain that as a person deteriorates their appetite and ability to swallow will decrease. Explain the needs of a dying person and suggest alternatives such as ice, sips and oral hygiene. Are carers aware what options are available when the patient is no longer able to swallow medications?
Changes to breathing	Changes to breathing patterns, especially Cheyne-Stokes breathing, can be very distressing for families. It can be helpful to compare such breathing patterns to 'snoring'. Explain that such breathing is more distressing for the family than the patient.

Table 14.2 (*Continued*).

Changes to bladder/ bowels	Explain that a reduction in dietary and fluid intake means that the person's bladder and bowel functions may slow down or be absent.
	Explain that due to frailty, the patient may be unable to use a toilet/ commode and as such there is a risk that the patient may be incontinent.
	Explore with the family how they may respond to this and what support/ resources are available to keep the patient dry and comfortable.
Confusion, restlessness and agitation	Explain that simply being present and talking to the person in a calm manner can reduce restlessness and agitation.
	Encourage family and friends to maintain a calm environment. If it becomes worse should medication be considered?
Changes to skin	Explain that the patient's skin may feel cold or their hands may swell—explain that this is normal and not painful.
Increased sleeping	As the patient becomes sleepier they may interact less with those around them.
	Explain that the patient can still hear and encourage the family to speak to the patient as 'normal'.
	It can be helpful to encourage loved ones to say things which are 'important' such as 'goodbye'. It can also be helpful for loved ones to give the patient 'permission to go'.
Meeting spiritual, religious or cultural needs	Are there particular religious or cultural needs surrounding the last acts of care that healthcare professionals should be aware of?
Waiting/ bedside vigils	During the final days and hours, families may commence a 'bedside vigil'.
	Explain that patients may 'choose' to die when loved ones leave the room/are not present.
When to get help	Do carers understand the difference between expected/normal changes in the patent's condition and a sudden, acute or unexpected deterioration?
	Who should the family contact if they are concerned, particularly out of hours?
The moment of death	How will family and carers know that the patient has died?
	Whilst diagnosis of death may seem obvious to healthcare professionals, it can be confusing and upsetting for family and carers.
What to do after a death	Does the family know who to contact when the patient dies?
	Who will carry out 'confirmation of death'?
	Who will issue the medical certificate of cause of death (MCCD) and how, where and when will the family collect it?

Source: Grey, 2015; Hospice UK, 2019; Marie Curie, 2019.

By spending time with family and carers and preparing them for the death of a loved one, healthcare professionals can reduce distress and upset. In addition, explaining simply what happens to an individual during the dying phase can help the reduce 'panic' calls to the healthcare team, particularly 'out of hours' services, and can also prevent inappropriate admissions to acute hospitals, thereby allowing the person to be cared for at home.

It is important to remember that many families and carers will be distressed, confused and feeling overwhelmed by events. Therefore, it is helpful to give families written information about the dying process, including who to contact for advice and support if they are concerned. NHS Inform, Marie Curie and Hospice UK all provide good resources for those caring for a dying loved one.

Anticipatory Grief

Anticipatory grief is complex and poorly understood, despite being recognised over 70 years ago (Rando, 1984; Costello, 2012). Put simply, anticipatory grief, preparatory grief or anticipatory mourning is a process of cognitive, physical and social responses made by both the person who is dying and those soon to be bereaved (Costello, 2012). Healthcare professionals can be actively attentive to the presentation of anticipatory grief, facilitating increased compassion, choice and communication for both the patient and the family members (Moon, 2016). However, there is little guidance on what interventions might be useful (Costello, 2012).

Whilst anticipatory grief differs from post-death grief in its duration and form, it may provide a potential opportunity for the grieving person to recognise their feelings for the dying person in advance of the death itself (Clukey, 2008). Whilst some preparation in advance of dying may be helpful for the person facing the end of their life, it may also provide an improved bereavement outcome for family members. Conversely, if the timescale between diagnosis and death is prolonged, complications may arise (Costello, 2012). Costello considers the different characteristics between anticipatory and post-death grief (Table 14.3), providing a useful insight for the healthcare team.

Table 14.3   Comparing anticipatory and post-death grief.

Anticipatory	Post-death grief
Patient and family member	Family members only
Can start at diagnosis and finishes when the patient dies	Grieving starts at time of death
Duration limited to time of death	Can last indefinitely
Emotional intensity increases as death approaches	Emotional intensity diminishes over time

Source: Costello, 2012.

It is noted that preparatory grief can be regarded as anticipatory grief in the dying. However, it must be remembered that whilst the dynamic may be similar to that of the family member, the dying person may face the potential to grieve for the separation of multiple persons, whereas individual family members will, in general, only grieve for the loss of one person (Moon, 2016). Research has identified five significant processes, shown in Table 14.4, with associated characteristics that can assist in helping to make the psychosocial transition during an expected loss.

Healthcare professionals caring for patients and families at the palliative and end stages of life are ideally positioned to help people navigate this complex transition of preparing to lose a loved one. With appropriate timely information and support concerning pain and symptom management, people can be helped to manage their expectations, and be given information as to how and who to contact when needed, and how to access complex care resources appropriately.

Table **14.4**   Processes which can aid psychosocial transition.

Characteristic	Description
Realisation	Acknowledgement Sharing with each other Attending to business Changing relationship
Caretaking	Provision of comfort Emotional and psychological support Managing physical aspects of illness Being able to manage the situation
Presence	Being supportive Being together Physical closeness Being there Sense of duty
Finding meaning	Spiritual belief Things as they should be Acceptance
Transitioning	Emotional shift Emotional numbing Fatigue

Source: Adapted from Clukey, 2008.

Complex/Unresolved Grief

Between 10% and 20% of people (Dyregrov et al., 2008) will experience adjustment difficulties after a death. This chapter explores how to recognise grief which is continuing and impeding life. Within the academic field of bereavement the debate over classification of prolonged grief disorder (PGD), persistent complex bereavement disorder, complicated grief, pathological grief or traumatic grief continues (Jordan et al., 2014; Boelen, 2017). However, the focus of this chapter is to provide insight to support practitioners in identifying people who may benefit from more focused psychological support to manage their grief.

It is normal for people to have intense feelings of loss, grief, sadness, anger or anxiety leading up to, and at the point of, the death of a loved one and the weeks/short months that follow. Usually the intensity of these feelings subsides and people report being more able to function on a day-to-day basis. Complications arise when grief is persistent and hinders normal functioning.

Grief in and of itself is not an illness; however, when grief impacts an individual's health and well-being it may be time to refer on to more specialist help. Characteristics of abnormal grief include the following (Dyregrov et al., 2008):

- Intrusive memories or delusions from the death continue to disturb the bereaved
- The bereaved continuously blames themself for what they could have done, thought or said, or refrained from doing, thinking or saying
- The bereaved has a strong sense of their own worthlessness
- The fear of another 'disaster' is strong and persistent
- The bereaved is not able to function at work or in their free time, cannot speak about their deceased at all or must avoid everything that reminds them of the deceased or the death
- The bereaved continues to brood and think about the death without room for other thoughts
- Bitterness, anger and other vengeful thoughts continue with undiminished intensity
- All talk about what has happened or about the deceased has ceased within the family
- After a child's death the parents are overly preoccupied with the deceased to such an extent that they do not manage to see the surviving children.

Factors linked to complex grief reactions
Care

Caring for a loved one with a terminal diagnosis is an exceptionally stressful and demanding experience. Tiredness, uncertainty, lack of sleep, social isolation and the ever-changing role within the relationship can erode one's ability to cope with caring for a loved one and face the inevitable death. When death occurs the bereaved may have limited internal resources to cope, which could prevent grief being acknowledged or processed.

Time

For those who have a short time from diagnosis to death there is a limit to the amount of time they have to process the information and prepare for loss. This can affect the bereaved later on when faced with decisions about funerals and their future life.

How the person died

If the death was traumatic, real or perceived, the bereaved may become fixed or locked in a trauma response. It plays as if it has just happened. Discussions with medical staff to debrief and gain understanding may be sufficient to help contextualise and narrate the event. However, if fixation continues, more focused bereavement support could be of help. Consider if the bereaved feels guilt for not being present and not having had the opportunity to say 'goodbye' and whether this is causing them significant distress.

The relationship with the deceased

The death of someone who has been abusive towards the bereaved may trigger memories and emotions of past events that can become enmeshed in the grieving process. If there was a deep level of dependence, the bereaved may lack the ability to cope with daily living or have feelings of grief, feeling extremely vulnerable and helpless (Worden, 2009). Often couples will say 'we never needed anyone else – we had each other'. Does this lifestyle choice leave the remaining spouse particularly vulnerable as a result of having little or no social support network?

Social isolation

Loneliness hinders a normal grieving process. It may be that bereavement groups can provide support and build a meaningful community, which can support the bereaved. However, individual work on a one to one basis may be required in order to meet specific emotional or psychological needs.

Health and well-being

If the bereaved has pre-existing mental health problems or significant concurrent life stressors, additional psychological support may be required to help negotiate the stormy waters of grief.

Where to signpost

Support will be variable depending on where you live. There are various support groups who may be able to signpost to counselling or psychological support:

- Private counselling – the British Association of Counselling and Psychotherapy (BACP) website can help people to find a private counsellor (www.bacp.co.uk).
- Local hospice – if the patient was cared for by a local hospice they may offer bereavement support as part of their service.
- Maggie's – has centres across the country and may run bereavement support services with those who are bereaved through cancer.
- Cruse Bereavement Care – a national network with bereavement support workers and counsellors (www.cruse.org.uk).

If you have concerns that bereavement or grief may be having an adverse affect on a person's mental health, or are concerned that there may be indications of complex/ unresolved grief, consideration should be given in relation to referral to local psychological services or to community psychiatric mental health nurses for assessment/additional support.

Family

Bereavement support for families should be included as a part of end-of-life care for all individuals (WHO, 2017; Scottish Government, 2015). Individuals are generally also part of a family or social group system and do not always grieve in separation from that. The dual-process model of grief has more recently been extended to take into account family processes (Stroebe et al., 2015), thereby recognising the inter-relationship between individual and family adjustment to the subjective and concrete changes which inevitably follow a death.

Family-centred care or working with the family unit rather than solely focusing on providing care to the patient is recognised in palliative care as one of the greatest challenges faced by practitioners (Kissane, 2017). Firstly, whilst the family may be legally, biologically and/ or relationally determined, cultural and societal variations can lead to self-definition by members without necessarily requiring consensus. This means that health staff will often find themselves coping with longstanding relationship issues about 'who belongs' that are not directly related to the current situation, but which impact upon it. This is particularly the case with former partners who are co-parents, or parents of married adults who have not managed to accept the changed status of their 'child'.

Secondly, families have pre-existing experiences of change, loss and trauma and may have established styles of communicating, coping and ascribing authority (Kissane et al., 1996; Kissane et al., 2016; Nadeau, 1998; Walsh, 2003). The death of a member can overwhelm these, highlight weaknesses or prevent some key individuals being allowed access to information and support. Working out who to talk to and how to approach this can be something of a minefield. As much as possible, seeking consent from patients about how to resolve these difficulties is essential. Helping families to find ways of allowing members to have short private visits with patients rather than feeling they all have to be there all of the time can also help alleviate tensions.

Whilst most families are resilient in the face of loss, others demonstrate relational styles which leave them vulnerable to poor bereavement outcomes (Kissane et al., 1996; Kissane et al., 2016). Where possible, assessing reactions before the death to allow appropriate support to be offered during the dying process and immediately after the death is desirable. This is particularly important for family carers whose physical and psychological well-being may have been affected whilst fulfilling caring responsibilities; particularly immediately after death where grief may be compounded due to loss of 'purpose' and 'role'. The Carer Support Needs Assessment Tool (CSNAT, 2021) enables carers to prioritise areas where they need more support, and what they would find helpful. This might include emotional well-being during and after bereavement where, for example, family members who expect to experience the same grief may find themselves isolated within the family. Where working with the family as a system is not possible, offering individual support may help to ameliorate relationship difficulties, at least for the immediate task of dealing with the dying process and managing the funeral.

Supporting Bereaved Children and Young People

Current research suggests that around one in three bereaved children will benefit from professional support following a bereavement (Penny et al., 2015). That statistic means that, because grief is a natural process, most young people will find ways of grieving well without any intervention. The families and the professionals who encounter them before, at the time of death or afterwards, can by their words and actions positively influence a child's ability to cope and, in some cases, prevent the need for professional support (Ribbens McCarthy et al., 2005). Children experience similar emotions to adults following the death of a significant person in their lives. Feelings may include shock, denial, anger, guilt, confusion, sadness and fear. However, children frequently express these feelings differently to adults and can, unlike most adults, move quickly in and out of grief (Irish Hospice Foundation, 2013).

Give choices

Adults often wonder about how much a young person should be told. There is a natural impulse to try and protect the young from things that might hurt them, but the reality is that they cope best when they understand what is happening and have all the information they need to make informed choices. It is important to remember that children are naturally curious and resilient, and their imaginations can be much worse than the reality.

Preparation

It is always difficult to prepare a child[1] for the death of a loved one, particularly a parent, and this situation may be further complicated if the parent is a single parent or has been living apart from the child. It is important to remember that the parent may be struggling with their own illness and the need to care for their child whilst ensuring that appropriate arrangements are in place to care for the child following their death.

Honest, accurate and timely, age-appropriate information and conversations are essential in supporting children at this time (Winston's Wish, 2019). As adults, this may feel counter-intuitive in our desire to protect children. However, inaccurate information, half-truths or avoidance will lead to mistrust and potentially greater distress in the long term. Children of all ages benefit by being prepared in advance for the death of someone close to them (Warnick, 2019).

---

[1]Please note that a range of legislation in Scotland variously describes childhood: for example, from birth to 16 years, from birth to 18 years, from birth to 21 years and, in the case of Care Experienced individuals, up until age 26. For the purposes of this section, birth to 18 years has been selected as the most commonly accepted general understanding of childhood.

There is no absolute 'right time' to start to prepare a child for the loss of a loved one. The timing will depend on the family and their specific circumstances. However, there are some strategies families can use to help them decide when to share this information.

These include (Warnick, 2019):

- Asking the child to describe what they already know about the situation. Many adults are surprised to learn that some children have already considered the likelihood of the loved one dying.

- Recognising that it's unnecessary to delay telling children until all of the medical information is obtained. Many adults think they shouldn't talk to children until they have more information (more test results, a more accurate prognosis).

- Asking the child how much information they want. Some children need more information than others and benefit from being told about the prognosis as soon as possible. It's also important to let children know that they can change their minds later on if they would like more or less information.

- Creating an environment where the child feels safe to ask questions. Adults can invite children to ask any questions they have about the illness and prognosis. It can be a relief for children to hear that adults may not have all the answers to their questions. Adults can provide reassurance that even though they do not have all the answers it is still important to talk about these difficult things together.

- Reassuring the child that talking about the likelihood of death does not increase the chances of the death occurring. Children often engage in 'magical thinking'. This can make them feel responsible for good and bad outcomes, despite not actually having any control over them. Providing children with facts and concrete explanations can help them focus on things that are actually within their control (such as how to spend time with their family member). Knowing what to expect can help them let go of things beyond their control (such as worrying about when the person will die).

Following death

Families will often seek advice from professionals to find out if it is appropriate for a child to see the deceased or to attend the funeral. It can be a meaningful and important experience for children to have the opportunity to say goodbye to the person who died, in a way that feels right for them. The key to doing this well is to make sure that things are properly explained. In general terms, children and young people do not fear death or dead bodies as much as adults think they do.

If a child chooses to see the deceased, they need to know what they may see and feel beforehand. If a child decides they do not want to view the body, they should be supported and affirmed in their decision.

For the funeral, the family's tradition and views should be respected but, where possible, children should be helped to understand what happens at a funeral and given the choice of whether to attend or not. They might also be involved in the ritual in other ways, for example be given a copy of the eulogy, choose flowers, write something to be read at the service or have something put in the coffin.

Language

The words we use need to be understood by the child and it is helpful to remember that some words familiar to adults are not yet in some children's vocabulary. Words like cancer, coffin, funeral or hearse might not be understood by a young child and euphemisms like 'lost' or 'passed away' might be confusing. While it might appear harsh to use 'die' or 'dead', these words are more sensible to the child and help avoid confusion. For instance, images such as 'gone to sleep' might, in future, generate a fear of sleeping in the young person.

It's important to be honest with children. They don't need to know every detail about an illness or a death but they need truthful answers and information. The final choice over what they are told lies with their families and carers but professionals can help by modelling the language that they might use. In light of this, it is key for a child to know, for instance, that a loved one took his or her own life rather than finding out later that their conception of the death was misconstrued. When this happens, a new grief process can commence, often with anger and significantly decreased trust towards those who had concealed the truth. Children require honest communication, opportunities to ask questions and reassurance that they have not caused the death.

In addition, adults can encourage children to share their feelings safely and without judgement. It is helpful to avoid using words such as 'should' or 'should not' when talking to children about loss or impending loss. Adults can also encourage compassion and support among other people in the child's life.

Age is important

The following is an introduction to how bereavement is experienced by children of different ages. The ages may vary depending on the development of the child but this is a rough guide.

0–2 years:

- No concept of death
- Babies and toddlers experience loss as separation
- Little language to express their loss
- Reactions are physical and emotional
- Will sense parental feelings of grief and changes in routine
- May fear separation from close family members.

Especially at this age, minimise disruptions and changes. Keep the comfort of familiar routines based around the five senses. Talking and remembering the person is important as the child grows and, additionally, keeping physical reminders (belongings) for them when they are older might be helpful.

2–5 years:

- Death viewed as temporary and reversible – like sleep
- Dead people are elsewhere
- Dead people have sensorial feelings and bodily functions, as well as thoughts and feelings
- Understand the concept of death, but not the finality
- May expect the deceased to reappear
- Magical thinking
- Can become confused by words and expressions
- May require the story of what has happened to be told over and over again.

Children may believe that something they did or said caused the death to occur. It is important to remind them that nothing they said, thought or did caused the person to die.

5–9 years:

- Sixty percent of 5-year-olds have an almost complete concept of death
- Seven-year-olds understand that death is irreversible and final and may begin to fear death
- Most 8-year-olds have a fully developed concept of death and understand external causes
- Begin to understand the difference between people who are alive and people who are dead
- Able to understand that a dead person cannot feel, speak, hear or see
- By age 7, most children know that death is final and that it can happen to anyone. Although able to express thoughts and feelings, they may also hide them.

Give children of this age the opportunity to ask questions and explain what is happening in an age-appropriate way.

10 years–adolescence:

- The concept of death becomes more abstract
- There is an understanding of the long-term consequences of loss
- Personal implications of death are being appreciated
- Some teenagers may challenge beliefs and explanations given to them by others
- Many teenagers feel more comfortable talking to their peers rather than a close family member

- Not unusual for teenagers to seem more insecure and to behave more like younger children
- Emotions are felt intensely, may become easily angry and display aggression
- Change is a factor at this age: their own relationships, those of a surviving parent, change of schools, housing and so on can all be difficult as young people struggle for control and normality after a death in their lives
- Self-harming, suicidal thoughts and substance misuse also appear more often in this age group.

Understand that changed behaviours in children of this age may be related to the death, so keep routine where possible, encourage communication and help them to express their feelings.

Knowing when professional support will help

For the majority of children satisfactory support can be provided by their existing networks of family, friends and communities (including their geographical communities, communities of interest, schools and further education providers).

Keeping life as normal as possible is important and so is sticking to usual routines. Although the pain of grief is difficult to witness, it is natural.

For some children who require additional support, listening groups and voluntary bereavement services may be helpful. GPs and social work services should be able to signpost to these services locally. A very small number of children will require specialist mental health support from child psychology services, Community Adolescent Mental Health Services (CAMHS) and/or specialist bereavement counselling services. Children who need this level of support may suffer from persistent anxiety and/or aggression, social withdrawal, persistent self-blame or guilt and self-destructive behaviours including self-harm or expressing a wish to die. Referrals to specialist services can be made via GPs.

Specialist help would normally only be sought after some months have passed and some of the changes subsequent to the bereavement have begun to settle. Consider allowing the young person 4 to 6 months after the bereavement for a sense of normality to take place. Indications that a child might benefit from support would be one or more of the following:

- The young person is unable to find a safe way of expressing their loss or coping with their feelings
- A marked change in behaviour or attendance at school or at home
- The presence of anxiety or depression
- Physical symptoms, not sleeping or nightmares
- Reliving sights and sounds connected with the death.

All of the above can be a part of normal grief but when they intensify through time, are causing worry, or are particularly distressing for the child then it might be time to consider whether professional advice or support should be sought.

Specific bereavements

The specific challenges facing children who have lost a parent include (Hardie-Williams, 2016):

- Accepting the significance of the loss (it changes them forever)
- Allowing the grief process to unfold on their own terms as they work through painful feelings
- Transitioning into an environment where the family member is no longer physically present.

Surviving parents have the unique challenge of supporting their child as well as processing their own grief. Some parents may feel that they need to grieve in private, believing it is in the child's best interests to shield them from displays of pain. However, it is appropriate to allow children to see adults grieving as it indicates that it is normal to feel the impact of the loss and to openly express their own grief.

Where a loved one has suffered from long-term conditions or disability, such as cancer, chronic obstructive pulmonary disease (COPD) or multiple sclerosis (MS), the child may have taken on caring responsibilities and, as such, is entitled to request support from their local authority (council) (*Carers (Scotland Act) 2016*).

Children may not identify themselves as carers, however young carers are defined in legislation as people under 18 years who spend time looking after someone who is ill, regardless of diagnosis. This care may be practical, for example helping with dressing, shopping or taking medication, or psychological. Young carers can feel isolated from their peers, with limited time or energy to spend with friends, and may be disadvantaged educationally due to the impact of their caring responsibilities.

Practical help and support is available as any young carer (or an adult acting on their behalf) can ask for a 'young carer statement' from social work services to find out what support can be offered and is acceptable to the family (further information on young carers' rights and available support can be found at www.carers.org).

Help and support for young carers can also be provided by third sector organisations such as Macmillan Cancer Support, the Children's Society, Carers UK, Barnardo's and Crossroads Caring Scotland. Healthcare professionals may be in the best position to recognise that a child is providing unpaid caring and, with the child's permission, can act on their behalf to request a referral to social work services or a relevant third sector partner. Young carers may require additional bereavement support.

Voluntary Sector

With people now living longer and a healthcare system focused on prevention and cure, death and supporting the bereaved can pose a challenge for healthcare professionals in terms of time, resources and potential ongoing health-related issues. In addition, it can be argued that changes within society, including family and community structures, over the past 50 years mean that society and individuals have become reliant on professional services to 'fix' things. Indeed, the modern medicalisation of dying has developed from the roots of the longer and broader history of community-based care. Such medicalisation has resulted in the care we provide for each other as ordinary citizens in the wider community being completely overlooked at times. As the reach and complexity of healthcare systems widen, the social and economic costs of providing bereavement care are not sustainable. In addition if we claim that grief and bereavement are not illnesses then we must question if health and social care professionals are the most appropriate groups to provide bereavement care.

Healthcare professionals should consider looking beyond the traditional statutory services (both primary and secondary care), in the context of bereavement, to initiate collaborative partnerships with local voluntary organisations. The social awkwardness and difficulties around talking about grief may be one of the barriers to the bereaved seeking help. Voluntary or third sector organisations often seek to create a positive social impact, therefore adding to the social capital within a community. Working alongside local and national voluntary organisations specialising in bereavement has the potential to improve both community and individual resilience, whilst easing the pressure on primary and secondary services. Voluntary organisations have a significant contribution to make in positively supporting the bereaved, and have the time and expertise to help navigate the process of grief.

Voluntary models of support can be easily accessed by those requiring them. These models have the time, skills and knowledge to facilitate the bereaved person to take responsibility for their own support in transitioning and moving forward when they are able to do so. In addition, many organisations use the assets and experiences of members who have experienced similar deaths to provide an empathetic and compassionate service. Organisations which provide bereavement support offer a number of different service models, including self-help groups, one to one, listening services and digital resources available to suit the individual requirements of the bereaved person.

There are a wide range of organisations offering bereavement support at both local and national levels, many of whom offer support to those who have experienced specific types of bereavement. These include SANDS (for those who have experienced a pregnancy loss or death of a baby), The Compassionate Friends (death of a child or a sibling), SOBS (following a suicide), Petal (following a homicide), as well as those offering more general support, such as Maggie's (for those affected by cancer) and CRUSE Scotland (general bereavement care). Belief communities and religious groups can also be helpful in supporting people who experience difficulties after bereavement. The majority of these organisations are more than happy to provide leaflets/information for use by the healthcare team. It is therefore suggested that healthcare teams are aware of appropriate organisations and know how to access/refer to services as appropriate. Healthcare professionals need to consider how they develop working relationships or connections with this developing sector, which is well positioned to support individuals experiencing the pain and distress of grief. For more information about the third sector see Chapter 10 – Complementary Resources.

Scenario Recap

Timely and appropriate information and support can reduce anxiety and fears and help families to 'cope with' the death of a loved one. Identifying specific problems and areas of concern, and allowing individuals to explore such fears/concerns, can reduce the possibility of complex/unresolved grief. There is little that healthcare professionals can do to 'make it better', however, those experiencing grief require support and time to 'process' the experience, thereby developing new 'bonds' with the deceased and a 'new life' where they are no longer present.

Useful Links/Sources of Information

Barnardo's

The UK's largest children's charity helps children in poverty, supports young carers and helps families looking to foster or adopt a child. See also: www.barnardos.org.uk

Carers Trust

A major charity (a third sector organisation) which provides advice and support for carers of all ages across the UK. See also: www.carers.org

Cruse Bereavement Care Scotland

This organisation exists to promote the well-being of bereaved people in Scotland. It provides help to anyone experiencing bereavement to understand their grief and cope with their loss. Working primarily through volunteers, it provides free care to bereaved people. See also: www.crusescotland.org.uk

Macmillan Support Line 0808 808 00 00

This helpline is staffed by trained experts who can offer people with cancer and their loved ones practical, clinical, financial and emotional support.

***When Dinosaurs Die* by Laurie Krasny Brown and Mark Brown**

A straight-talking book that could help you explain what is going on to a 4–7-year-old.

Winston's Wish Freephone National Helpline 08088 020 021

The helpline is run by extremely experienced practitioners who can talk about a specific situation and provide support in talking to children about the prognosis. The helpline is for children, young people, parents/carers and professionals. See also: www.winstonswish.org

References

Boelen PA (2017) Disturbed grief: prolonged grief disorder and persistent complex bereavement disorder. *British Medical Journal*, 357: j2016.

Buglass E (2010) Grief and bereavement theories. *Nursing Standard*, 24(41): 44–47.

Clukey L (2008) Anticipatory mourning: processes of expected loss in palliative care. *International Journal of Palliative Nursing*, 14(7): 316–325.

Costello J (2012) End of life care and bereavement. In *Grief, Loss and Bereavement: Evidence and Practice for Health and Social Care Practitioners*. Wimpenny P and Costello J (eds.). London: Routledge, pp. 71–90.

Carers (Scotland Act) 2016 (asp 9) Available at: https://www.legislation.gov.uk/asp/2016/9/contents/enacted Edinburgh: Scottish Government.

CSNAT (2021) Carer Support Needs Assessment Tool. Available at: https://csnat.org/

Dyregrov K and Dyregrov A (2008) *Effective Grief and Bereavement Support: The Role of Family, Friends, Colleagues, Schools and Support Professionals*. London: Jessica Kingsley Publishers.

Grey A (2015) What to expect when someone important to you is dying. For the National Council for Palliative Care, Hospice UK and Sue Ryder. Available at: https://www.rowcrofthospice.org.uk/wp-content/uploads/Rowcroft-Hospice-What-to-expect-when-someone-important-to-you-is-dying.pdf

Hardie-Williams K (2016) How to help children grieve the death of a parent. Available at: https://www.goodtherapy.org/blog/how-to-help-children-grieve-death-of-parent-1212165

Hospice UK (2019) Changes in the last days of life. Available at: https://www.hospiceuk.org/what-we-offer/clinical-and-care-support/what-to-expect/what-happens-when-someone-is-dying/changes-in-the-last-days-of-life

Irish Hospice Foundation (2013) Hospice Friendly Hospitals Programme. Available at: http://palliativecare.issuelab.org/resources/19130/19130.pdf

Jordan A and Litz HB (2014) Prolonged grief disorder: diagnostic, assessment and treatment considerations. *Professional Psychology, Research and Practice*, 45c: 180–187.

Kissane DW et al. (1996) The Melbourne family grief study, I: perceptions of family functioning in bereavement. *American Journal of Psychiatry*, 153(5): 650–658.

Kissane DW et al. (2016) Randomized controlled trial of family therapy in advanced cancer continued into bereavement. *Journal of Clinical Oncology*, 34(16): 1921–1927.

Kissane DW (2017) Under-resourced and under-developed family-centred care within palliative medicine. *Palliative Medicine*, 31(3): 195–196.

Marie Curie (2019) Signs that someone is in their last days of life. Available at: https://www.mariecurie.org.uk/professionals/palliative-care-knowledge-zone/final-days/recognising-deterioration-dying-phase

Moon PJ (2016) Anticipatory grief: a mere concept. *American Journal of Hospice and Palliative Medicine*, 33(5): 417–420.

Nadeau JW (1998) *Families Making Sense of Death*. Thousand Oaks, CA: Sage.

Stevenson A (ed.) (2010) Oxford Dictionary of English, third edition. Oxford: Oxford University Press.

Penny A and Stubbs D (2015) Bereavement in childhood: what do we know in 2015? London: The Childhood Bereavement Network.

Rando TA (1984) *Grief, Dying, and Death: Clinical Interventions for Caregivers*. Champaign, IL: Research Press Publishers.

Ribbens McCarthy J with Jessop J (2015) The impact of bereavement and loss on young people. Available at: https://www.jrf.org.uk/report/impact-bereavement-and-loss-young-people

Royal College of Psychiatrists (2015) Bereavement. Available at: https://www.rcpsych.ac.uk/mental-health/problems-disorders/bereavement

Scottish Government (2015) Strategic framework for action on palliative and end of life care 2016–2021. Edinburgh: Scottish Government.

Scottish Government (2021) Annual death totals in Scotland for the last 5 years: FOI release. Available at: https://www.gov.scot/publications/foi-202000128465/

Scottish Palliative Care Guidelines (2019) Care in the Last Days of Life. Available at: https://www.palliativecareguidelines.scot.nhs.uk/guidelines/end-of-life-care/care-in-the-last-days-of-life.aspx

Stroebe M et al. (2017) Grief is not a disease but bereavement merits medical awareness. *The Lancet*, 389(10067): 347–349.

Stroebe MS and Schut HAW (2015) Family matters in bereavement: toward an integrative intra-interpersonal coping model. *Perspectives on Psychological Science*, 10(6): 873–879.

Tol W et al. (2014) World Health Organization guidelines for management of acute stress, PTSD, and bereavement: key challenges on the road ahead. *PLOS Medicine*, 11(12): e1001769.

Walsh F (ed.) (2003) *Normal Family Processes: Growing Diversity and Complexity,* 3rd edition. New York: Guilford Press.

Warnick A (2019) When to tell the children; preparing children for the death of someone close to them. Available at: http://www.virtualhospice.ca/en_US/Main+Site+Navigation/Home/Topics/Topics/Communication/When+to+Tell+the+Children_+Preparing+Children+for+the+Death+of+Someone+Close+to+Them.aspx

WHO (World Health Organisation) (2017) WHO definition of palliative care. Available at: http://www.who.int/cancer/palliative/definition/en/

Winston's Wish (2019) How to prepare a child for the death of a parent by cancer. Available at: http://www.winstonswish.org/prepare-death-by-cancer/

Worden JW (2009) *Grief Counselling and Grief Therapy: A Handbook for the Mental Health Practitioner*, 2nd edition. Abingdon: Routledge.

Conclusion

When we offer care, we should remember that our patients did not choose us — we chose them. We could have chosen another profession, but we did not. We have accepted the responsibility to provide compassionate, realistic and holistic care for people at a time which, for most, is the most challenging, frightening, and unpredictable of their lives. We must give to our patients the best care possible by preparing ourselves with current knowledge, honing our clinical skills, offering empathetic communication, and focusing on their individual needs.

At the end of each journey, we should feel that the patient, their family and carers had received nothing but the very best.

Index